Skin and Systemic Disease

Skin and Systemic Disease: A Clinician's Guide, Second Edition is a revised and updated new edition of an essential clinical guide for health care providers to diagnose and treat patients presenting with skin symptoms that may indicate systemic disease. Information on each disorder's etiopathogenesis and clinical and systemic manifestations is presented, with guidance on evaluation and management of the disorder. This edition includes new entries, additional differential diagnoses and workups, improved images, and new images from patients with different skin types.

Skin and Systemic Disease

A Clinician's Guide

Second Edition

Joseph C. English III, MD
Professor of Dermatology
University of Pittsburgh, Pennsylvania, USA

Timothy J. Patton, DO
Assistant Professor of Dermatology
University of Pittsburgh, Pennsylvania, USA

CRC Press
Taylor & Francis Group
Boca Raton London New York

CRC Press is an imprint of the
Taylor & Francis Group, an **informa** business

Designed cover image: Authors

Second edition published 2026
by CRC Press
2385 NW Executive Center Drive, Suite 320, Boca Raton FL 33431

and by CRC Press
4 Park Square, Milton Park, Abingdon, Oxon, OX14 4RN

CRC Press is an imprint of Taylor & Francis Group, LLC

ISBN: 9781032762814 (hbk)
ISBN: 9781032795485 (pbk)
ISBN: 9781003492665 (ebk)

DOI: 10.1201/9781003492665

Typeset in Times
by KnowledgeWorks Global Ltd.

Dedication

The authors dedicate this book to their families; past, current, and future dermatology residents; and to our patients, past, present, and future, for whom we strive to deliver the best dermatologic healthcare possible.

In memory of Lisa Grandinetti, MD (1976–2015).

Contents

List of Abbreviations

For laboratory tests and other studies

ACA	Anti-centromere antibodies
ACTH	Adrenocorticotropic hormone
AMA	Anti-mitochondrial antibodies
ANA	Anti-nuclear antibodies
ANCA	Anti-neutrophilic cytoplasmic antibodies
APLA	Anti-phospholipid antibodies (anti-cardiolipin and anti-β 2 glycoprotein antibodies)
BMI	Body mass index
C3/4	Complement 3 and 4
CA-125	Cancer antigen 125
CA 19-9	Cancer antigen 19-9
CADM-140	Anti-clinically amyopathic dermatomyositis -140 antibodies
Ca^{2+}	Calcium ion
CBC	Complete blood count with platelets and differential
CCP	Anti-cyclic citrullinated protein antibodies
CEA	Carcinoembryonic antigen
CELIAC	Anti-gliadin, endomysial, transglutaminase antibodies
CMP	Comprehensive metabolic panel
CPK	Creatinine phosphokinase
CRP	C-reactive protein
CRYO	Cryoglobulin
CS	Colonoscopy
CT	Computed tomography scan
CXR	Chest X-ray
DHEA-s	Dehyroepiandrosterone sulfate
DLCO	Diffuse Lung Capacity Carbon Monoxide
dsDNA	Anti-double stranded DNA antibodies
EGD	Esophagogastroduodenoscopy
ESR	Erythrocyte sedimentation rate
FBG	Fasting blood glucose
FLip	Fasting lipids
FSH	Follicular stimulating hormone
GH	Growth Hormone
HA1c	Hemoglobin A1c
HCG	Human chorionic gonadotropin
Hep B	Hepatitis B panel (HBsAg, anti-HBc antibodies)
Hep C	Anti-hepatitis C antibodies
HIV	Human Immunodeficiency virus
HLA	Human leukocyte antigen
HTLV	Human T-lymphotrophic virus
HyProg	17-hydroxyprogesterone
HIAA	5-hydroxy indoleacetic acid
IRON	Iron panel with Ferritin
Jo-1	Anti-Jo-1 antibodies
LAC	Lupus Anticoagulant

LFT	Liver function tests (AST, ALT, LDH, Total/Direct bilirubin)
LH	Luteinizing hormone
META	Metanephrines
MDA-5	Anti-melanoma differentiation associated protein 5 antibodies
Mi-2	Anti-Mi-2 antibodies
MMGX	Mammography
MRI	Magnetic resonance imaging
MTHFR	Methyltetrahydrofolate reductase
p155	Anti-p155 antibodies
PO_4	Phosphate
PFT	Pulmonary function test
PRL	Prolactin
PPD	Purified protein derivative
PT/PTT	Prothrombin time/Partial thromboplastin time
PTH	Parathyroid hormone
Ro/La	Anti-Ro/SSA and Anti-La/SSB antibodies
RF	Rheumatoid Factor
RFT	Renal function tests (BUN/Creatinine)
RPR	Rapid Plasma Reagin
RNP III	Anti-RNA polymerase III antibodies
Scl70	Anti-scl 70 (toposimerase) antibodies
SHGB	Sex hormone binding globulin
Sm	Anti-smith antibodies
SPEP/SIFE	Serum protein electrophoresis/serum immunofixation electrophoresis
TCR	T-cell receptor
TFT	Thyroid function tests (TSH/fT4)
Test	Testosterone (free/total)
TG	Anti-thyroglobulin antibodies
TPO	Anti-thyroid peroxidase antibodies
U1RNP	Anti-U1 nuclear ribonucleoprotein antibodies
UA	Urinalysis
UPEP/UIFE	Urine protein electrophoresis/urine immunofixation electrophoresis
U/S	Ultrasound

1

Skin Findings with Systemic Associations

Acanthosis Nigricans and Acrochordon

Etiopathogenesis

Acanthosis nigricans (AN) and acrochordons have been commonly associated with insulin resistance (IR) and metabolic syndrome. AN can be seen in other disorders, including Cushing syndrome, polycystic ovaries, thyroid diseases, hirsutism, Addison disease, acromegaly, genetic syndromes, and malignancy. The mechanism of IR is complex, but essentially, it is a disorder where target cells in the body do not respond to circulating insulin. This leads to compensatory hyperinsulinemia, which causes an upregulation of insulin-like growth factor type 1 (IGF-1). Increased IGF-1 leads to keratinocyte and fibroblast proliferation, which clinically manifests as AN and acrochordons. Malignancy-associated AN is believed to be due to stimulation of keratinocytes by secreted factors from the associated tumor, including transforming growth factor-α (TGF-α).

Clinical Manifestations

AN is characterized by hyperpigmented, symmetrical, and velvety to verrucous patches and plaques, commonly on the posterior neck, axillae, antecubital/popliteal fossae, umbilicus, and the groin, although it can occur anywhere (**Figures 1.1–1.8**). Malignancy-related AN is rare, usually abrupt in onset, exuberant, and involves mucous membranes (buccal mucosa, lips) and palms (tripe palms). Acrochordons are common, pedunculated, flesh-colored to hyperpigmented papules that frequently occur in similar sites as AN (**Figure 1.9**). Acrochordons (**Figure 1.10**) can occur in the general population; however, multiple skin tags (>8) are generally regarded as a sign of IR.

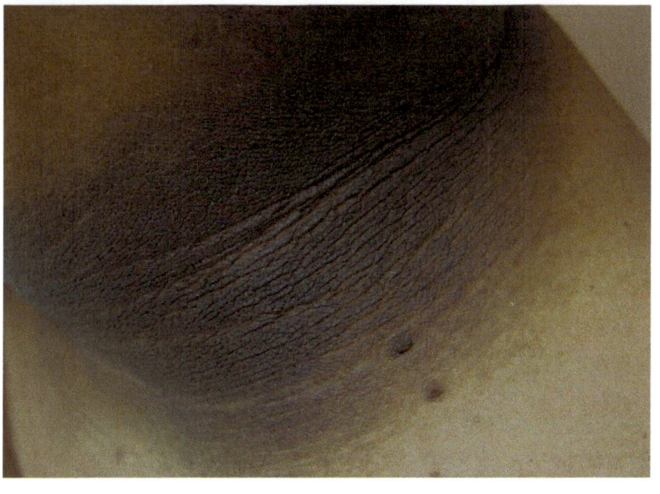

FIGURE 1.1 Acanthosis nigricans: Neck.

DOI: 10.1201/9781003492665-1

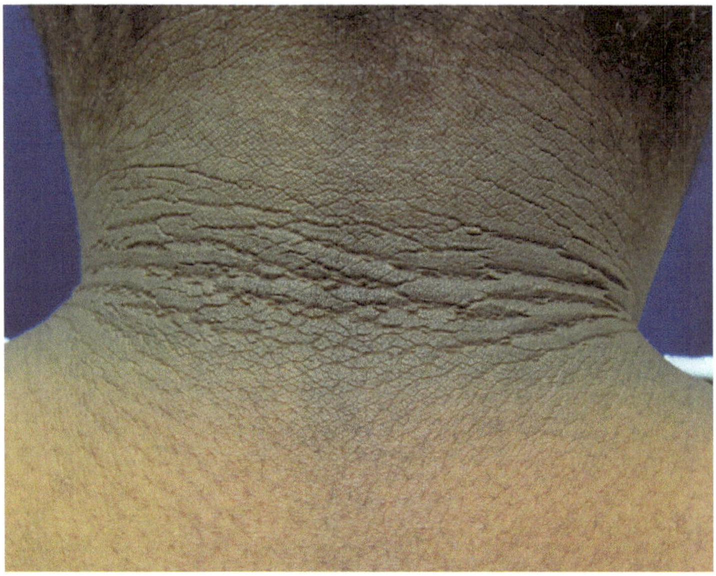

FIGURE 1.2 Acanthosis nigricans: Posterior neck.

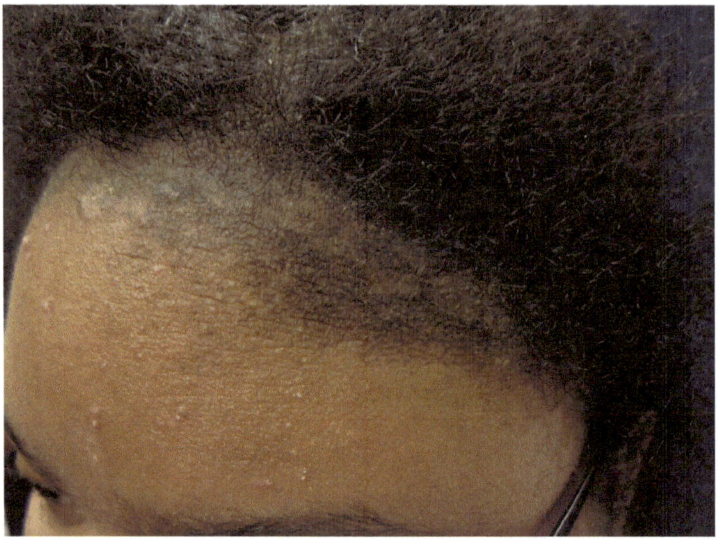

FIGURE 1.3 Acanthosis nigricans: Forehead.

Systemic Manifestations

AN has been classified into obesity/endocrinopathy/syndromic/medication-related AN and malignancy-related AN. Obesity-related AN is the most common type affecting children and adults. It can coexist with other cutaneous manifestations of IR and diabetes mellitus, such as scleredema or diabetic dermopathy. Medications that induce AN include agents such as systemic steroids, nicotinic acid, estrogen, insulin, and oral contraceptives. Malignancy-associated AN is most frequently reported as occurring with gastric, breast, and lung adenocarcinomas.

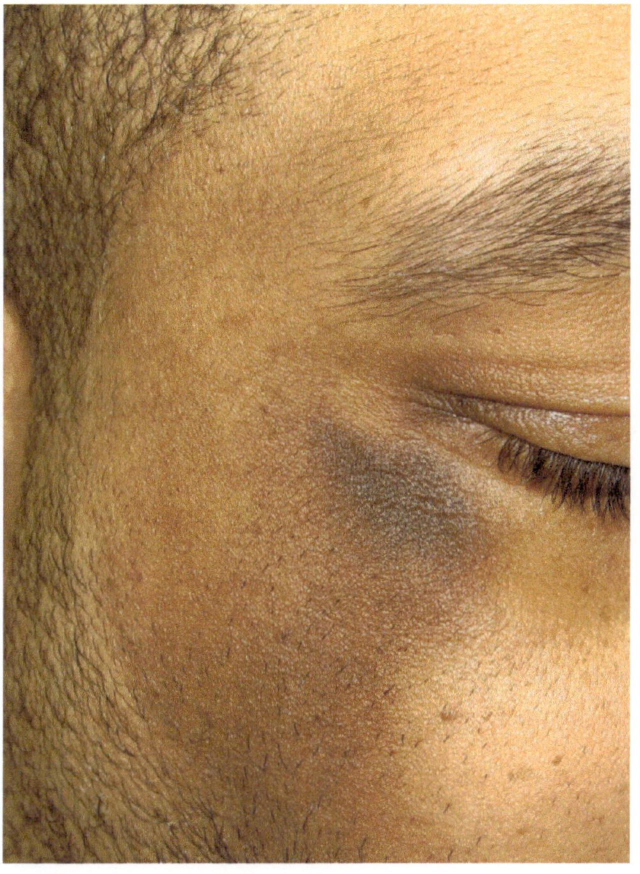

FIGURE 1.4 Acanthosis nigricans: Zygomatic arch.

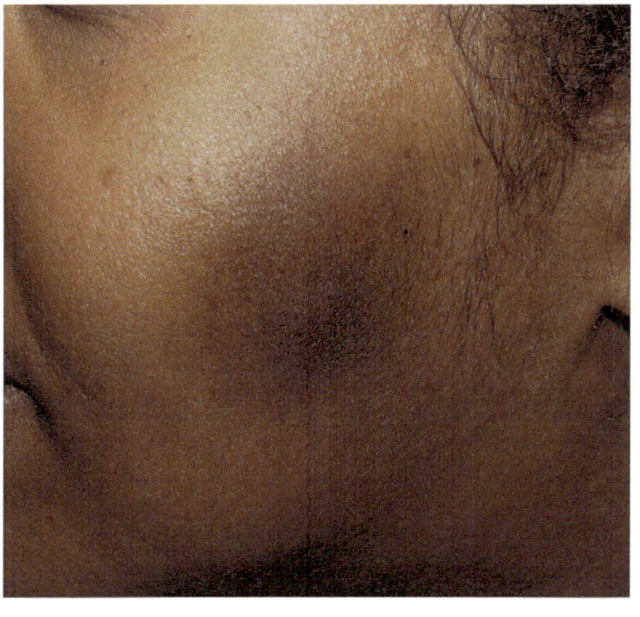

FIGURE 1.5 Acanthosis nigricans: Cheek.

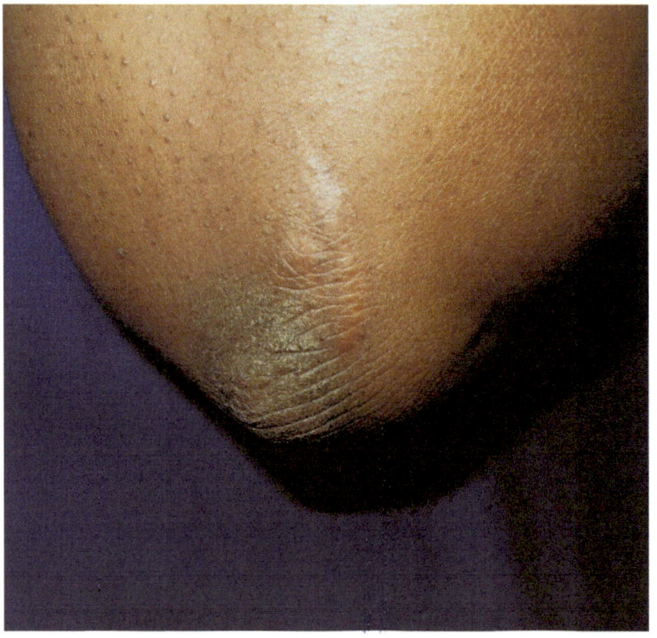

FIGURE 1.6 Acanthosis nigricans: Elbow.

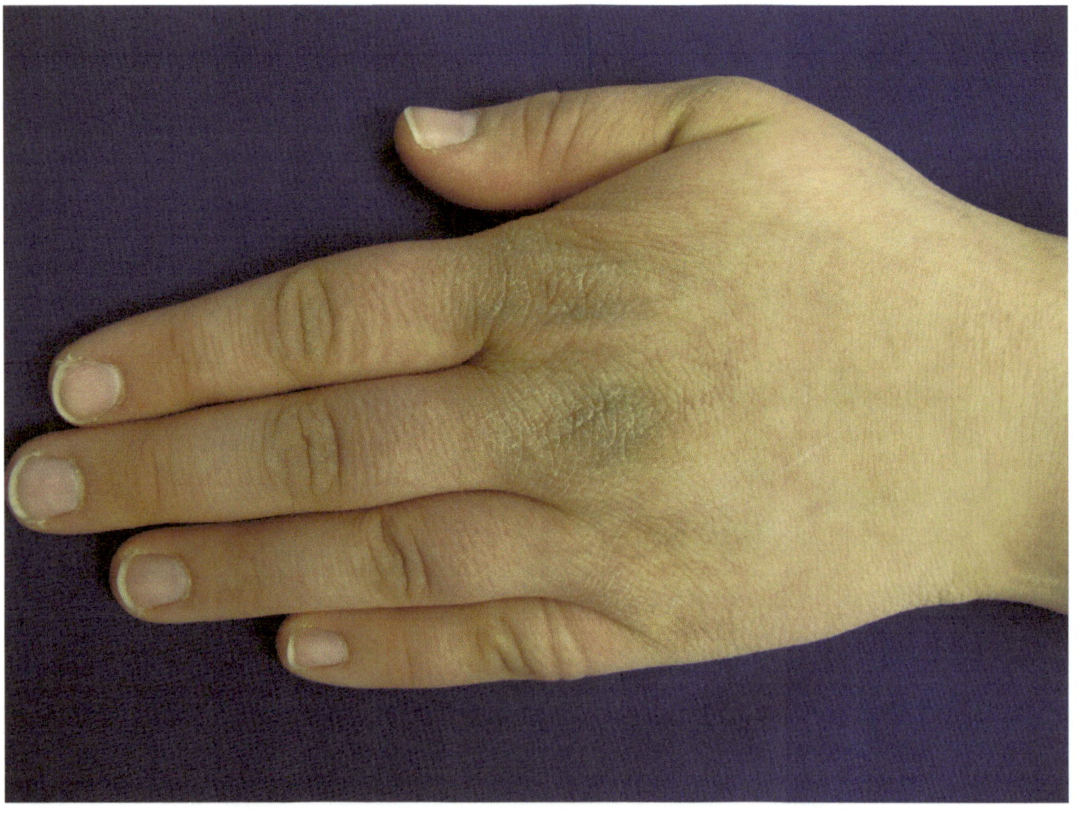

FIGURE 1.7 Acanthosis nigricans: Knuckle.

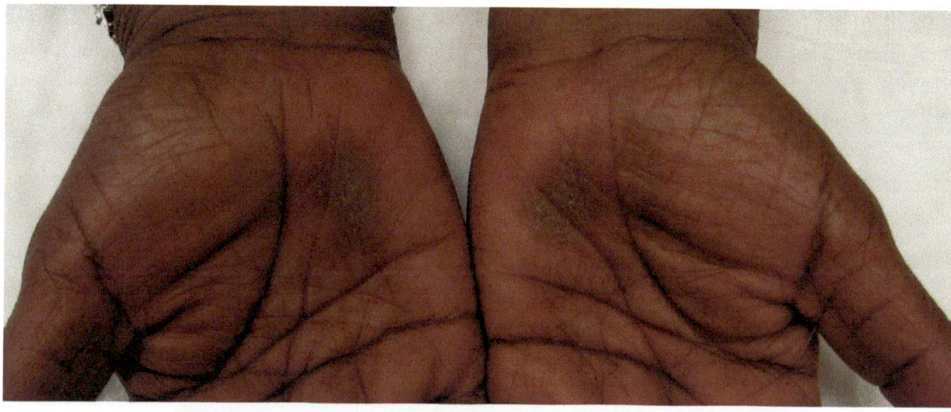

FIGURE 1.8 Acanthosis nigricans: Palmar (nonmalignant).

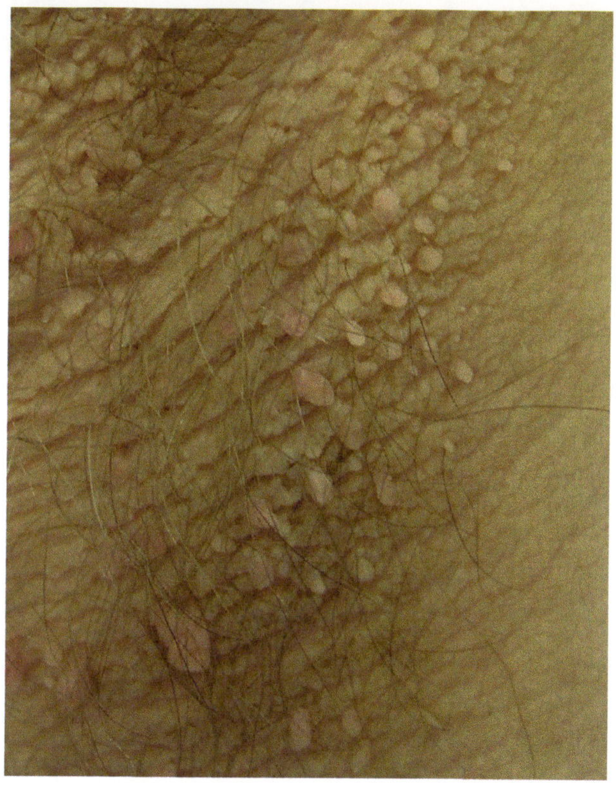

FIGURE 1.9 Acanthosis nigricans and acrochordons: Axilla.

Evaluation and Management

Recognizing the connection between AN, multiple acrochordons, and IR is of great importance for health-care providers. Patients should be evaluated for obesity, hypertension, dyslipidemia, and glucose intolerance—all components of metabolic syndrome (**Table 1.1**, see Chapter 8). Referral and evaluation by endocrinology may be indicated in certain patients with abnormal findings. Abrupt onset and exuberant AN should raise suspicion of underlying malignancy. Esophagogastroduodenoscopy/colonoscopy (EGD/CS), mammography (MMGX), and chest X-ray/computed tomography (CXR/CT) scans can help initiate the evaluation. Resolution of AN is primarily achieved by improved lifestyle, discontinuation of any associated medication, and weight loss. Other reported therapies include metformin, topical/oral retinoids, topical calcipotriol/calcipotriene, and laser therapy. Acrochordons can be treated with electrodesiccation, scissor-snip excision, or local cryotherapy.

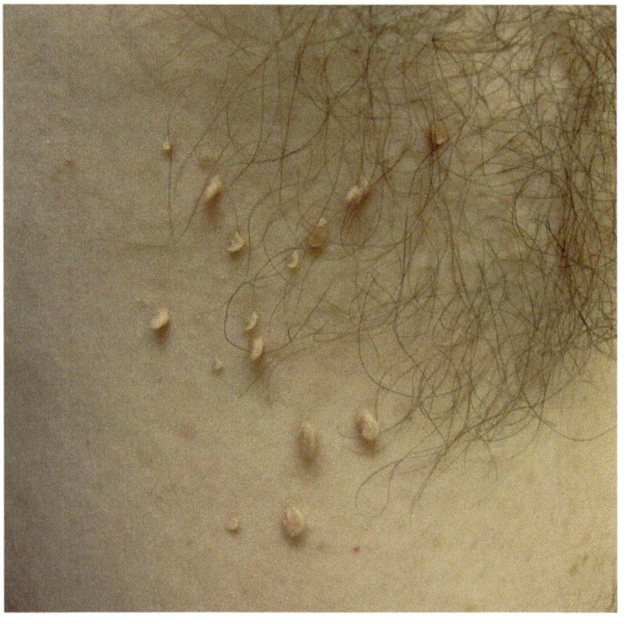

FIGURE 1.10 Acrochordons: Axilla.

TABLE 1.1

Laboratory Evaluation of Acanthosis Nigricans and Acrochordons
Fasting lipids
Fasting blood glucose
Fasting insulin
Hemoglobin A1c
Liver function test

BIBLIOGRAPHY

Byard R. Manifestations and etiology of cutaneous findings in cases of morbid obesity. Forensic Sci Med Pathol 2023. https://doi.org/10.1007/s12024-023-00721-3

Das A, Datta D, Kassir M, et al. Acanthosis nigricans: A review. J Cosmet Dermatol 2020;19:1857–1865.

Leung AK, Lam JM, Barankin B, et al. Acanthosis nigricans: An updated review. Curr Pediatr Rev 2022;19(1):68–82.

Acrocyanosis

Etiopathogenesis

Acrocyanosis is the purplish discoloration of the distal extremities as a result of arterial/arteriolar vasoconstriction, capillary/venous vasodilation, and pathologically low blood flow from autonomic dysfunction. There is no association of gender, race, or geography with primary acrocyanosis. Secondary acrocyanosis occurs more frequently in women, most likely related to its association with anorexia nervosa and connective tissue disease.

Clinical Manifestations

Typically, acrocyanosis will develop in the adolescent to young adult age group (teens–30s). The discoloration is best described as a blue/purple to violaceous discoloration of acral skin that is persistent (may worsen with cold but persists with rewarming), dependent, symmetrical, blanchable, painless, and has normal pulses. These features distinguish acrocyanosis from Raynaud phenomenon (RP) and erythromelalgia. In addition to discoloration, the involved skin is typically moist, and hyperhidrosis may be a concomitant complaint. Ulcerations are indicative of a secondary cause.

Systemic Manifestations

Primary acrocyanosis (**Figure 1.11**) is considered benign and is typically devoid of other systemic findings. Secondary acrocyanosis (**Table 1.2**) may result from hematologic disorders (**Figure 1.12**), many connective tissue disorders (**Figure 1.13**), medications, paraneoplastic phenomenon neurologic disorders, and malnutrition. Some disease processes develop acrocyanosis prior to a purpuric component (endocarditis, cryoglobulinemia, cholesterol emboli, infection) or may have both simultaneously (cryoglobulinemia; antiphospholipid antibodies [APLA] syndrome). Abnormal vital signs can point toward a diagnosis related to hypoxemia (**Figure 1.14**) or infectious disorder such as endocarditis, gonococcemia, or meningococcemia. Prior vascular procedures with the development of a purple digit should raise suspicion for cholesterol emboli. Association with decreased or absent peripheral pulses is concerning for peripheral vascular disease with or without thrombosis. Differentiating conditions from RP (**Figures 1.15–1.17**) and erythromelalgia (**Figure 1.17**) is important. RP, a vasospastic process, may be associated with scleroderma, systemic lupus erythematosus (SLE), Sjögren syndrome, dermatomyositis, and rheumatoid arthritis. Erythromelalgia, a small nerve fiber neuropathy, can be associated with polycythemia, thrombocythemia, and neurologic and autoimmune disorders.

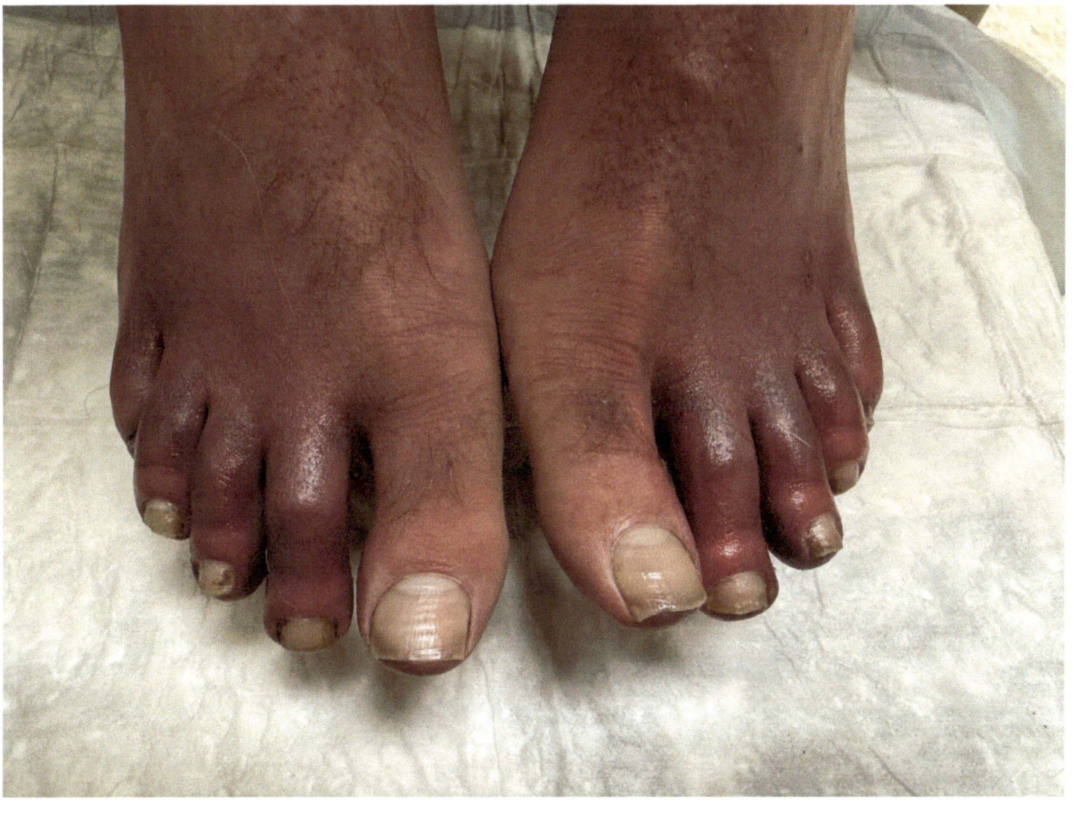

FIGURE 1.11 Primary acrocyanosis.

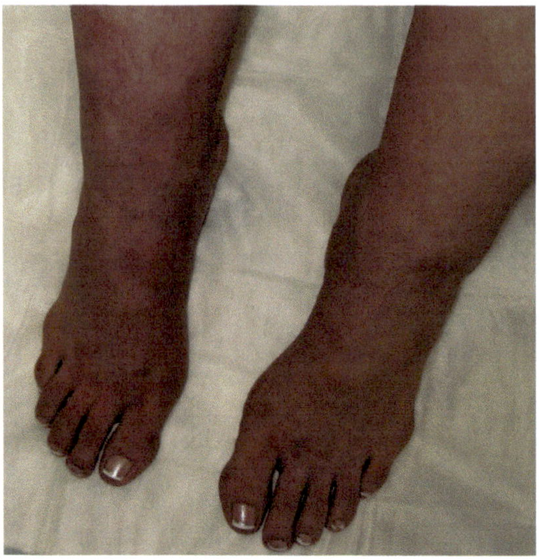

FIGURE 1.12 Secondary acrocyanosis: Cryoglobulinemia.

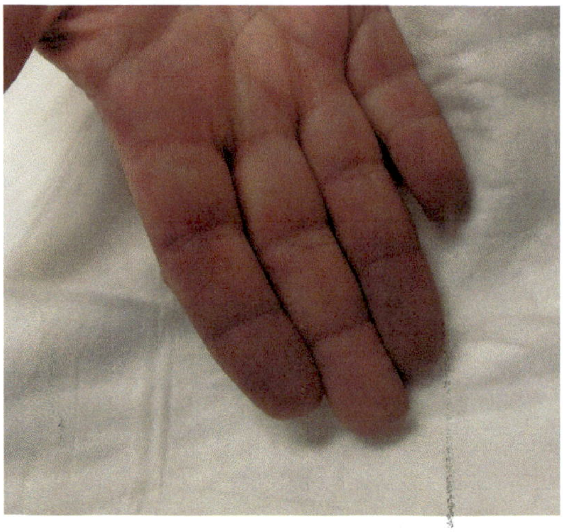

FIGURE 1.13 Secondary acrocyanosis: Systemic lupus erythematosus.

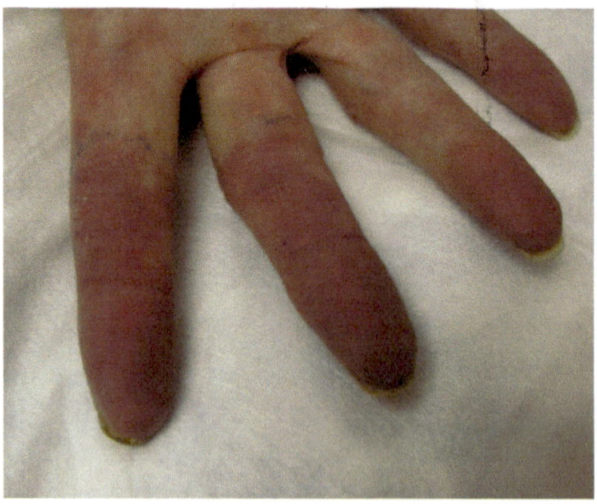

FIGURE 1.14 Secondary acrocyanosis: Hypoxia.

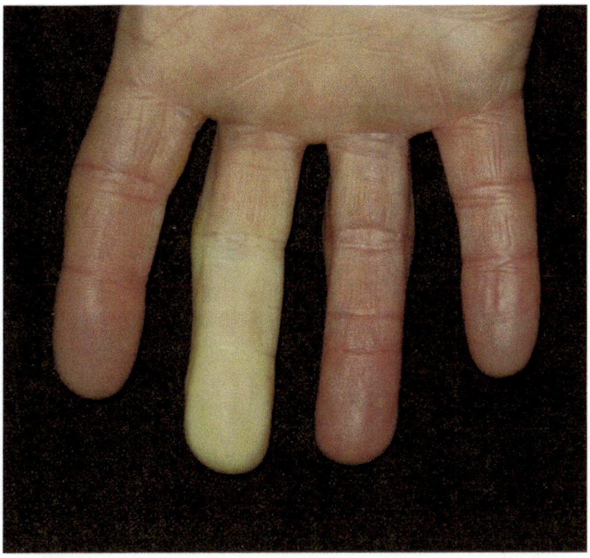

FIGURE 1.15 Raynaud phenomenon.

Evaluation and Management

Primary acrocyanosis is considered a benign phenomenon. Evaluation for secondary acrocyanosis may include laboratory testing for cryoglobulin (CRYO), lupus anticoagulant (LAC), antiphospholipid antibodies (anticardiolipin and anti-β2 glycoprotein antibodies) (APLAs), antinuclear antibodies (ANAs), prealbumin, and radiographic studies such as CT. Additional testing to differentiate from RP and erythromelalgia may include ANAs, anti-Scl 70 antibodies (Scl70), anti-Ro/SSA and anti-La/SSB antibodies (Ro/La), rheumatoid factor (RF), complete blood count (CBC) with platelets and differential, serum protein electrophoresis/serum immunofixation electrophoresis (SPEP/SIFE), and urine protein electrophoresis/urine immunofixation electrophoresis (UPEP/UIFE). The use of Doppler ultrasound can help differentiate causes. Treatment of secondary acrocyanosis is based on any underlying disorder that is identified.

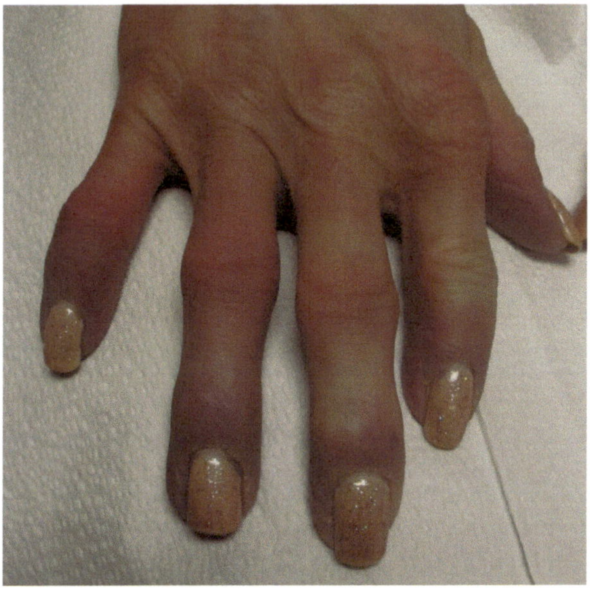

FIGURE 1.16 Raynaud phenomenon with acrocyanosis.

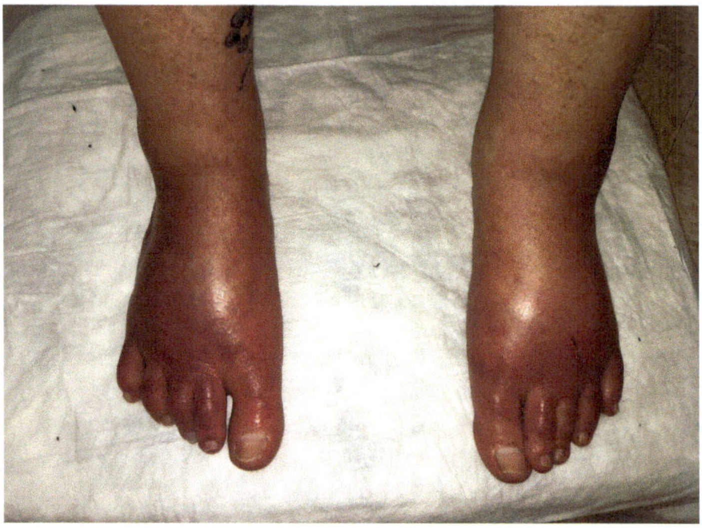

FIGURE 1.17 Acral erythromelalgia.

TABLE 1.2

Differential Diagnosis of Secondary Acrocyanosis

Hematologic disorders

- Cryoglobulinemia
- Antiphospholipid antibody syndrome
- Myeloproliferative disorders

Connective tissue disease

- Systemic lupus erythematosus

Medications

- Interferon
- Vasopressors
- Chemotherapy
- Biologic agents

Paraneoplastic phenomenon

- Lymphoma
- Ovarian cancer
- Esophageal cancer
- Breast cancer

Neurologic disorders

- Spinal cord injury
- Neuropathy
- Schizophrenia
- Mental retardation

Malnutrition

- Eating disorders

BIBLIOGRAPHY

Bergersen TK, Walloe L. Acral coldness – Severely reduced blood flow to fingers and toes. Handb Clin Neurol 2018;157:677–685.

Brown PJ, Zirwas MJ, English JC III. The purple digit: An algorithmic approach to diagnosis. Am J Clin Dermatol 2010;11(2):103–116.

Casanegra AI, Shepard RF. Raynaud phenomenon and other vasospastic disorders. Cardiol Clin 2021;39(4):583–599.

Raja A, Karch J, Shih AF, et al. Part II cutaneous manifestations of peripheral vascular disease. J Am Acad Dermatol 2023;89(2):211–226.

Zhang D, Slaven K, Shields BE. Cutaneous signs of malnutrition secondary to eating disorders. Cutis 2023;111(5):231–238.

Alopecia

Etiopathogenesis

Alopecia is the loss of hair, and the most commonly encountered form of alopecia associated with systemic disease is telogen effluvium (TE). TE, a nonscarring and genetically unrelated alopecia, is due to an increase of the intrinsic physiologic hair shedding of normal clubbed (telogen) hairs in a response to an emotional or physical stressor. Three months after a given stimulus, noticeable loss of hair shafts occurs due to an excessive shift of anagen (fixed/growing) to telogen (resting/shedding) hairs. This is differentiated from androgenetic alopecia (hormonal miniaturization of follicles) and alopecia areata (CD8+ and natural killer (NK) T-cell-induced loss of immune tolerance).

Clinical Manifestations

Patients are usually anxiety ridden from sudden onset of abnormal hair shedding with bathing/grooming, noticeable decrease in hair volume, and a "Hair Bag" sign (collection of lost hairs presented in a plastic bag [**Figure 1.18**]). Physical examination reveals no primary scalp dermatoses, but visible bitemporal hair thinning (**Figures 1.19** and **1.20**). A gentle hair pull test, grasping 2.5 cm width of hair (±25–50 hairs) and gently pulling from scalp to hair tip, which removes greater than two telogen hairs, is positive from the temporal scalp. A false negative test may occur due to bathing/grooming prior to the appointment. Androgenetic alopecia (**Figures 1.21** and **1.22**) is a more gradual onset of diffuse thinning without noticeable hair shedding. Alopecia areata (**Figure 1.23**) may be a rapid loss of hair but is usually diffuse and irregular.

Systemic Manifestations

TE is precipitated by psychogenic and physical ailments approximately 3 months before hair loss. Daily emotional stressors, anxiety, depression, and obsessive-compulsive disorder may commonly induce TE. Systemic diseases associated with TE include iron-deficiency anemia, hypoferritinemia, hyper/hypothyroidism, vitamin deficiency (vitamin D, zinc), weight gain/loss, anorexia/bulimia, malnutrition, starting/stopping medications, and any illness or condition (fever, pregnancy, trauma, COVID-19). TE associated with trichodynia can be due to secondary vitamin B12/folate deficiency or scalp dysesthesia from sensory nerve impingement.

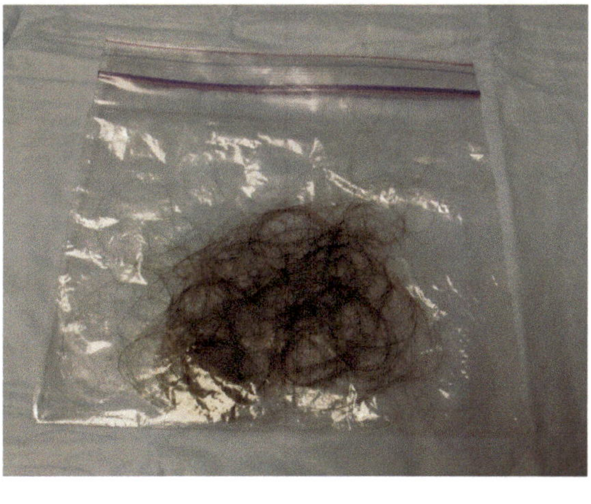

FIGURE 1.18 Telogen effluvium: Hair bag sign.

Early age of onset and diffuse disease in androgenetic alopecia (both sexes) has been reported as an independent predictor of mortality in diabetes and heart disease. Black men with early-onset androgenetic alopecia have a significant association with developing prostate cancer. Young women with androgenetic alopecia may have hyperandrogenic states. Alopecia areata may occur in relation to autoimmune thyroiditis, diabetes, and pernicious anemia.

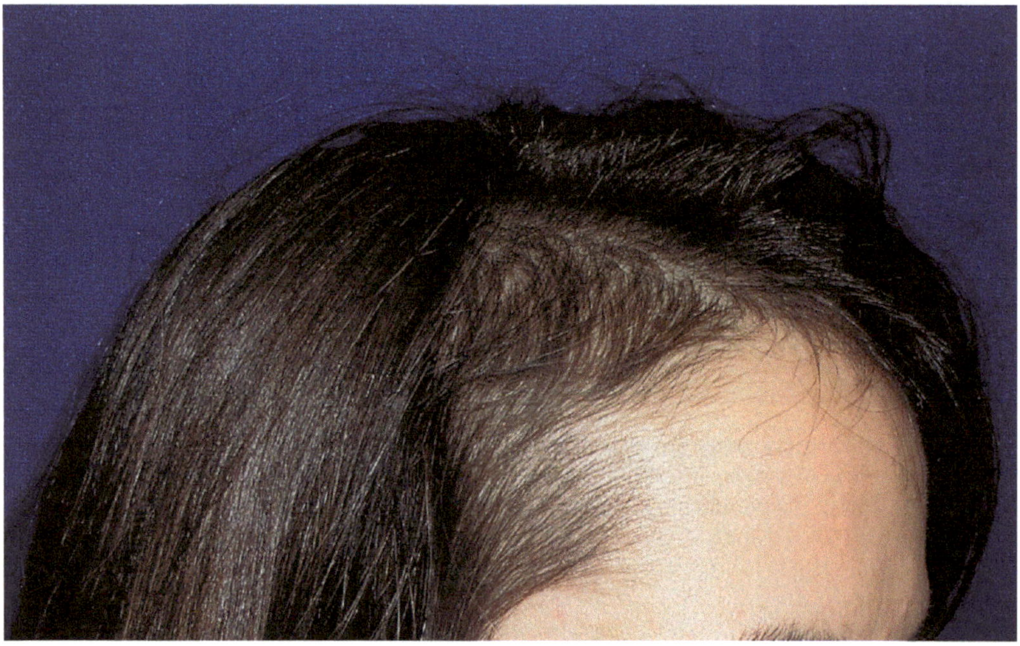

FIGURE 1.19 Telogen effluvium.

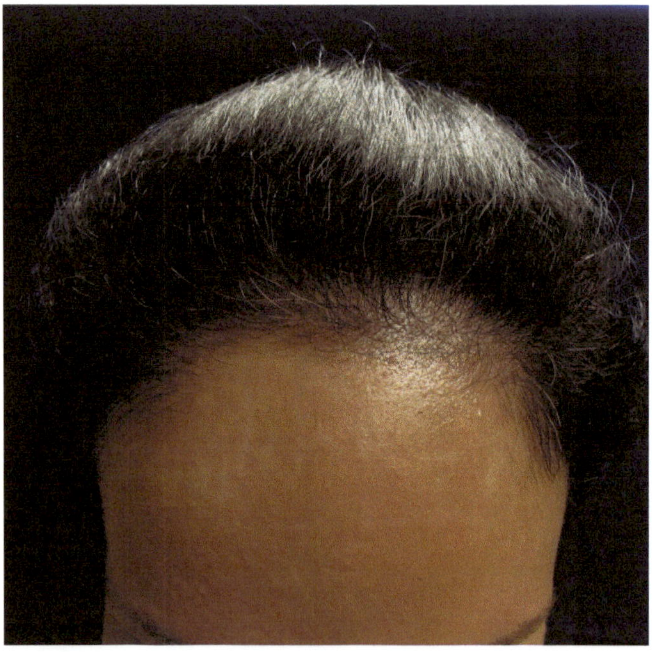

FIGURE 1.20 Telogen effluvium.

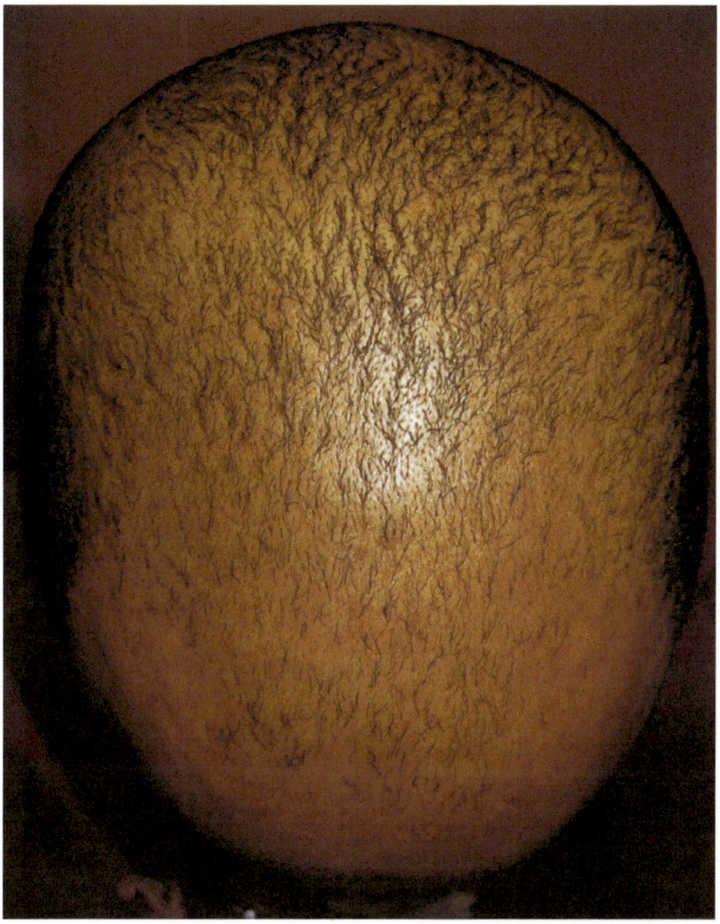

FIGURE 1.21 Androgenetic alopecia: Male.

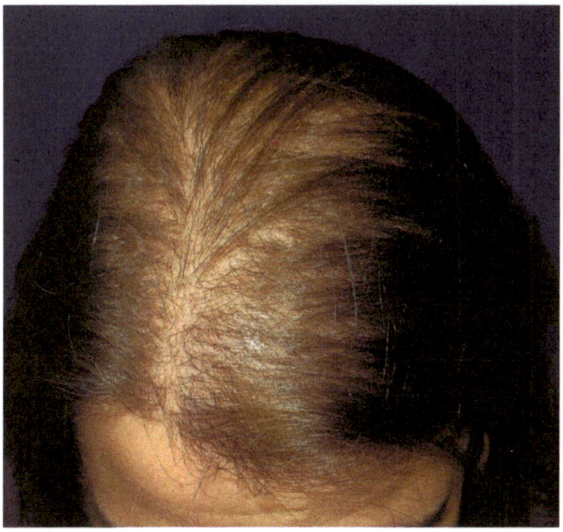

FIGURE 1.22 Androgenetic alopecia: Female.

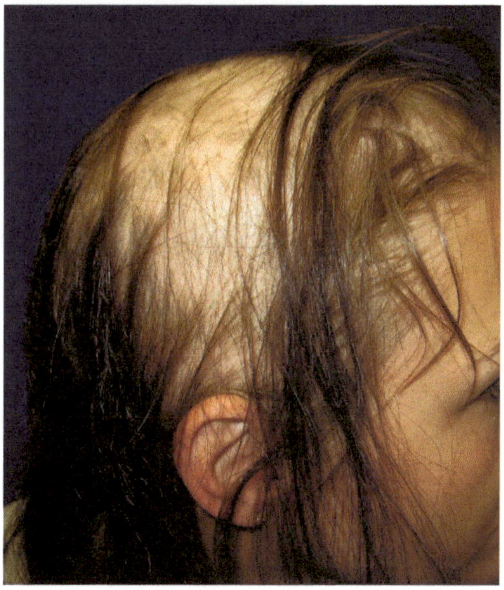

FIGURE 1.23 Alopecia areata: Diffuse.

Evaluation and Management

Laboratory testing recommendations are reviewed in **Table 1.3**. Management of TE includes reassuring/educating the patient, topical minoxidil and antiandrogens for androgenetic alopecia, and IL-steroids, immunotherapy, or oral immunosuppressants (methotrexate, cyclosporine, baricitinib) for alopecia areata.

TABLE 1.3

Laboratory Testing to Consider for Alopecia

Telogen effluvium

- Complete blood count with platelets and differential
- Iron panel with ferritin
- Thyroid stimulating hormone and free T4
- Vitamin D
- Zinc
- Vitamin B12/Folate (if trichodynia)
- Pre-albumin
- Albumin
- Anti-nuclear antibody (if signs/symptoms of connective tissue disease)
- Anti-thyroglobulin and thyroid peroxidase antibodies (if abnormal thyroid function)

Androgenic alopecia

Female

- Prolactin
- Follicular stimulating and luteinizing hormones
- Thyroid stimulating hormone and free T4
- Dehydroepiandrosterone sulfate
- 17 Hydroxyprogesterone
- Free and total testosterone
- Sex hormone binding globulin

Male and female

- Fasting lipid panel
- Fasting glucose
- Hemoglobin A1c

Alopecia areata

- Thyroid stimulating hormone and free T4
- Fasting glucose
- Hemoglobin A1c
- Complete blood count

BIBLIOGRAPHY

Asfour L, Cranwell W, Sinclair R, et al. Male androgenetic alopecia. In: Endotext [Internet]. South Dartmouth (MA): MDText.com; 2000.

Bertoli MJ, Saoughifar R, Schwartz RA, et al. Female pattern hair loss: A comprehensive review. Dermatol Ther 2020;33:e14055.

Sterkens A, Lambert J, Bervoets A. Alopecia areata: A review on diagnosis, immunological etiopathogenesis and treatment options. Clin Exp Med 2002;21:215–230.

Yin GOC, Siong-See JL, Wang ECE. Telogen effluvium – A review of the science and current obstacles. J Dermatol Sci 2021;101:156–163.

Clubbing

Etiopathogenesis

Primary hypertrophic osteoarthropathy (HOA) is an autosomal dominant disorder linked to a defect affecting the prostaglandin transporter encoded by the gene *SLCO2A1* and the gene coding for 15-hydroxyprostaglandin dehydrogenase. It consists of clubbing, pachyderma, and periostosis. Isolated phenotypical expressions of primary HOA account for isolated clubbing ("familial" clubbing), whereas secondary HOA may also have a full or partial expression of findings (isolated acquired clubbing). Clubbing in secondary HOA may be unilateral (neurologic/vascular abnormalities) or bilateral. Bilateral clubbing is associated with disorders of other organ systems, including pulmonary, cardiac, gastrointestinal (GI), endocrine, and psychiatric. Infectious and malignant causes have also been described. No one mechanism of action can explain all secondary associations, but the abnormal presence of megakaryocytes or megakaryocyte remnants and elevated vascular endothelial growth factor cytokines likely promote tissue growth, resulting in increased tissue mass of the finger.

Clinical Manifestation

The volume of the distal phalanx is increased, the nailbed becomes softened, and the nail plate becomes convex (**Figures 1.24** and **1.25**). The alteration of fingertip anatomy can be measured in many different ways: the profile sign (Lovibond sign), modified profile sign, hyponychial angle, and the ratio of distal phalangeal to interphalangeal depth. Obliteration of the diamond shape, typically present when the dorsal surfaces of opposite fingernails are placed together (Schamroth sign), serves as a simple and reliable indicator of clubbing (**Figures 1.26** and **1.27**). Patients may have cutis verticis gyrata (**Figure 1.28**) and long bone pain.

Systemic Manifestation

Clubbing in the context of malignancy has been described in pulmonary malignancies, nasopharyngeal cancer, and lymphoma. Other pulmonary disorders with digital clubbing include cystic fibrosis, interstitial prominent fibrosis, and sarcoidosis. GI and hepatic diseases (chronic hepatitis, primary biliary cirrhosis, inflammatory bowel disease) often feature clubbing. Thyroid disease, especially those with thyroid dermopathy, often features thyroid acropachy (clubbing). Infectious disorders associated with clubbing include chronic parasitic infections, human immunodeficiency virus (HIV), infectious endocarditis, and tuberculosis.

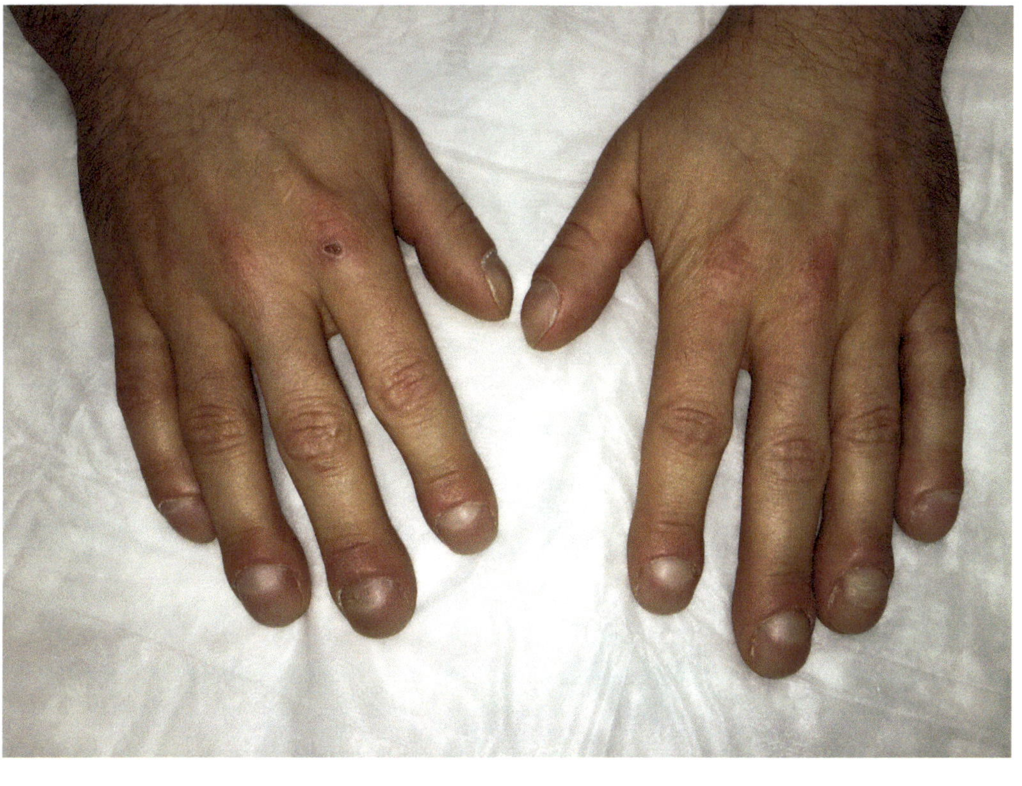

FIGURE 1.24 Clubbing: Fingers.

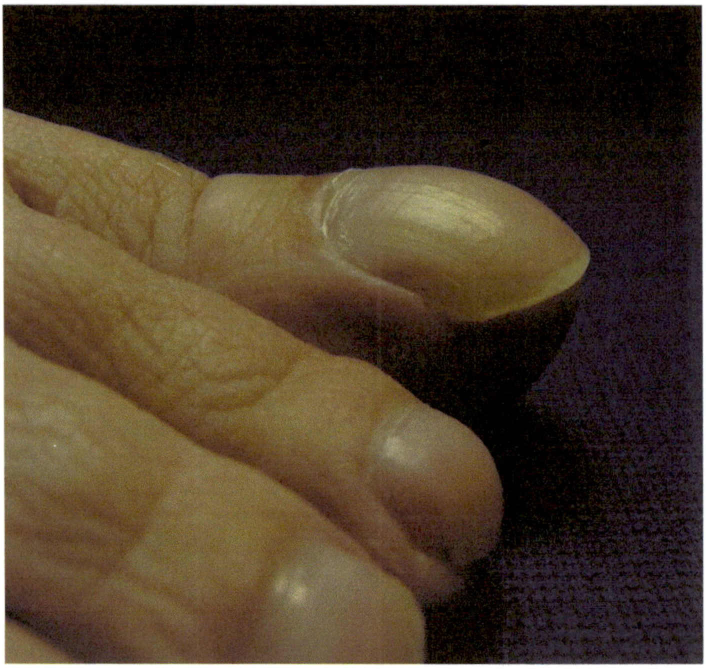

FIGURE 1.25 Clubbing: Toes.

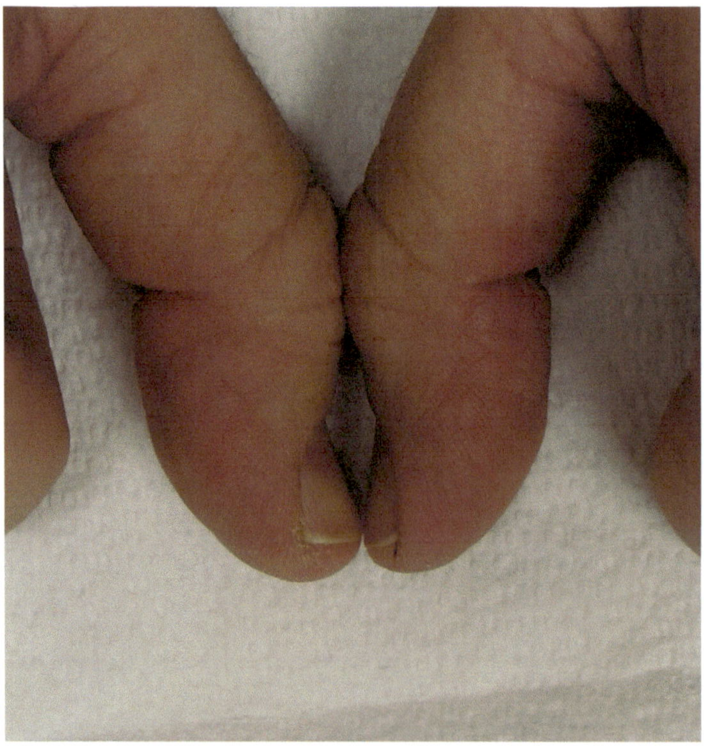

FIGURE 1.26 Schamroth sign negative: Normal nails.

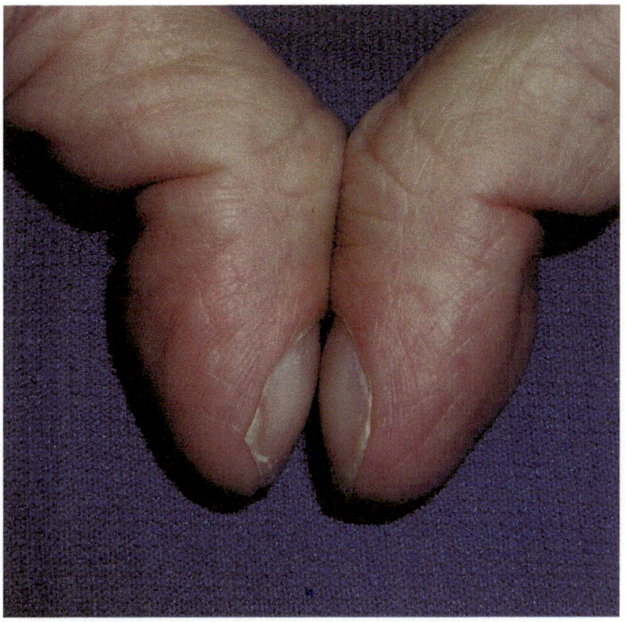

FIGURE 1.27 Schamroth sign positive: Clubbed nails.

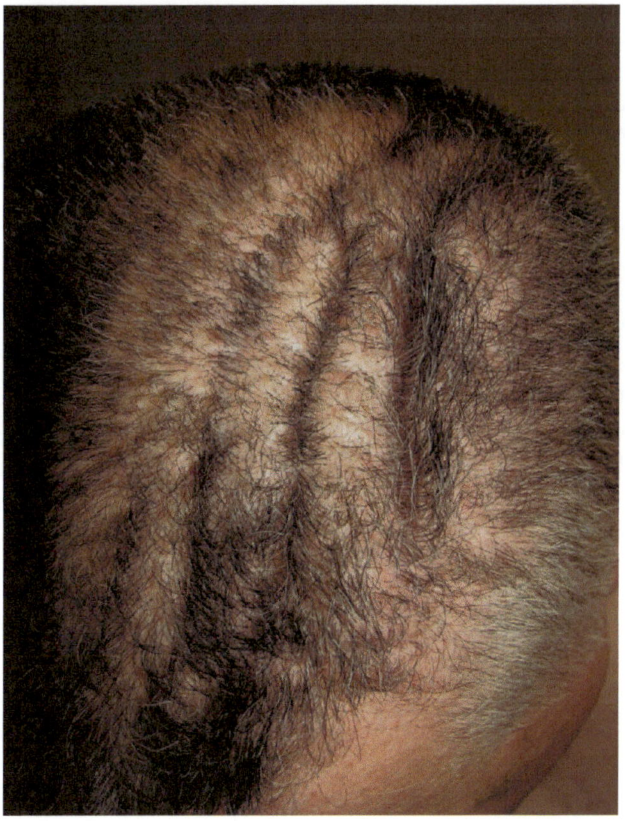

FIGURE 1.28 Cutis verticis gyrata.

Evaluation and Management

Confirmation of digital clubbing with a Schamroth sign or careful measurement of the various depth ratios or angles of the distal digit is a good first step. This should be followed with a thorough review of systems and careful medical, family, social, sexual, and travel history. Investigative testing is summarized in **Table 1.4**.

TABLE 1.4

Investigative Testing for Patients with Clubbing

Laboratory

- Complete blood count with platelets and differential
- Liver function tests
- Viral hepatitis serology
- HIV
- Thyroid function and thyroid antibodies
- Quantiferon gold
- Blood cultures

Diagnostic

- Chest X-ray
- Pan CT scan
- Pulmonary function tests
- Transesophageal echocardiogram

BIBLIOGRAPHY

Burcovschii S, Aboeed A. Nail clubbing. In: StatPearls [Internet]. Treasure Island, (FL): StatPearls Publishing; 2022.

Matinez-Lavin M. Hypertrophic osteoarthropathy. Best Pract Res Clin Rheumatol 2020;34(3):101507.

Spicknall KE, Zirwas MJ, English JC III. Clubbing: An update on diagnosis, differential diagnosis, pathophysiology, and clinical relevance. J Am Acad Dermatol 2005;52:1020–1028.

Zhang Z, He JW, Fu WZ, et al. Mutations in the SLCO2A1 gene and primary hypertrophic osteoarthropathy: A clinical and biochemical characterization. J Clin Endocrinol Metab 2013;98(5):E923–E933.

Dyschromia

Etiopathogenesis

The pathogeneses of skin pigment changes are varied: from a normal or exaggerated physiologic finding, sequelae of inflammation, or by deposition of compounds within the skin. Acquired forms of dyschromia (**Table 1.5**). can be due to melanin overproduction, underproduction, or other pigment deposition (drug, hemosiderin). Yellowish skin discoloration will be discussed in the Xanthoderma section.

Clinical Manifestations

Cutaneous hyper- or hypopigmentation may be localized or generalized. Lesions are routinely macular in nature and range in size from 1 to 2 mm in diameter to lesions that can involve the entire skin surface. Often, patients may have a mixture of both spectrums of pigmentation

Systemic Manifestations

Physiologic hyperpigmentation is common in pregnancy (**Figure 1.29**). Diffuse hyperpigmentation with systemic complaints of fatigue, weight fluctuations, and muscle weakness can be associated with Addison disease, Cushing disease, diabetes, and the polyglandular autoimmune syndrome. Diffuse hyperpigmentation with flushing, abdominal cramping, and diarrhea should suggest hyperthyroidism, carcinoid syndrome, pheochromocytoma, or vitamin deficiency. The bronze diabetic should raise concern for hemochromatosis. End-stage renal disease patients often develop generalized hyperpigmentation. Dyschromia with symptoms of joint pain and photosensitivity in association with erythematous eruption or induration could suggest a connective tissue disorder (scleroderma [**Figures 1.30** and **1.31**] or lupus erythematosus [**Figure 1.32**]). Generalized melanosis is also a very rare form of metastatic melanoma and hereditary hemochromatosis (**Figure 1.33**). Leopard skin changes indicate chronic graft-versus-host disease (GVHD) in bone marrow transplant patients (**Figure 1.34**). Some medications can also result in skin pigmentation, including minocycline (**Figure 1.35**), hydroxychloroquine, gold, and silver (**Figure 1.36**). Vitiligo (**Figure 1.37**), or cutaneous depigmentation, has been associated with autoimmune thyroiditis, pernicious anemia, and diabetes.

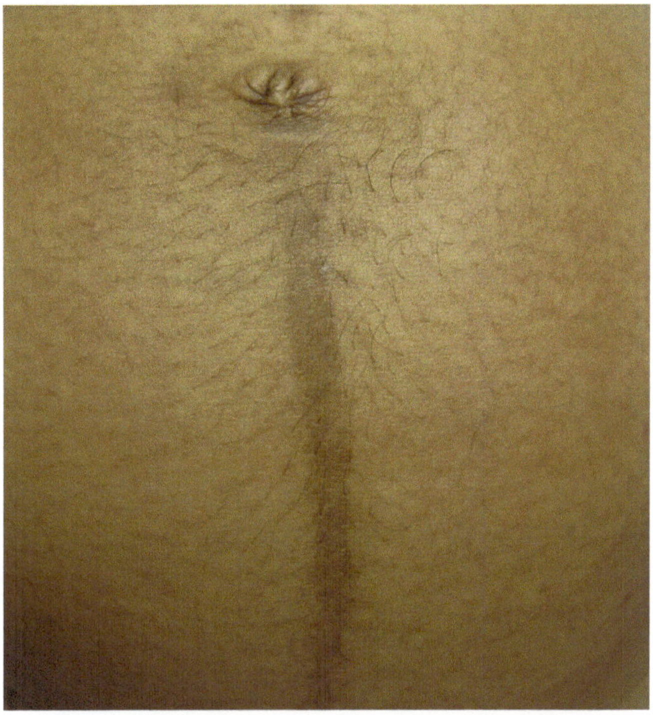

FIGURE 1.29 Dyschromia: Linea nigra of pregnancy.

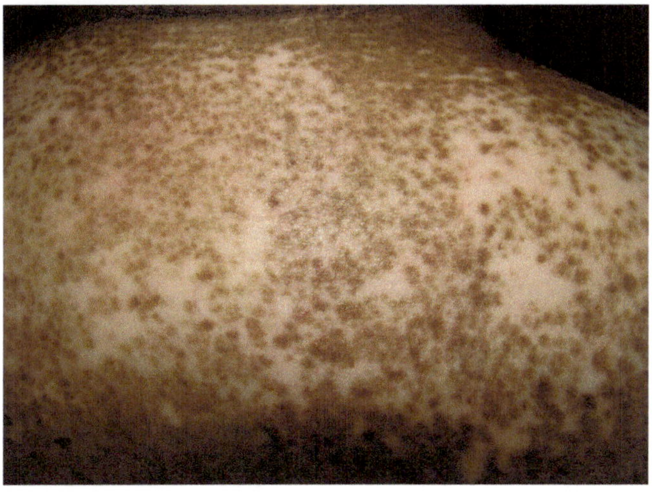

FIGURE 1.30 Dyschromia: Scleroderma.

Evaluation and Management

Given the wide range of conditions and exposures that can cause dyschromia, a careful history, review of medications, and physical examination should be performed to establish a thorough differential diagnosis. Skin biopsy is helpful to determine whether the pigment abnormality is melanin or nonmelanin in etiology. Laboratory testing may include fasting blood glucose (FBG), hemoglobin A1c (HA1c), thyroid function tests (TFTs), a.m. cortisol, adrenocorticotropic hormone (ACTH) stimulation or dexamethasone-suppression test, CBC, liver function tests (LFTs), iron, hemochromatosis gene studies, serum/24-hour urine metanephrines (META), 24-hour urine for 5-hydroxy indoleacetic acid (5HIAA), antinuclear antibodies (ANAs), anticardiolipin antibodies (ACAs), Scl70 antibodies, anti-U1 nuclear ribonucleoprotein antibodies (U1RNP), and anti-RNA polymerase III antibodies (RNP III). For melanin hyperpigmentation, use of hydroquinone, topical retinoids, azelaic acid, kojic acid, niacinamide, and tranexamic acid can be helpful in diminishing hyperpigmentation. For melanin and nonmelanin hyperpigmentation, laser ablation can be considered. Cosmetic camouflage can be considered for focal hypo- or depigmented skin. Use of phototherapy (**Figure 1.38**), topical Janus kinase (JAK) inhibitors, and topical calcineurin inhibitors may be used in vitiligo. For extensive depigmentation in vitiligo patients, a decision to use monobenzylether of hydroquinone can be considered to depigment the remaining skin. The treatment of any underlying disease state may or may not cause the skin to return to normal.

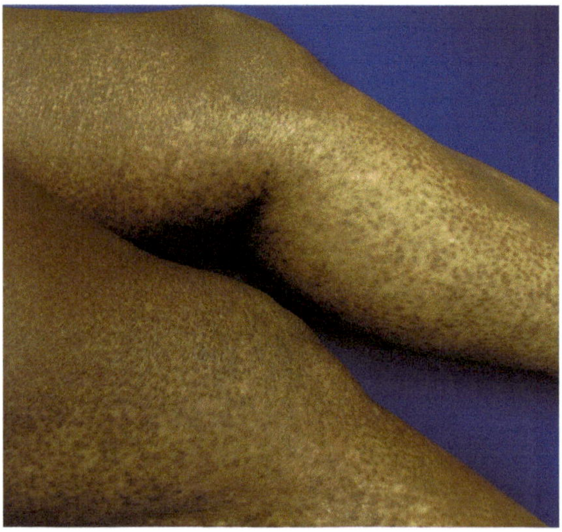

FIGURE 1.31 Dyschromia: Scleroderma.

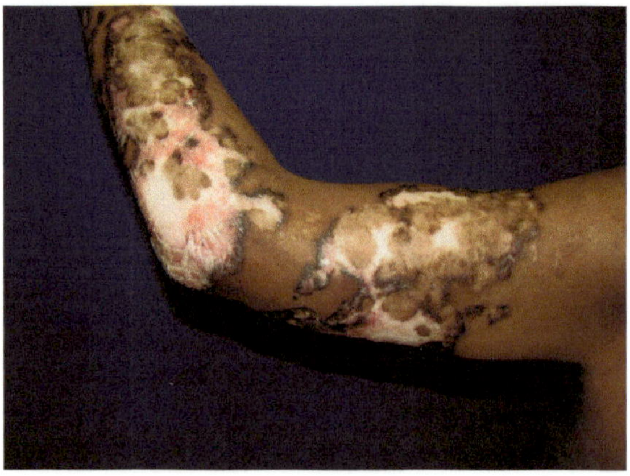

FIGURE 1.32 Dyschromia: Chronic cutaneous lupus.

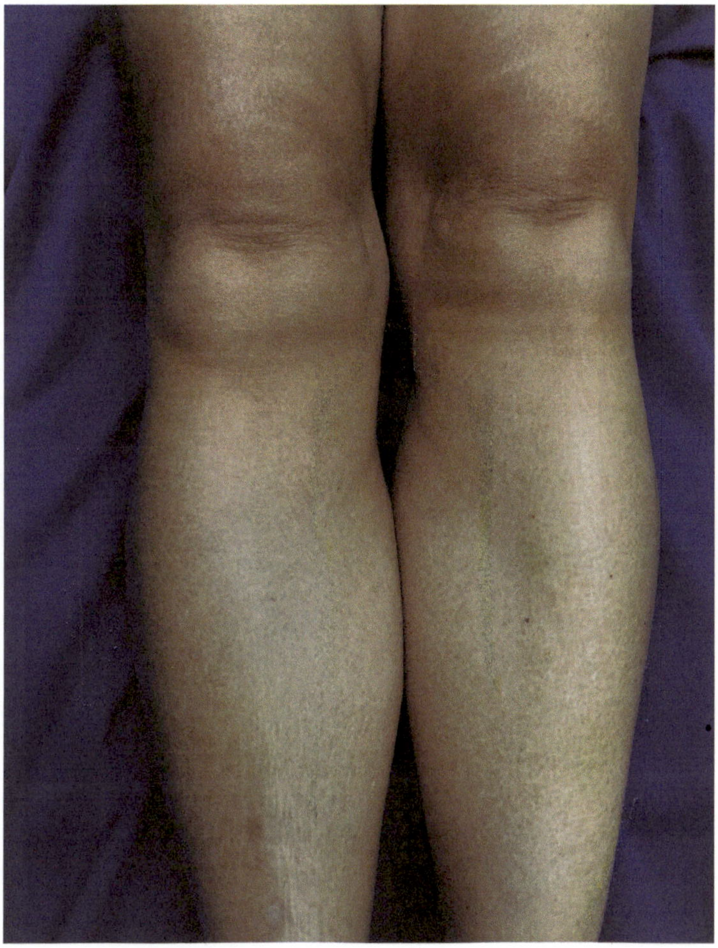

FIGURE 1.33 Dyschromia: Hemochromatosis.

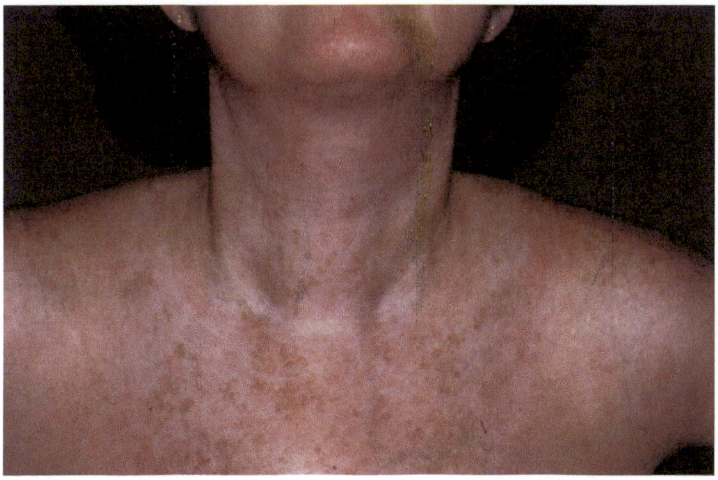

FIGURE 1.34 Dyschromia: Chronic GvHD.

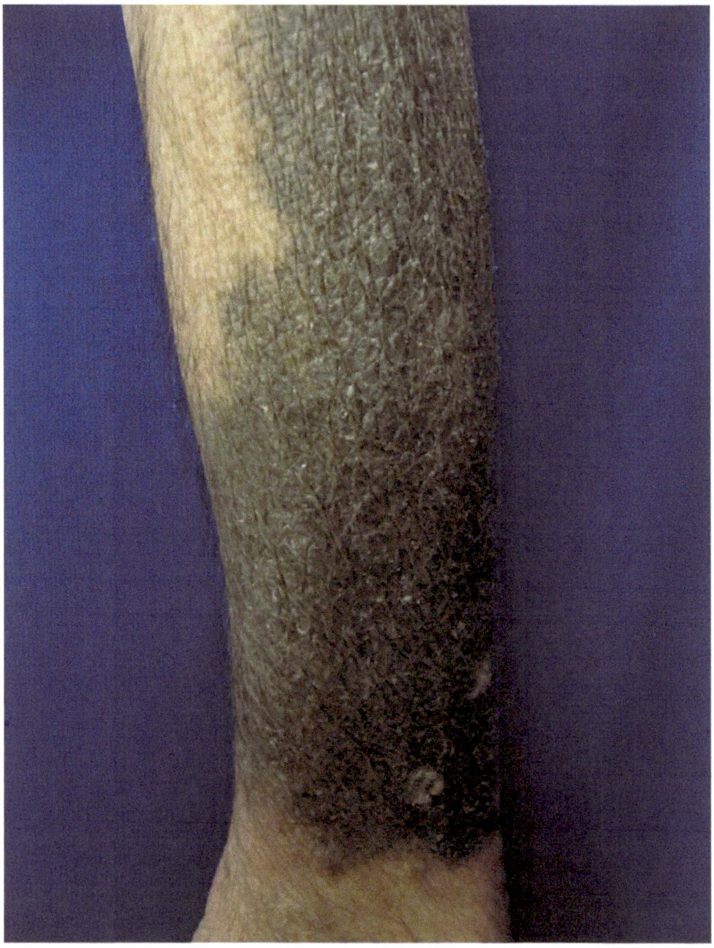

FIGURE 1.35 Dyschromia: Minocycline.

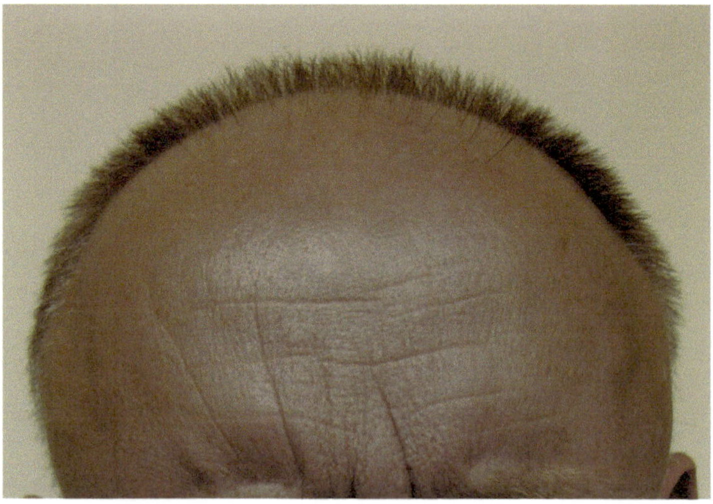

FIGURE 1.36 Dyschromia: Silver (argyria).

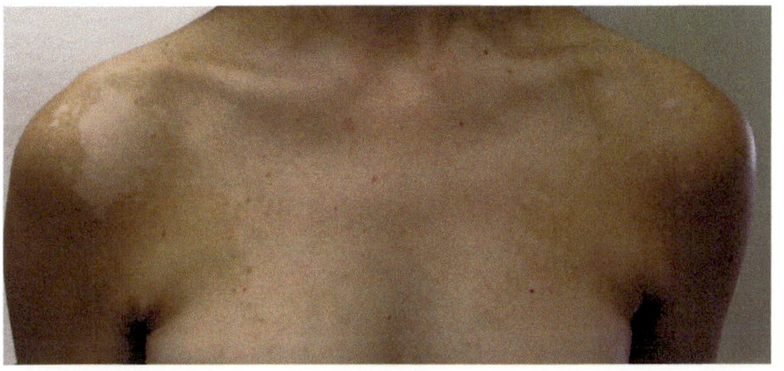

FIGURE 1.37 Dyschromia: Vitiligo with autoimmune thyroiditis.

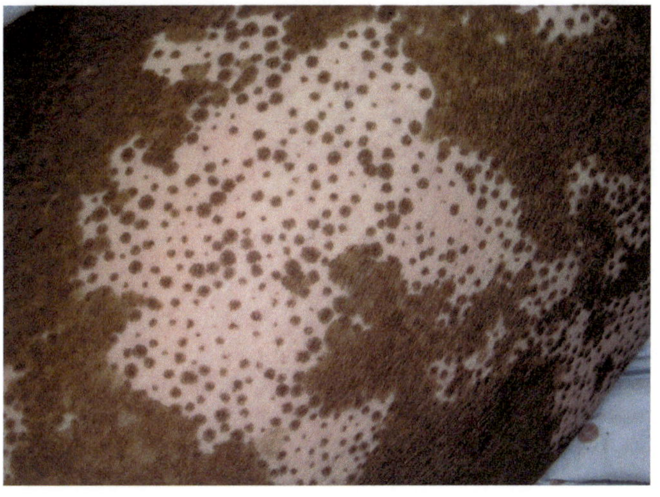

FIGURE 1.38 Dyschromia: Re-pigmenting vitiligo from phototherapy.

TABLE 1.5

Systemic Conditions Associated with Hyperpigmentation

Systemic Condition	Clinical Features	Associated Symptoms	Diagnosis
Pregnancy	Linear hyperpigmentation along the medial abdomen (linear nigra), reticulated hyperpigmentation of the cheeks and forehead (melasma), hyperpigmentation of the areola	Morning sickness, fatigue, breast tenderness	Serum or urine human chorionic gonadotropin (HCG)
Addison disease or Cushing disease	Generalized hyperpigmentation, most prominent in sun-exposed skin, elbows, PIP and MIP joints, knees. Mucosal and nail bed hyperpigmentation	Malaise, weakness, weight loss, nausea, vomiting, diarrhea	Serum cortisol, ACTH ACTH stimulation test (Addison) Dexamethasone suppression test (Cushing)
Diabetes	Thickening and hyperpigmentation of the skin folds (acanthosis), atrophic brown macules on the anterior lower legs (diabetic dermopathy)	Polyuria, excessive thirst	Fasting glucose, hemoglobin A1C
Hemochromatosis	Bronze or gray pigmentation in the skin, accentuated in sun-exposed skin	Diabetes, liver disease	Serum ferritin, liver biopsy, genetic studies
Scleroderma	"Salt and pepper" hyper- and hypopigmentation	Skin thickening, dyspnea, renal disease	Skin biopsy, serum antibodies, pulmonary testing
Lupus erythematosus	Annular and polycyclic hyperpigmentation and depigmentation	Fatigue, arthritis and myalgias, renal disease	Skin biopsy, serum antibody testing

BIBLIOGRAPHY

Giménez García RM, Carrasco Molina S. Drug-induced hyperpigmentation: Review and case series. J Am Board Fam Med 2019;32(4):628–638.

Kaufman BP, Aman T, Alexis AF. Post-inflammatory hyperpigmentation: Epidemiology, clinical presentation, pathogenesis and treatment. Am J Clin Dermatol 2018;19(4):489–503.

Rosmarin D, Passeron T, Pandya AG, et al. Two phase 3, randomized, controlled trials of ruxolitinib cream for vitiligo. N Engl J Med 2022;387(16):1445–1455.

Dysesthesia

Etiopathogenesis

Dysesthesia is an abnormal sensation in the skin that is most often described as itching, burning, tingling, bugs crawling, pain, or numbness without a primary dermatosis. It can be generalized or dermatomal (local). The etiology of such sensations may be due to central or peripheral nervous system pathology. Neuropathic disorders and psychogenic disorders often overlap. Dermatome-related (local) dysesthesia is most commonly due to a sensory nerve impingement. Pruritus is discussed separately.

Clinical Manifestations

Patients with neuropathic dysesthesia most often present with a complaint of abnormal sensations of a unilateral nature, but bilateral distribution may also occur. Clinical presentations vary, based on anatomical location: scalp (scalp dysesthesia), mouth (burning mouth syndrome), face (trigeminal trophic syndrome [**Figure 1.39**]), arms (brachioradial pruritus [**Figure 1.40**]), torso (notalgia paresthetica [**Figure 1.41**]), thigh (meralgia paresthetica [**Figure 1.42**]), and anogenital area (dysesthetic anogenital syndrome [**Figure 1.43**]). Secondary skin findings can include excoriations, prurigo nodularis, and dyschromia from macular amyloidosis. Patients often deny these lesions are self-induced but can be performed subconsciously and/or while sleeping. Neurogenic dysesthesia will often coexist with a loss of pain sensation, so excoriations may present as deep erosions/ulcerations to underlying tissue (i.e., soft tissue and bone).

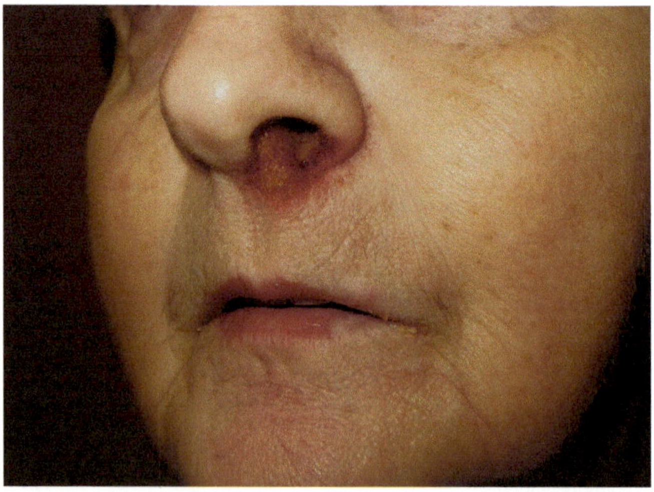

FIGURE 1.39 Trigeminal trophic syndrome: Stroke.

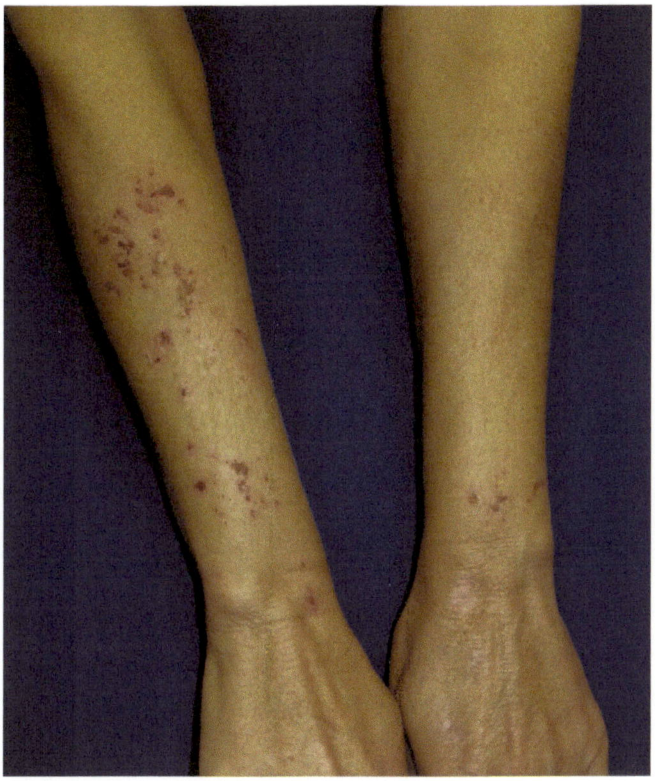

FIGURE 1.40 Brachioradial pruritus: C5-7 spine degenerative disc disease.

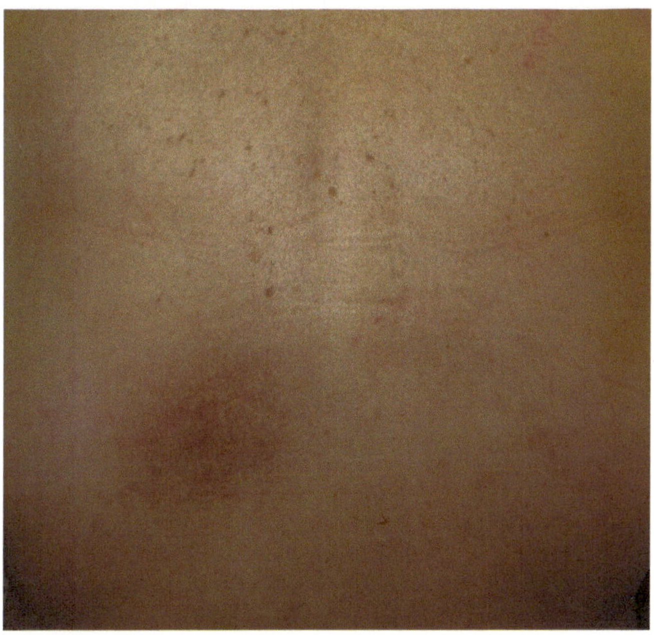

FIGURE 1.41 Notalgia paresthetica with macular amyloidosis.

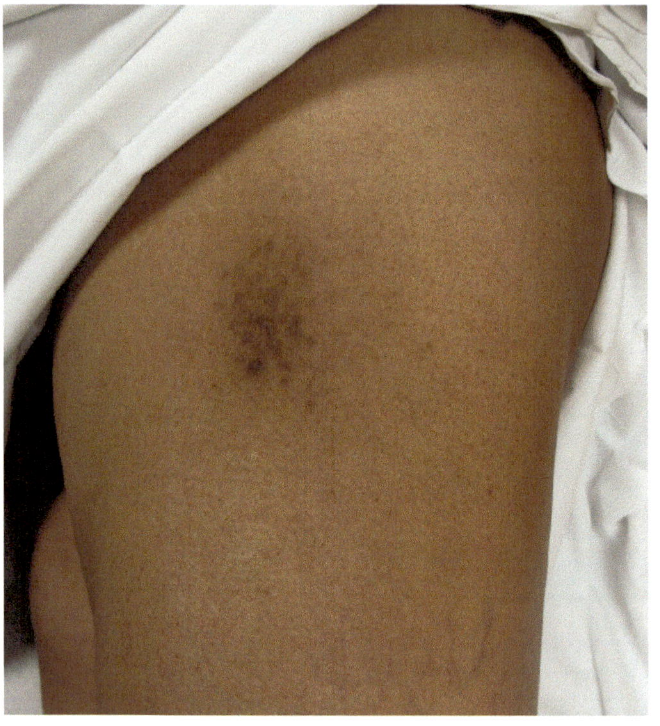

FIGURE 1.42 Meralgia paresthetica with prurigo nodules.

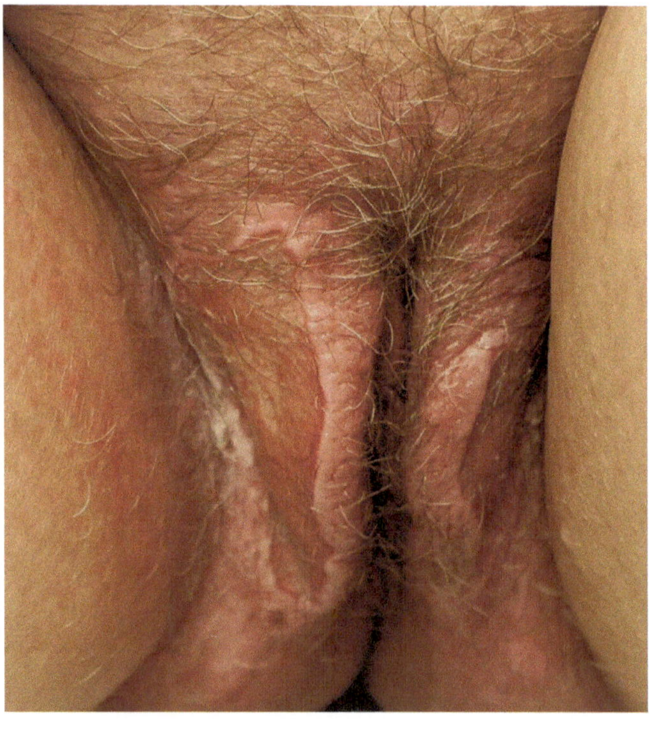

FIGURE 1.43 Dysesthetic anogenital syndrome.

Systemic Manifestations

Diseases affecting the central nervous system (tumors [**Figure 1.44**], strokes, infection, multiple sclerosis), spinal cord (hemangiomas, syringomyelia), and peripheral nervous system (small nerve fiber neuropathy [**Figure 1.45**] not from diabetes [neurotrophic ulcers], vitamin deficiencies, exposure to toxins and plasma cell dyscrasias), and radiculopathy from nerve impingement/entrapment from degenerative discogenic disease (**Figures 1.46–1.48**) requiring surgery summarize the etiologies of neurogenic dysesthesia.

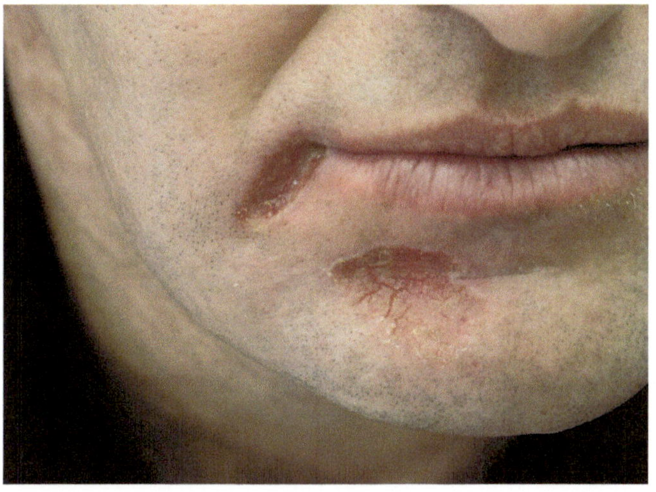

FIGURE 1.44 Trigeminal trophic syndrome: Meningioma resection.

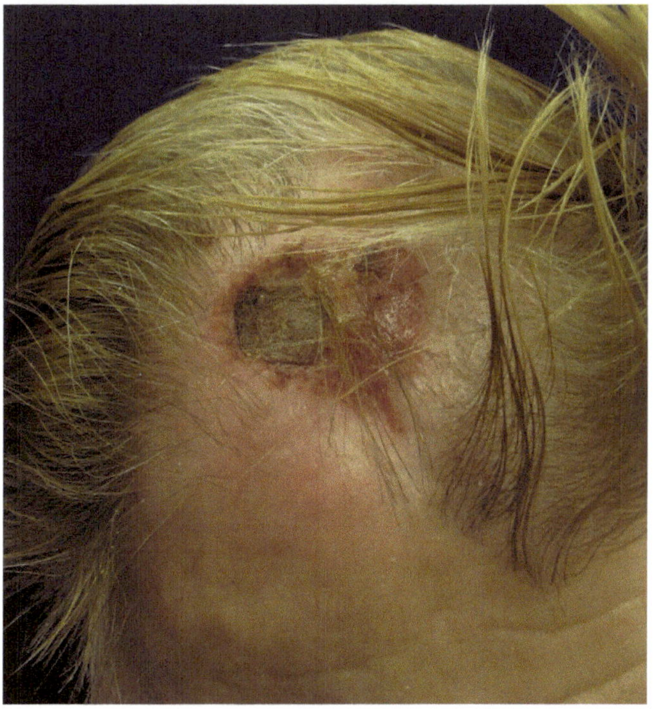

FIGURE 1.45 Trigeminal trophic syndrome: Trigeminal neuralgia.

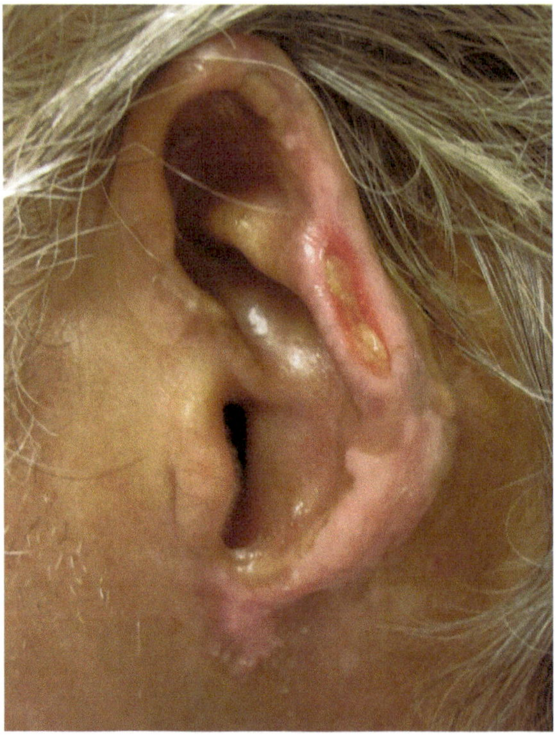

FIGURE 1.46 Neuropathic excoriations: C2 spine fusion.

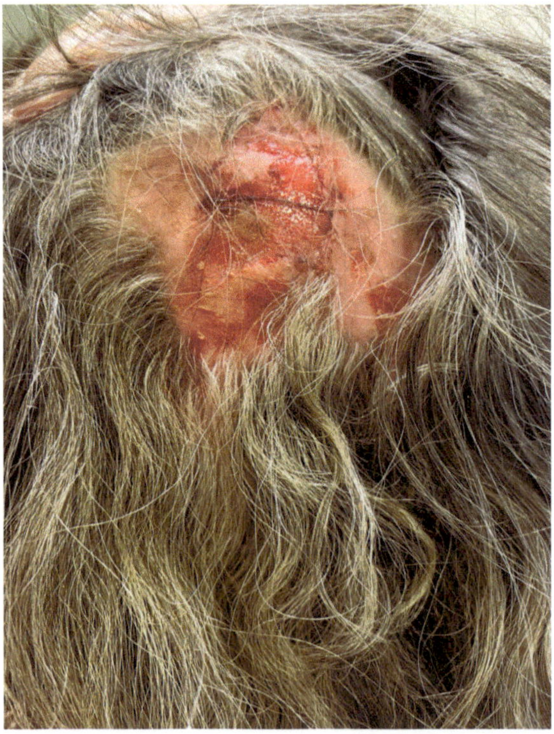

FIGURE 1.47 Scalp dysesthesia with excoriation.

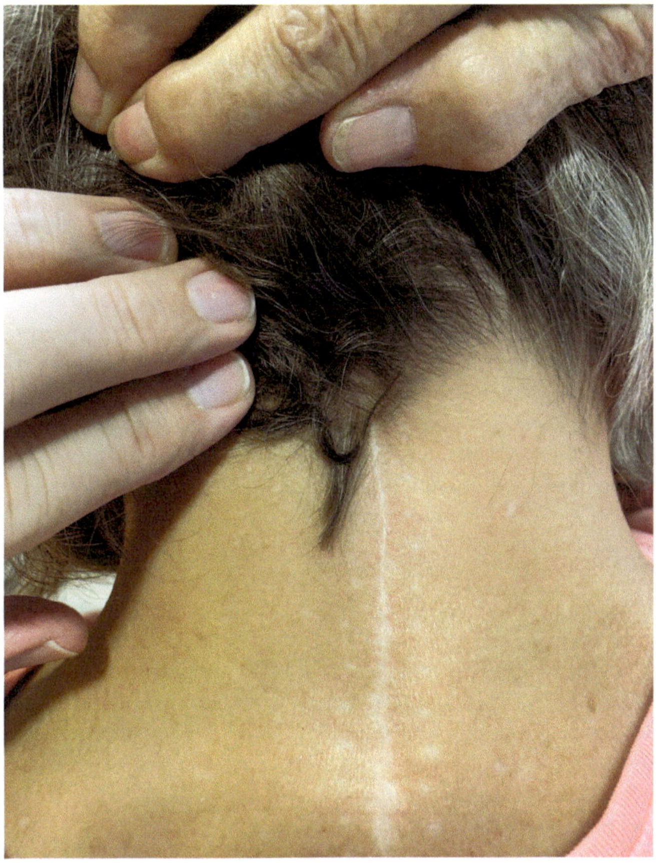

FIGURE 1.48 Scalp dysesthesia with excoriations: C-spine fusion surgery.

Evaluation and Management

A history and physical examination and appropriate radiographic imaging are required. Plain films followed by magnetic resonance imaging (MRI) of the brain and spinal column are most beneficial to determine an etiology. Nerve conduction studies may be normal and due to their lack of sensitivity, do not preclude the diagnosis of a neurogenic cause. Laboratory testing may include B vitamins, SPEP/SIFE, and UPEP/UIFE. The use of topical anesthetics (pramoxine, lidocaine) and/or oral nerve agents (gabapentin) with physical modalities such as physical therapy, chiropractic care, acupuncture, and surgery may be required.

BIBLIOGRAPHY

Auyeung KL, Jenkins BA, Kim BS. Clinical management of neuropathic itch. JAMA Dermatol 2023;159(12):1391–1392.

Labib A, Burke O, Nichols A, et al. Approach to diagnosis, evaluation, and treatment of generalized and nonlocal dysesthesia: A review. J Am Acad Dermatol 2023;89(6):1192–1200.

Lee JJ, Morillo-Hernandez C, Agarwal V, et al. Cervical spine imaging and treatment outcomes in scalp dysesthesia: A retrospective cohort study. J Am Acad Dermatol 2023;88(3):655–656.

Shumway NK, Cole E, Fernandez KH. Neurocutaneous disease: Neurocutaneous dysesthesias. J Am Acad Dermatol 2016;74(20):215–228; QUIZ 229–30.

Dyshidrosis

Etiopathogenesis

Sweating via eccrine glands is a means to regulate body temperature and is mediated by temperature control areas of the brain. Sweating can also occur in certain situations associated with stress. Hyperhidrosis, or excessive sweating, can be focal or generalized and can be either due to an underlying disease or medication (secondary hyperhidrosis) or due to unexplained sympathetic overactivity (primary hyperhidrosis).

Clinical Manifestations

Primary focal hyperhidrosis is much more common than secondary hyperhidrosis and usually occurs symmetrically in particular anatomical regions such as the axilla (**Figures 1.49** and **1.50**), palms, soles, or face, independent of temperature. When compared to primary hyperhidrosis, patients with secondary hyperhidrosis tend to be older and more often will have sweating that is asymmetric or generalized. Although secondary hyperhidrosis can occur in typical areas such as the axilla, palms, or soles, it more commonly occurs in atypical locations such as the trunk, head and neck, or groin.

Systemic Manifestations

Secondary hyperhidrosis can be due to underlying diseases or medications. Diseases that have been reported in patients with secondary hyperhidrosis include endocrine abnormalities such as diabetes (**Figure 1.51**), hyperthyroidism (**Figure 1.52**), pheochromocytoma, and carcinoid syndrome. Neurologic conditions, such as peripheral nerve injuries, reflex sympathetic dystrophy, spinal cord injuries, or RP (**Figure 1.53**) can also lead to sweating abnormalities. Night sweats can be triggered by certain infections and lymphoproliferative malignancies. Medications such as selective serotonin reuptake inhibitors and tricyclic antidepressants are rare causes of secondary hyperhidrosis, along with systemic infections and cardiovascular and respiratory failure.

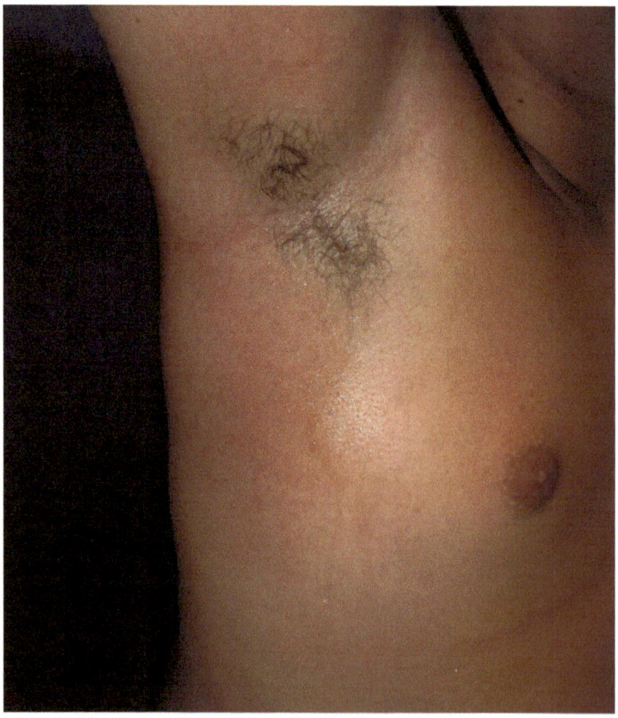

FIGURE 1.49 Hyperhidrosis: Axillary glistening.

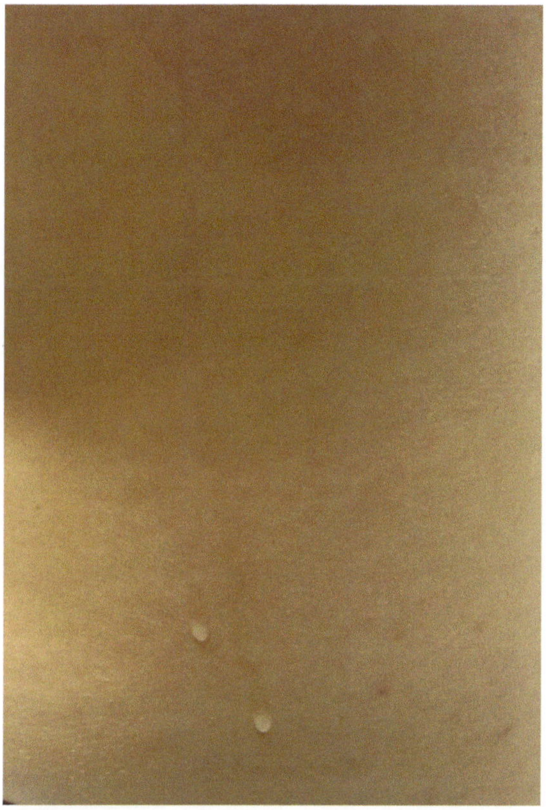

FIGURE 1.50 Hyperhidrosis: Beads of sweat.

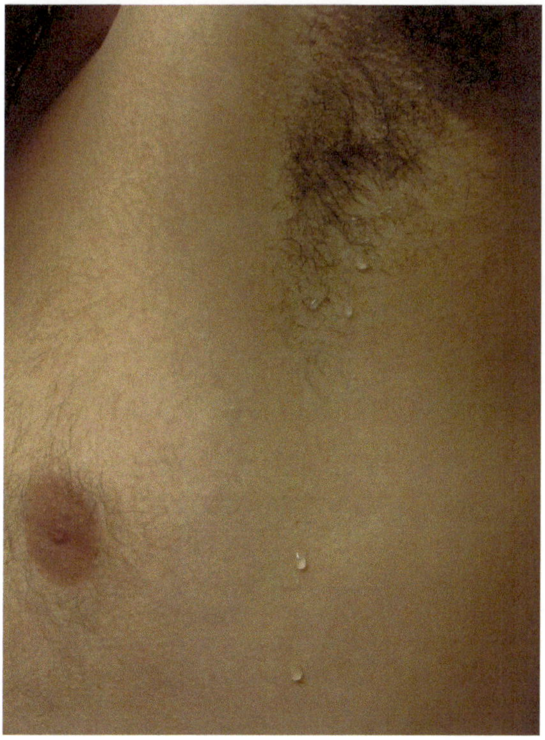

FIGURE 1.51 Hyperhidrosis: Diabetes mellitus.

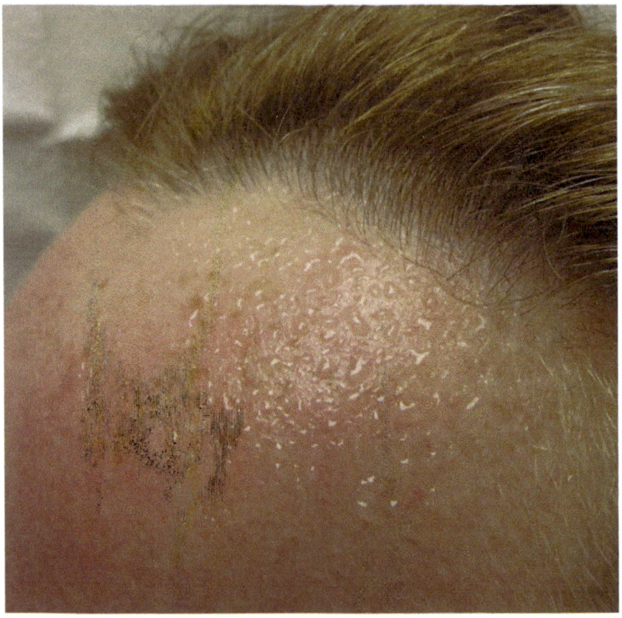

FIGURE 1.52 Hyperhidrosis: Hyperthyroidism.

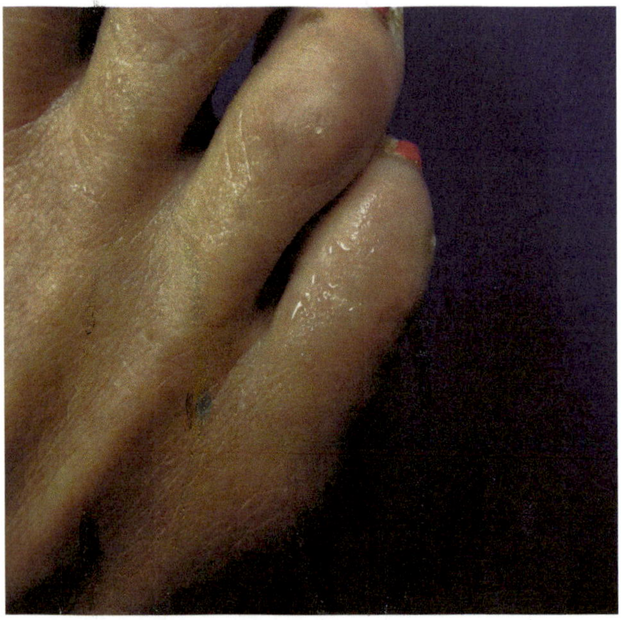

FIGURE 1.53 Hyperhidrosis: Acral with Raynaud phenomenon.

Evaluation and Management

A history of excess sweating is usually sufficient for making a diagnosis of hyperhidrosis. In patients with primary focal hyperhidrosis, excess sweating in the region of the axilla, palms, soles, or forehead may be apparent on physical examination. In patients who are older, with hyperhidrosis that is asymmetric or generalized, or in atypical areas, a secondary cause should be considered, and ordering an FBG, HA1c, TFTs, TGs, TPOs, serum metanephrines, and 24-hour urine for 5-HIAA are suggested. Localized therapy for focal disease, such as topical aluminum chloride or glycopyrrolate, intradermal botulinum toxin, or tap-water iontophoresis, can be tried. Generalized hyperhidrosis can be treated with systemic anticholinergic medications such as oral glycopyrrolate or oxybutynin. In severe cases of palmar hyperhidrosis, a thoracic sympathectomy can be performed. For secondary hyperhidrosis, management of the underlying secondary causes identified may be beneficial.

BIBLIOGRAPHY

Glaser DA, Hebert AA, Nast A, et al. A 44-week open-label study evaluating safety and efficacy of topical glycopyrronium tosylate in patients with primary axillary hyperhidrosis. Am J Clin Dermatol 2019;20(4):593–604.

Henning MAS, Bouazzi D, Jemec GBE. Treatment of hyperhidrosis: An update. Am J Clin Dermatol 2022;23(5):635–646.

Nawrocki S, Cha J. The etiology, diagnosis and management of hyperhidrosis: A comprehensive review: Etiology and clinical work-up. J Am Acad Dermatol 2019;81(3):657–666.

Zhong Y, Zhu Y, Li J, et al. Efficacy and safety of radiofrequency ablation versus surgical sympathectomy in palmar hyperhidrosis. Sci Rep 2024;14(1):7620.

Erythroderma

Etiopathogenesis

Erythroderma is defined as erythema and scaling that occurs over 90% of the body surface area (**Figures 1.54** and **1.55**). In most cases, erythroderma is idiopathic or the result of the worsening of a primary dermatosis. The more common underlying dermatoses include psoriasis and atopic dermatitis, whereas rare causes of erythroderma can include pityriasis rubra pilaris, crusted scabies, immunobullous diseases, cutaneous T-cell lymphoma, solid malignancy, or a medication reaction (**Figure 1.56**, **Table 1.6**).

Clinical Manifestations

In addition to scaling and erythema, patients with erythroderma can present with pruritus, fevers, chills, nail changes, alopecia, and lymphadenopathy, irrespective of the underlying cause. Some clinical findings may help to identify the underlying cause of the erythroderma, such as islands of sparing in pityriasis rubra pilaris, scaling of encrusted scabies (**Figure 1.57**), or bullae in immunobullous disease, although most of the time, clinical findings alone cannot be used in distinguishing one cause of erythroderma from another.

Systemic Manifestations

Fluid loss, electrolyte imbalance, protein wasting, and an inability to regulate body temperature can occur in patients with erythroderma. Death as a result of erythroderma is rare, although it can occur, usually in the setting of malignancy, from high-output cardiac failure or secondary infection (sepsis).

Evaluation and Management

Because erythroderma often occurs as a result of the flare of an underlying primary dermatosis, knowing the dermatologic history of the patient is essential. A thorough medication history, including over-the-counter supplements and traditional medicines, must be taken. In patients without a clear history of a preceding dermatosis, a skin biopsy may provide the diagnosis. Although nonspecific findings on histology are common, direct immunofluorescence will delineate any immunobullous disorders (**Figure 1.58**). A more extensive workup, such as CT to rule out underlying malignancy, or flow cytometry on peripheral blood to rule out Sezary syndrome (leukemic cutaneous T-cell lymphoma [**Figure 1.59**]), can be considered in selected patients. Hospital admission may be required in patients with severe dehydration or electrolyte abnormalities. Occlusive dressings with topical corticosteroids can be administered with good results in most patients. More specific therapy for erythroderma is directed at the underlying cause if it can be identified. In cases of idiopathic erythroderma, systemic corticosteroids can be given initially, with transition to a nonsteroid agent for long-term management of the disease.

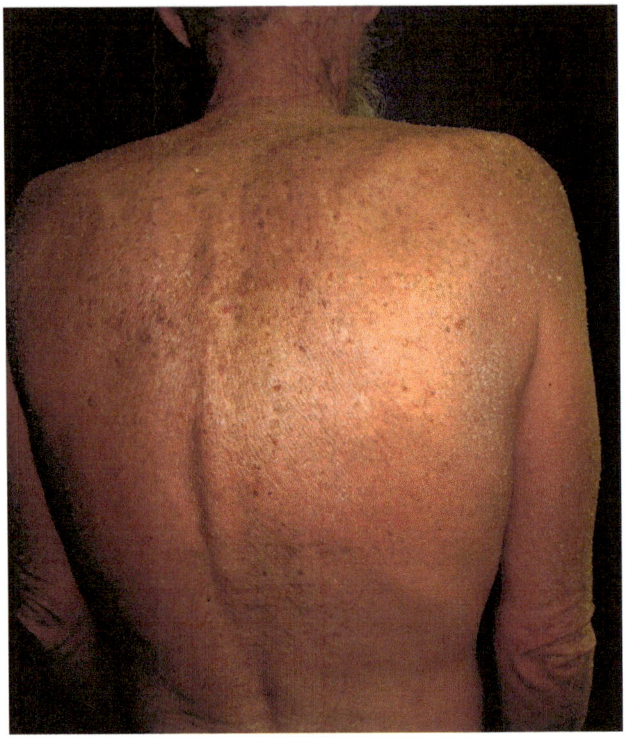

FIGURE 1.54 Erythroderma: Idiopathic.

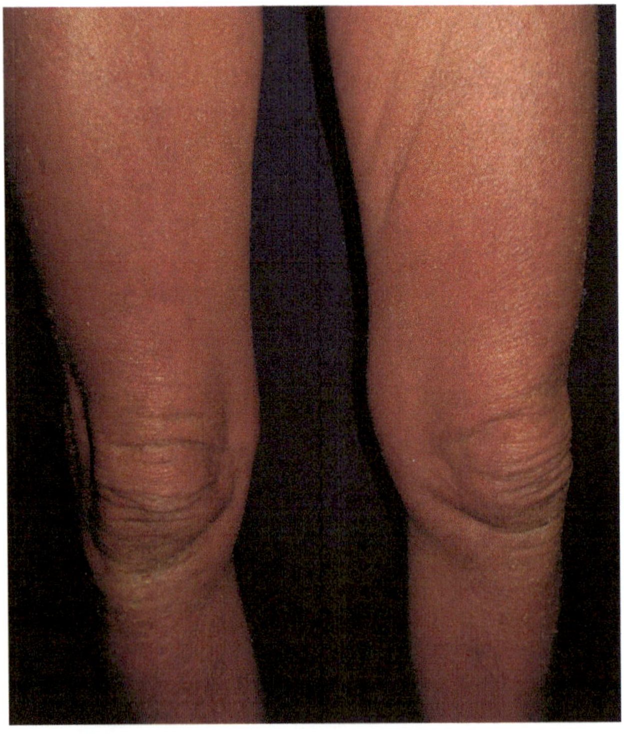

FIGURE 1.55 Erythroderma: Idiopathic.

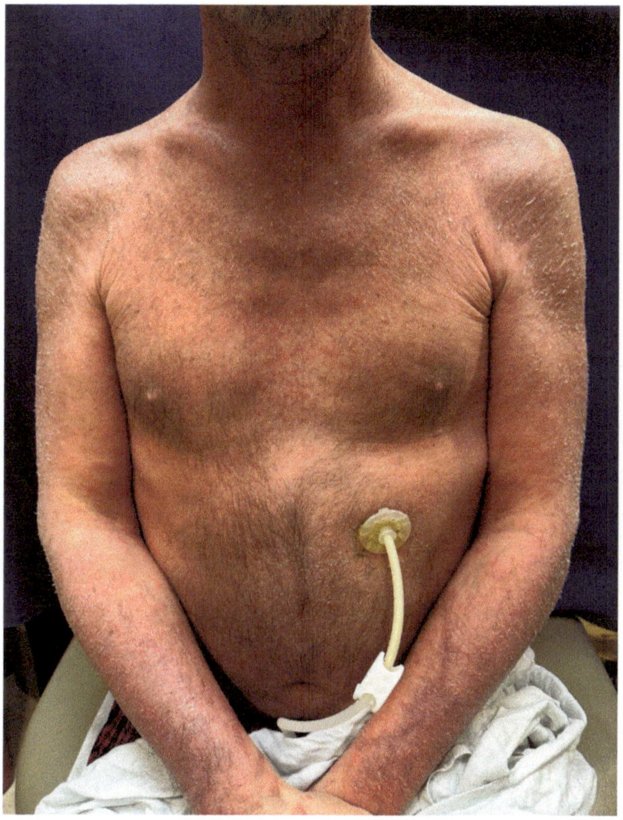

FIGURE 1.56 Erythroderma: Medication.

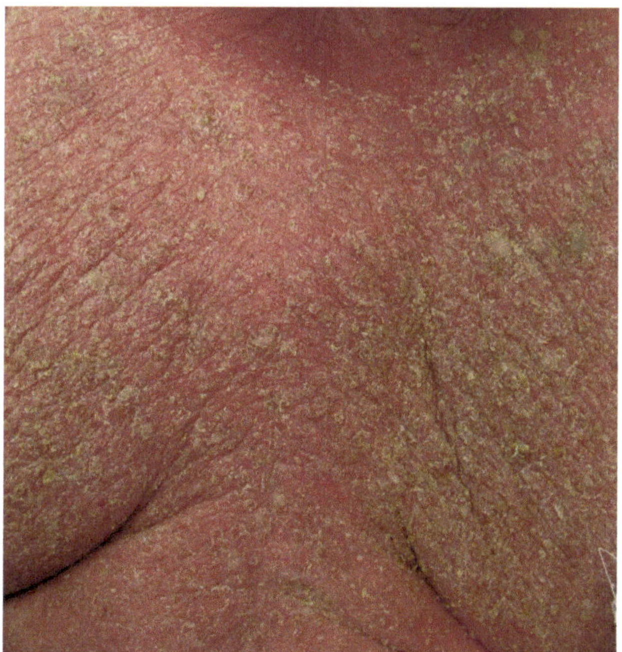

FIGURE 1.57 Erythroderma: Scabetic.

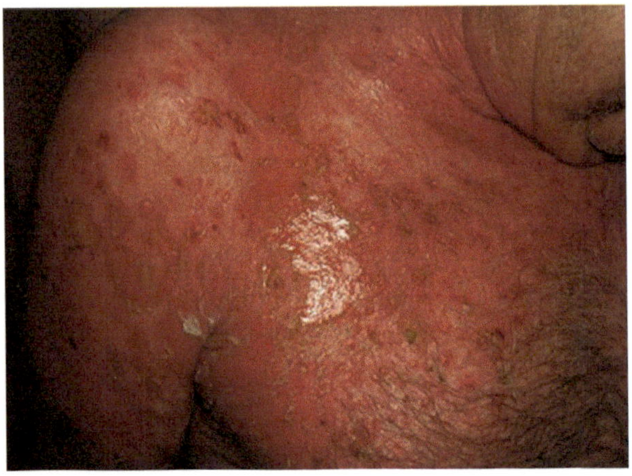

FIGURE 1.58 Erythroderma: Bullous pemphigoid.

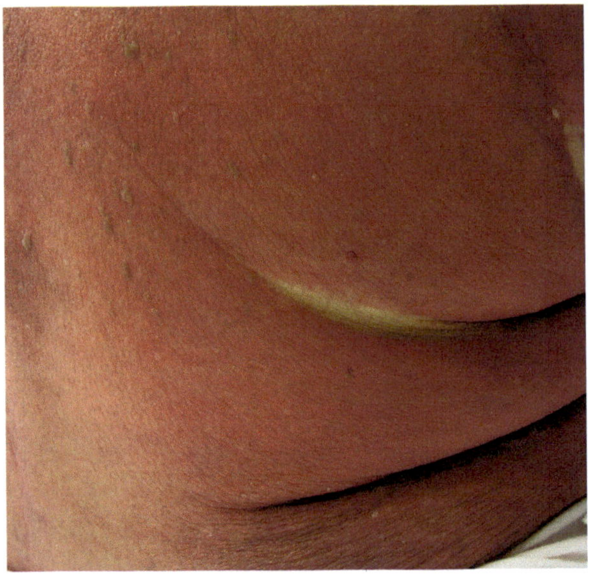

FIGURE 1.59 Erythroderma: Cutaneous T-cell lymphoma.

TABLE 1.6

Review of Erythroderma

Cause	History/Clinical Findings	Diagnosis
Psoriasis	History of psoriasis, recent psoriasis medication change, recent systemic corticosteroid treatment	Skin biopsy demonstrating microabscesses
Atopic eczema	Personal or family history of atopic diathesis, lichenification in antecubital and popliteal fossa	Skin biopsy demonstrating spongiosis
Medications	Recent medication changes	Diagnosis mostly through history, improvement with discontinuation of culprit medications
Cutaneous T-cell lymphoma	Associated B symptoms	Skin biopsy (may be nonspecific), peripheral blood flow cytometry studies
Pityriasis rubra pilaris	Islands of sparing, orange-red color, acral hyperkeratosis, follicular hyperkeratosis	Skin biopsy demonstrating classic "checkerboard" para- and ortho-keratosis

BIBLIOGRAPHY

Harper-Kirksey K. Erythroderma. Life-Threatening Rashes. 2018 Sep; 12:265–77.

Miyashiro D, Sanches JA. Erythroderma: A prospective study of 309 patients followed for 12 years in a tertiary center. Sci Rep 2020;10(1):9774.

Rothe MJ, Bernstein ML, Grant-Kels JM. Life-threatening erythroderma: Diagnosing and treating the "red man. Clin Exp Dermatol 2005;23(2):206–217.

Tso S, Satchwell F, Moiz H, et al. Erythroderma (exfoliative dermatitis). Part 1: Underlying causes, clinical presentation and pathogenesis. Clin Exp Dermatol 2021;46:1001–1010.

Flushing

Etiopathogenesis

Flushing is a common manifestation of cutaneous vasomotor activity. The causes of flushing are diverse and dependent on the underlying etiology. Regardless, they all share a common vasodilation pathway mediated by nerves or vasoactive mediators acting on vascular smooth muscle.

Clinical Manifestations

Flushing is characterized by rapid cutaneous vasodilation that manifests as sudden warmth and visible erythema of the skin (**Figures 1.60** and **1.61**), with occasional itching or tingling. It most often affects the head, neck, and upper portions of the chest, areas that are abundant in superficial cutaneous vasculature. Flushing can be episodic, usually lasting about 1 hour. When persistent, it can produce fixed facial erythema or a cyanotic hue.

Systemic Manifestations

Flushing can be secondary to physiologic stimuli (fever, emotion), or extrinsic agents such as medications (niacin, calcium channel blockers, betablockers, nitroglycerin, sildenafil citrate, angiotensin-converting enzyme (ACE) inhibitors, vancomycin, nonsteroidal anti-inflammatory drugs (NSAIDs), chemotherapeutic agents), foods (fish poisoning), alcohol, temperature changes, and hormonal/endocrine imbalance (climacterium). Symptoms such as flushing in association with increased GI motility, paroxysmal hypertension, palpitations, nausea and vomiting, abdominal/flank pain, or thyromegaly should prompt evaluation for conditions such as pheochromocytoma, carcinoid syndrome, systemic mastocytosis, pancreatic islet cell tumor (VIPoma), renal cell carcinoma, or medullary thyroid cancer.

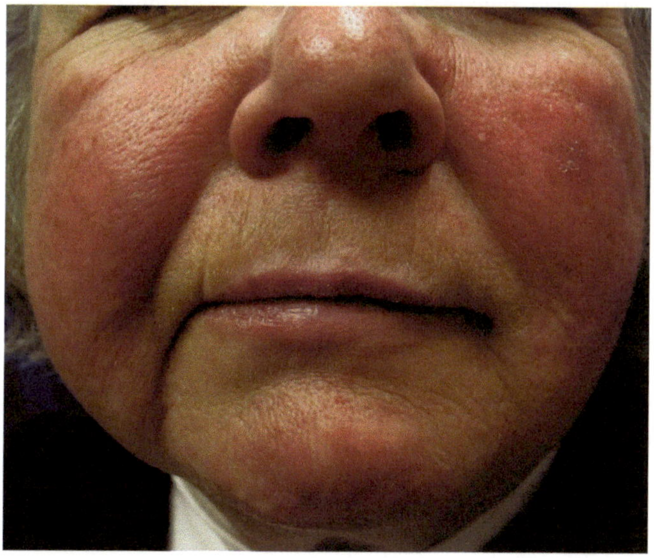

FIGURE 1.60 Flushing: Rosacea.

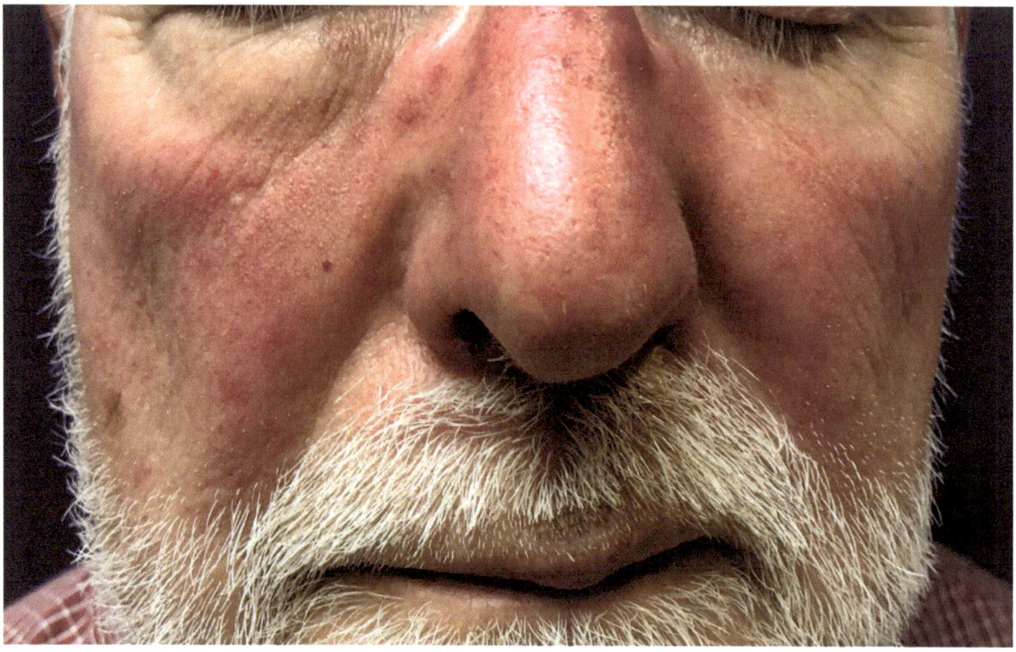

FIGURE 1.61 Flushing: Carcinoid syndrome.

Evaluation and Management

Given that flushing is a nonspecific finding associated with multiple entities, consideration of the patient's associated signs and symptoms and medications should help guide evaluation and management. Although rosacea is the most common, the rare and life-threatening causes of flushing should be considered if associated systemic symptoms are present. Flushing with systemic symptoms should lead to further investigation (**Table 1.7**). Subsequent appropriate imaging and referrals to specialists can be initiated if indicated. Treatment options are again based on the underlying etiology responsible for flushing.

TABLE 1.7

Evaluation of Malignant Causes of Cutaneous Flushing

Disease	Laboratory Tests
Carcinoid syndrome	24-h Urine for 5-HIAA
Pheochromocytoma	24-h urine or serum metanephrines
Medullary thyroid cancer	Calcitonin, carcinoembryonic antigen
Pancreatic neuroendocrine tumor	Vasoactive intestinal peptide
Systemic mastocytosis	Tryptase
Renal cell carcinoma	Urinalysis

BIBLIOGRAPHY

Hannah-Shmouni F, Stratakis CA, Koch CA. Flushing in (neuro) endocrinology. Rev Endrocr Metab Disord 2016;17(3):373–380.

Izikson L, English JC 3rd, Zirwas MJ. The flushing patient: Differential diagnosis, work-up and treatment. J Am Acad Dermatol 2006;55(2):193–208.

Sadeghian A, Rouhana H, Oswald-Stumpf B, et al. Etiologies and management of cutaneous flushing: Nonmalignant causes. J Am Acad Dermatol 2017a;77(3):391–402.

Sadeghian A, Rouhana H, Oswald-Stumpf B, et al. Etiologies and management of cutaneous flushing: Malignant causes. J Am Acad Dermatol 2017b;77(3):405–414.

Gingival Enlargement

Etiopathogenesis

Gingival enlargement (GE), or overgrowth of gingival tissue, has been associated with hematologic disorders, inflammatory disorders, adverse drug reactions (**Figure 1.62**), poor oral hygiene, genetic disorders, hormonal and nutritional states, or it can be idiopathic. The mechanism leading to gingival overgrowth is complex and involves the upregulation of numerous proteins, including transforming growth factor (TGF), endothelin-1, angiotensin II, IGF, and platelet-derived growth factor. Long-standing increases in the levels of circulating hormones and profibrotic mediators culminate in the development of GE.

Clinical Manifestations

Regardless of the etiology, GE (**Figures 1.62** and **1.63**) is clinically characterized by disproportional overgrowth of gingival tissues. This leads to subsequent inflammation, gingival bleeding, and discomfort when eating. "Strawberry" GE (**Figure 1.64**) has been reported in patients with granulomatosis with polyangiitis (GPA) and sarcoidosis.

Systemic Manifestations

GE has been associated with hematologic malignancies from leukemia (acute monocytic leukemia [M5] and acute myelomonocytic leukemia [M4]) to multiple myeloma. GE is the presenting sign of leukemia in approximately 5% of cases. Kaposi's sarcoma and metastatic cancer (**Figure 1.65**) may cause GE. Patients with epistaxis, purpura, and renal insufficiency with strawberry GE should be evaluated for GPA. If associated with shortness of breath, sarcoidosis needs to be considered. Of note, Crohn's disease, amyloidosis, acromegaly, scurvy, pregnancy, and puberty round out the differential diagnoses. Common causes of drug-induced GE are reviewed in **Table 1.8** and can have a synergistic effect if used in combination.

TABLE 1.8

Common Causes of Drug-Induced Gingival Enlargement

Anticonvulsants
• Phenytoin
• Valproic acid
• Phenobarbital
• Levetiracetam
• Carbamazepine
• Oxcarbazepine
• Lamotrigine
Immunosuppressants
• Cyclosporine
• Sirolimus
• Tacrolimus
Calcium channel blockers
• Nifedipine
• Felodipine
• Amlodipine
• Nisoldipine
• Verapamil
• Diltiazem

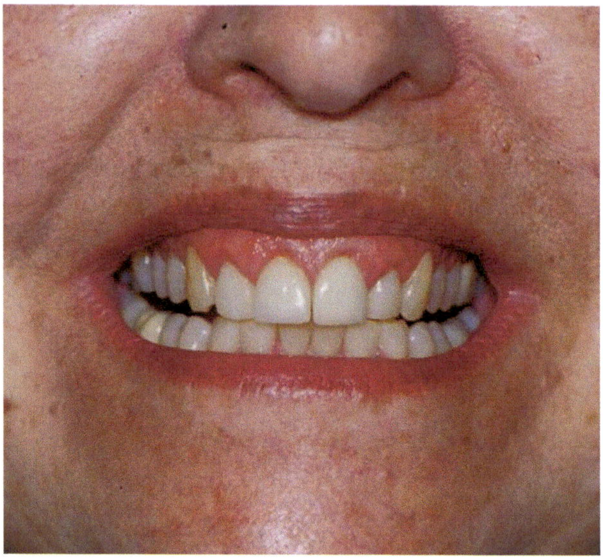

FIGURE 1.62 Gingival enlargement: Medication.

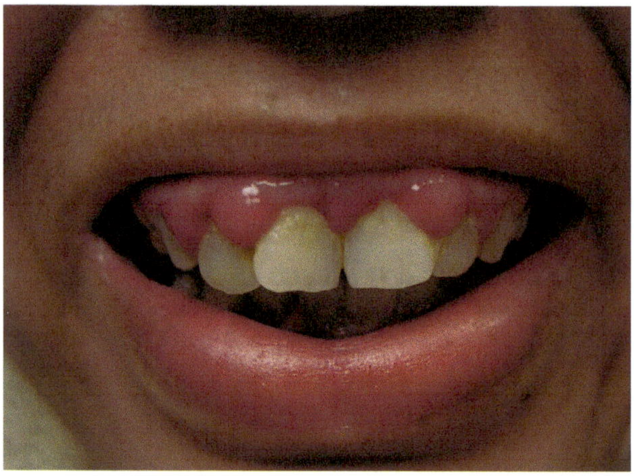

FIGURE 1.63 Gingival enlargement: Idiopathic.

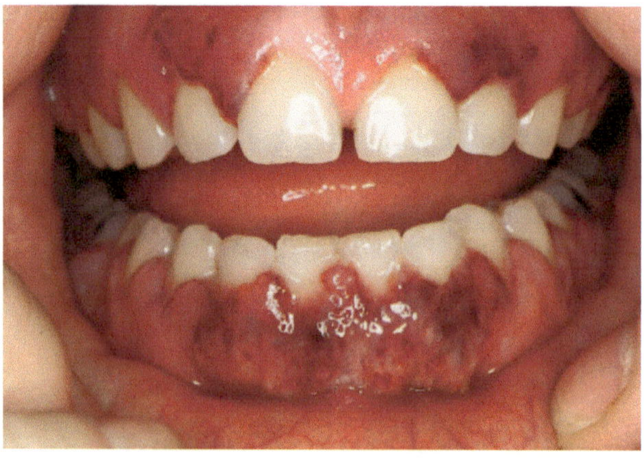

FIGURE 1.64 Gingival enlargement: Strawberry gums of granulomatosis with polyangiitis.

Evaluation and Management

The development of GE should prompt investigation into systemic causes. Gingival biopsy and other investigative studies may include CBC, comprehensive metabolic panel (CMP), urinalysis (UA), anti-neutrophilic cytoplasmic antibodies (ANCAs), HIV, SPEP/SIFE, UPEP/UIFE, vitamin C, and CXR. Consultation with a hematologist/oncologist and a bone marrow biopsy may be indicated. If any culprit drugs are noted, discontinuation and replacement with alternative therapy, if possible, may lead to some regression of the gingival tissue. This is most often reported with cyclosporine withdrawal. Additional treatment of cyclosporine-induced GE with a macrolide antibiotic has been reported to cause resolution. If drug substitutions cannot be done safely, then regular monitoring by a dentist at 3-month intervals is recommended. Conscientious oral hygiene is imperative. Despite this, gingivectomy is often required.

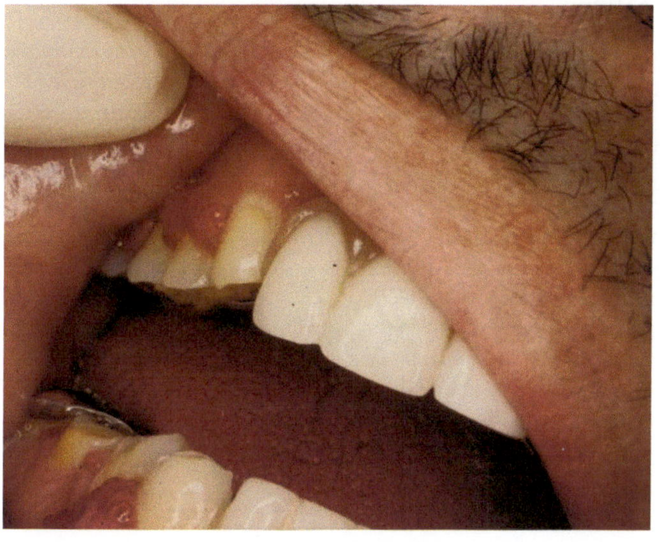

FIGURE 1.65 Gingival enlargement: Metastatic hepatocellular carcinoma.

BIBLIOGRAPHY

Bjkovec L, Mrzljak A, Likic R, et al. Drug-induced gingival overgrowth in cardiovascular patients. World J Cardiol 2021;13(4):68–75.

Gallo C, Bonvento G, Zagotto G, et al. Gingival overgrowth induced by anti-convulsant drugs: A cross-sectional study on epileptic patients. J Periodontal Res 2021;56(2):363–369.

Khera P, Zirwas MJ, English JC III. Diffuse gingival enlargement. J Am Acad Dermatol 2005;52(3 Pt 1):491–499.

Zisis V, Zisis S, Anagnostou E, et al. Gingival enlargement can constitute the only diagnostic sign of leukemia: Report of an unusual case. Cureus 2023;15 (10):e47959.

Glossitis and Stomatitis

Etiopathogenesis

Glossitis refers to inflammation of the tongue. Stomatitis refers to inflammation of the mouth and lips (cheilitis), whereas gingivostomatitis includes inflammation of the gums, mouth, and lip. The oral cavity can manifest a wide spectrum of localized or systemic diseases. Langerhans cells (antigen-presenting cells) are found throughout the structures of the mouth and play an important role in many inflammatory oral mucosal reactions.

Clinical Manifestations

Examination of the mouth should include the palate, buccal mucosa, floor of mouth, tongue, gingiva, and teeth. Clinicians may examine for color or pallor, loss of tongue papilla with erythema (atrophic glossitis), size and patterns (migratory [**Figure 1.66**]) of lesions on the tongue, gingival enlargement with friable erythema, buccal mucosal/hard palate cobblestoning, Wickham striae, keratotic papules (keratosis nicotina palatini) or plaques (leukoplakia), hemorrhage, or purpura. Ulcerations can manifest as punched-out ulcers with a ring of erythema or as large erosions with mucosal sloughing. The differential diagnoses include oral erosive lichen planus, autoimmune immunobullous disease, and recurrent aphthous stomatitis. Lesions may range from being asymptomatic to causing a burning sensation or producing severe pain.

Systemic Manifestations

Vitamin deficiencies can cause atrophic glossitis (**Figure 1.67**). Severe malnutrition compounded by infection results in acute necrotizing ulcerative gingivostomatitis (**Figure 1.68**). Diabetes and other immunosuppressed states may produce candidal gingivostomatitis (**Figures 1.69** and **1.70**) and median rhomboid glossitis (**Figure 1.71**). Anemia, thrombocytopenia, hemostatic disorders (von Willebrand disease), leukemia, and myelodysplasia may present with gingival bleeding, purpura, or enlargement. Aphthae (ulcers) can be idiopathic, recurrent, and range from minor to major (**Figures 1.72** and **1.73**). Aphthae can be a manifestation of oral lichen planus secondary to hepatitis C infection (**Figures 1.74** and **1.75**) or due to autoimmune blistering disorders such as mucous membrane pemphigus (**Figure 1.76**) and paraneoplastic pemphigus. Aphthae from erythema multiforme (**Figures 1.77** and **1.78**) may be minor (coexisting herpes simplex viruses or *Mycobacterium*-induced pneumonia) or major (drug). Severe oral disease with cutaneous findings is seen in Stevens–Johnson syndrome and toxic epidermal necrolysis drug reactions. They also may represent autoimmune disorders such as Behcet disease, inflammatory bowel disease such as pyostomatitis vegetans (**Figure 1.79**), or SLE. Macroglossia, or hypertrophy of the tongue, can be observed in systemic amyloidosis.

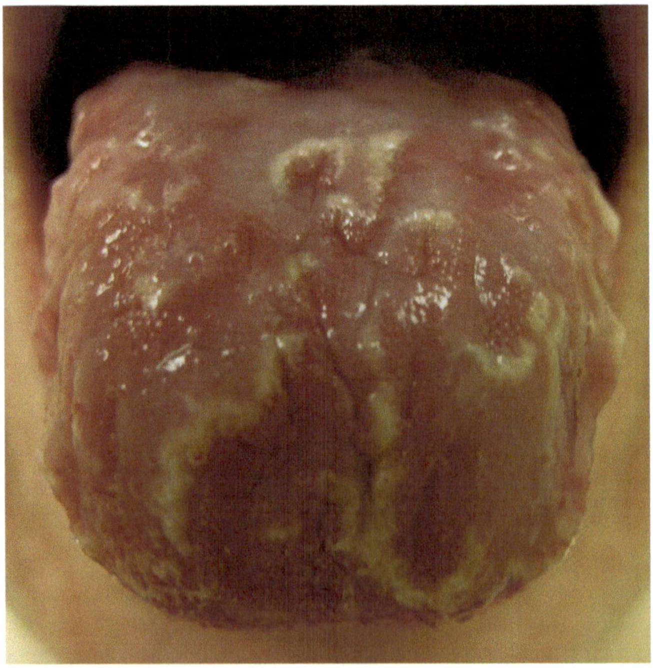

FIGURE 1.66 Glossitis: Migratory.

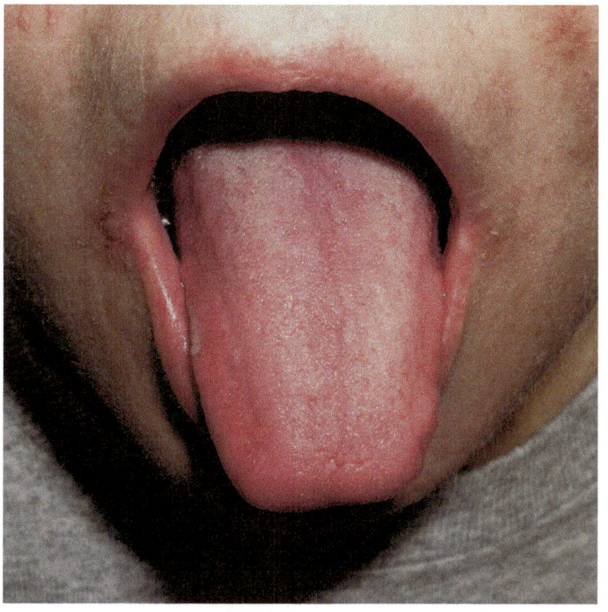

FIGURE 1.67 Glossitis: Zinc deficiency.

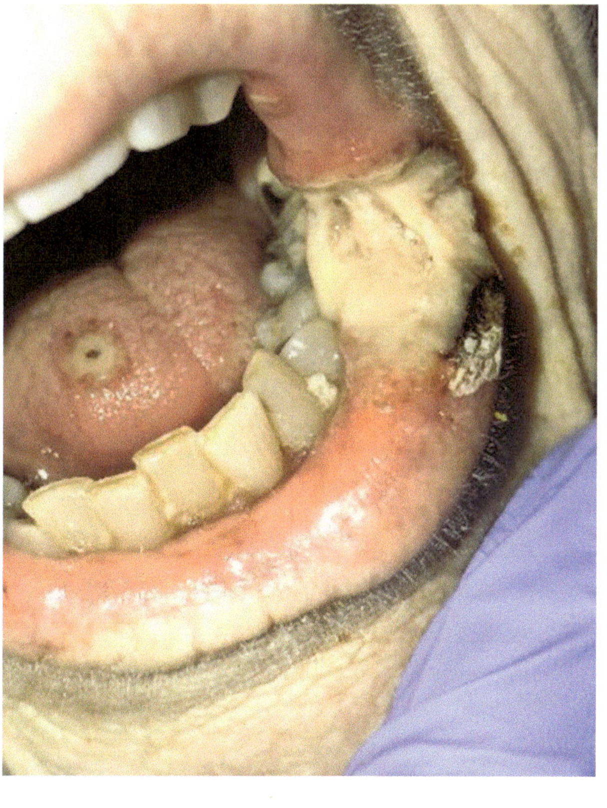

FIGURE 1.68 Necrotizing ulcerative gingivostomatitis from severe malnutrition.

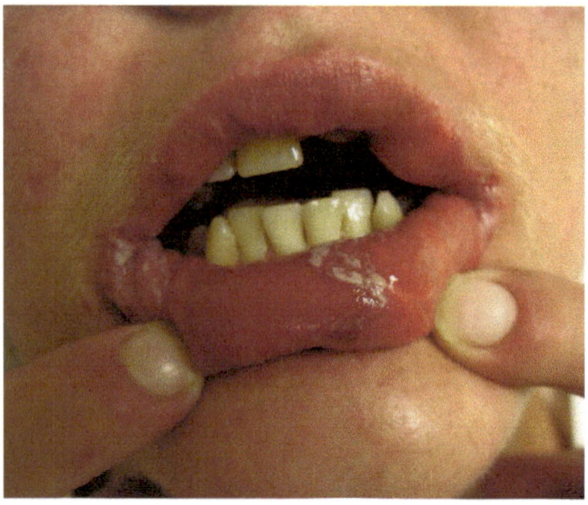

FIGURE 1.69 Stomatitis: Candidiasis from drug-induced immunosuppression for lupus.

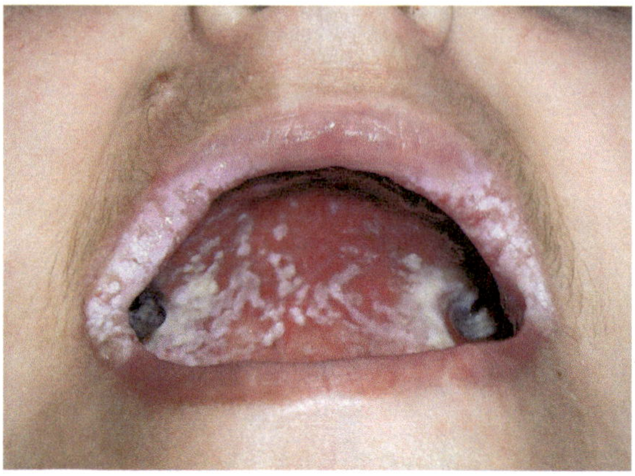

FIGURE 1.70 Stomatitis: Candidiasis from drug-induced immunosuppression for pemphigus.

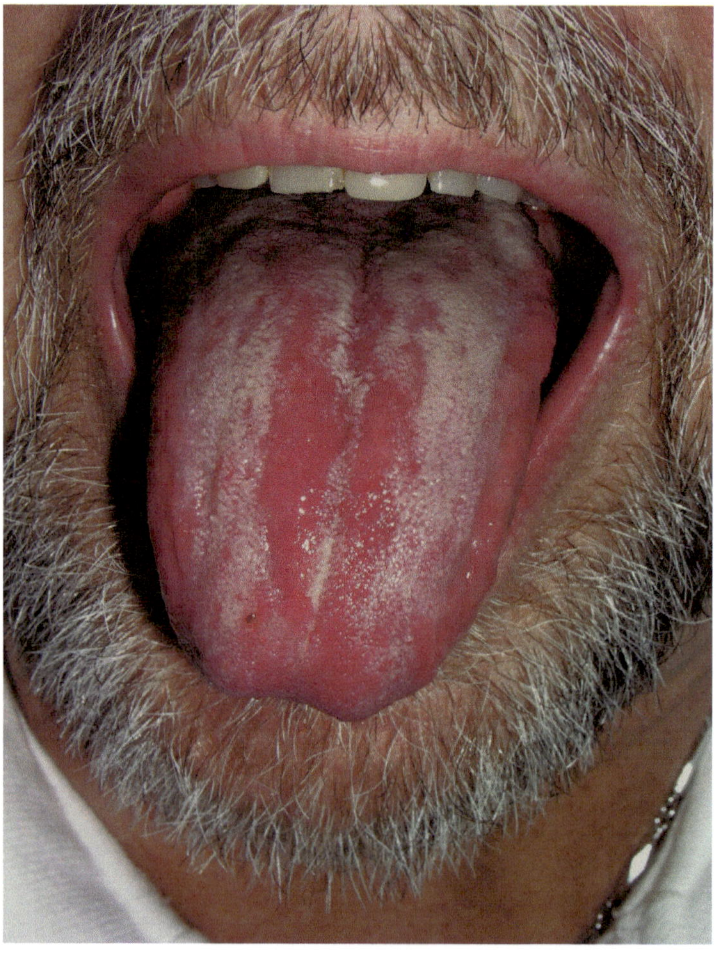

FIGURE 1.71 Glossitis: Median rhomboid.

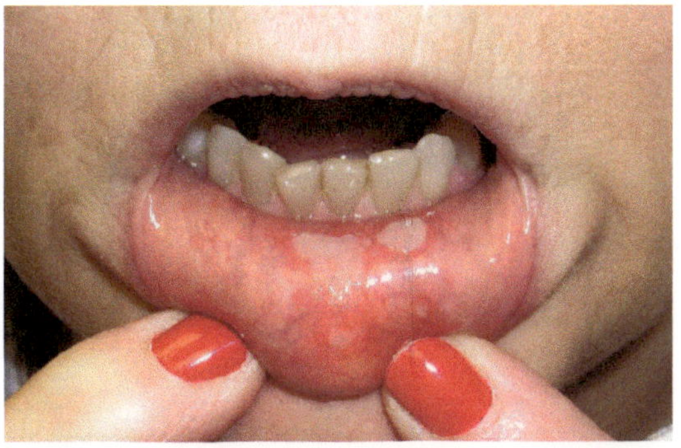

FIGURE 1.72 Stomatitis: Minor recurrent aphthae.

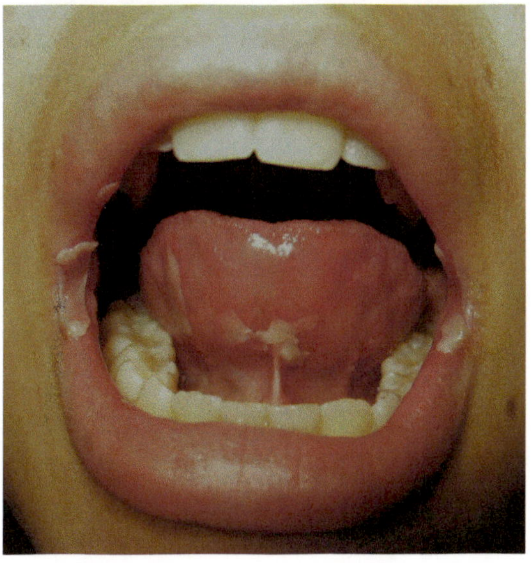

FIGURE 1.73 Stomatitis: Major recurrent aphthae.

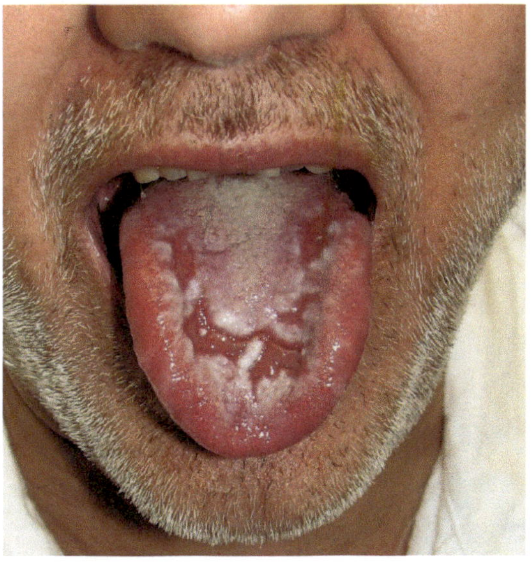

FIGURE 1.74 Glossitis: Ulcerative lichen planus.

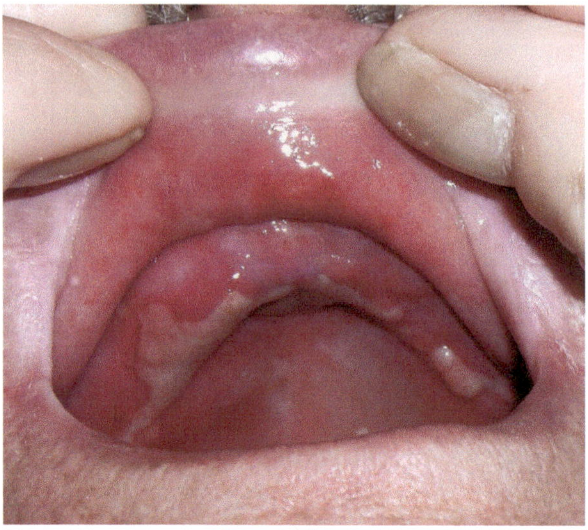

FIGURE 1.75 Stomatitis: Ulcerative lichen planus.

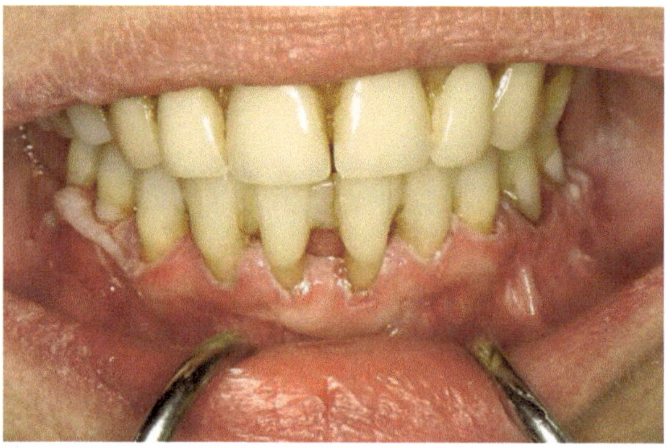

FIGURE 1.76 Gingivostomatitis: Mucous membrane pemphigus.

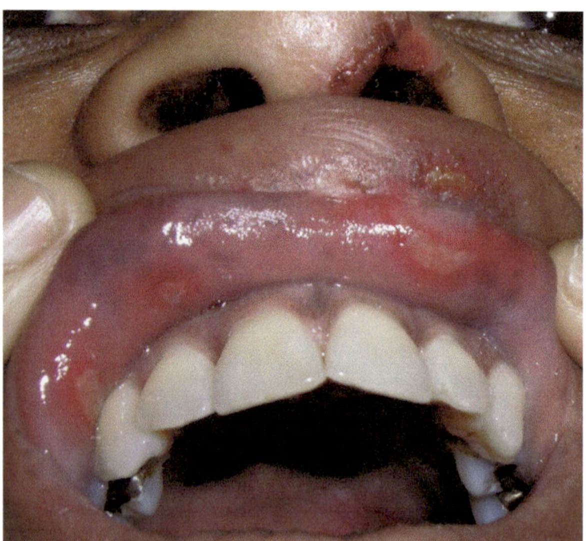

FIGURE 1.77 Stomatitis: Erythema multiforme minor from herpes infection.

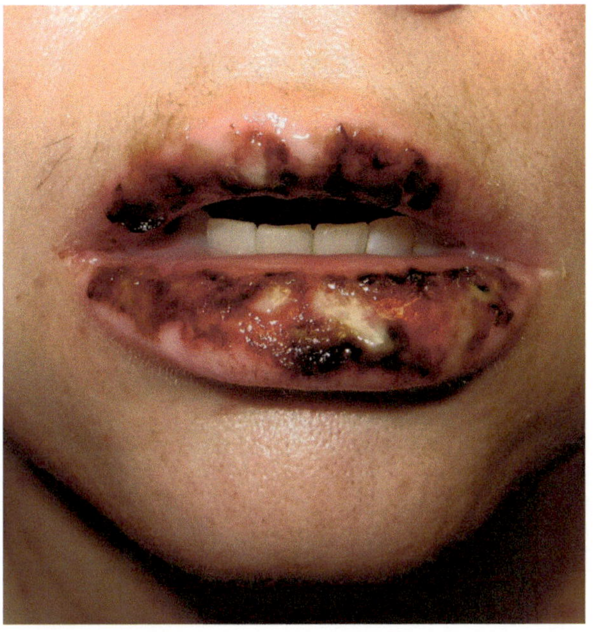

FIGURE 1.78 Stomatitis: Erythema multiforme major from drug reaction.

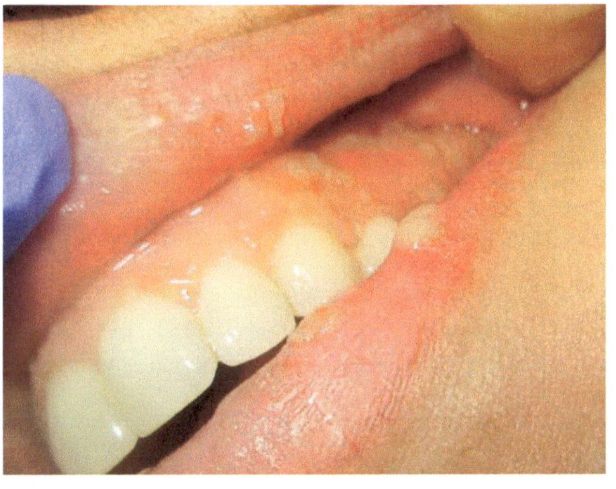

FIGURE 1.79 Pyostomatitis vegetans due to inflammatory bowel disease.

Evaluation and Management

Thorough history, review of systems, and examination of the oral mucosa should be coupled with screening for other systemic diseases or coexisting infections. Mucosal biopsy with direct immunofluorescence and skin biopsy of any associated cutaneous lesions can aid in diagnosis. Laboratory testing may include CBC, prothrombin time/partial thromboplastin time (PT/PTT), SPEP/SIFE, UPEP/UIFE, FBG, HA1c, vitamin and mineral levels (B, D, folate, iron, zinc), ANAs, and Hep C. Treatment will rely on accurate diagnosis of the underlying disease. For symptomatic treatment, exquisite oral hygiene, oral chlorhexidine rinses, and topical anesthetics/barrier formulations (e.g., viscous lidocaine, steroid, or diphenhydramine mixed with a barrier agent such as aluminum/magnesium hydroxide, or sucralfate) may be used.

BIBLIOGRAPHY

Lau CB, Smith GP. Recurrent aphthous stomatitis: A comprehensive review and recommendations on therapeutic options. Dermatol Ther 2022;35(6):e15500.

Napenas JJ, Brennan MT, Elad S. Oral Manifestations of systemic disease. Dermatol Clin 2020;38(4):495–505.

Narayanan D, Rogge M. Cheilitis: A diagnostic algorithm and review of underlying etiologies. Dermatitis 2024;35(5):431–442.

Saccucci M, DiCarlo G, Bossu M, et al. Autoimmune diseases and their manifestations on the oral cavity: Diagnosis and clinical management. J Immunol Res 2018. https://doi.org/10.1155/2018/6061825

Gyrate Erythema

Etiopathogenesis

Erythema annulare centrifugum (EAC) is a reactive dermatosis that can occur idiopathically or secondary to infections, drugs, and malignancies. Some sources use the terms *gyrate erythema* and *EAC* interchangeably, whereas other sources will define EAC as one of a number of gyrate erythema types, which can also include erythema gyratum repens, erythema chronicum migrans, and erythema marginatum. The TNF-α cytokine pathway has been suggested as being involved in the pathogenesis of this inflammatory pattern.

Clinical Manifestations

The superficial form of EAC (**Figures 1.80**, **1.81**, and **1.82**) appears as relatively flat, erythematous, annular patches with central clearing and a superficial scale that is present just inside the rim of erythema (the so-called trailing scale). The deep form (**Figure 1.83**) of EAC presents as indurated, annular plaques with central clearing and no scaling. Lesions may be multiple, occur anywhere on the body, spread centrifugally, persist, spontaneously resolve, or occur cyclically.

Systemic Manifestations

The etiology of EAC will vary considerably from patient to patient. Systemic manifestations may suggest the underlying cause in individual patients, but clinically significant systemic diseases are absent in most patients. Streptococcal and *E. coli* infections, tinea pedis or corporis, superficial candidiasis, and medications (interferon, rituximab, diuretics, oral contraceptives) are often initiating factors. Although not common, the presence of night sweats, fevers, and unintended weight loss should raise concern for an underlying lymphoproliferative malignancy because a paraneoplastic EAC eruption has been reported as well as EAC during pregnancy.

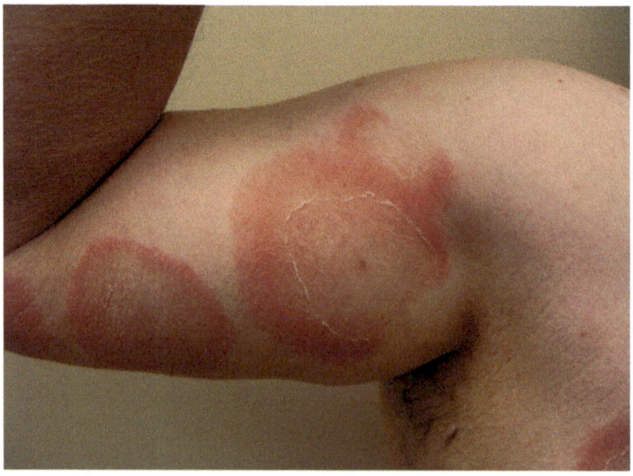

FIGURE 1.80 Erythema annulare centrifugum.

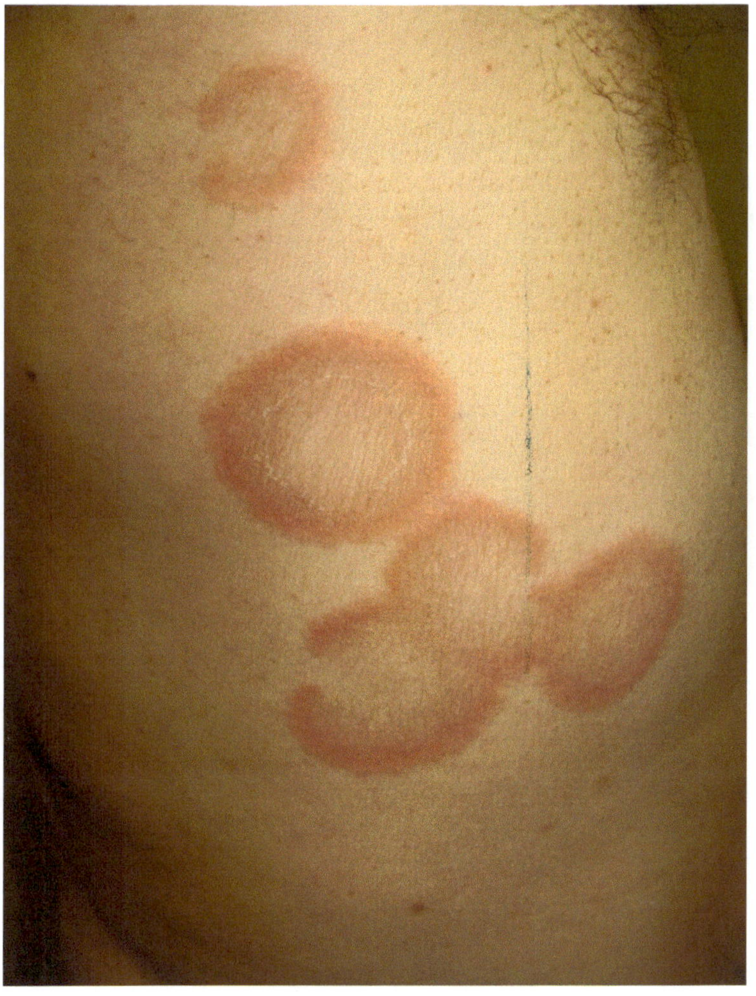

FIGURE 1.81 Erythema annulare centrifugum.

Evaluation and Management

EAC can be differentiated from other gyrate erythema (**Table 1.9**) such as erythema chronicum migrans of Lyme disease (**Figures 1.84**), erythema marginatum of rheumatic fever, and erythema gyratum repens of a rare paraneoplastic phenomenon can be ruled out with history, physical examination, blood work, and biopsy. Similarly, tinea, sarcoidosis, pityriasis rosea, mycosis fungoides, or cutaneous lupus can be eliminated from the differential diagnosis by biopsy. Histologic findings in the superficial form of EAC are that of focal spongiotic dermatitis, with superficial perivascular inflammation consisting of lymphocytes, eosinophils, and occasionally neutrophils. The deep form of EAC demonstrates little to no epidermal change and a more prominent superficial and deep lymphocytic infiltrate that demonstrates "cuffing" around dermal vessels. Once a definitive diagnosis of EAC has been established, searching for an underlying cause is the appropriate next step. If lymphoma is suspected, a CBC, CMP, SPEP, and CT may be obtained. Topical or oral steroids and nonsteroidal immunosuppressants may be required to help resolve the eruption in idiopathic cases.

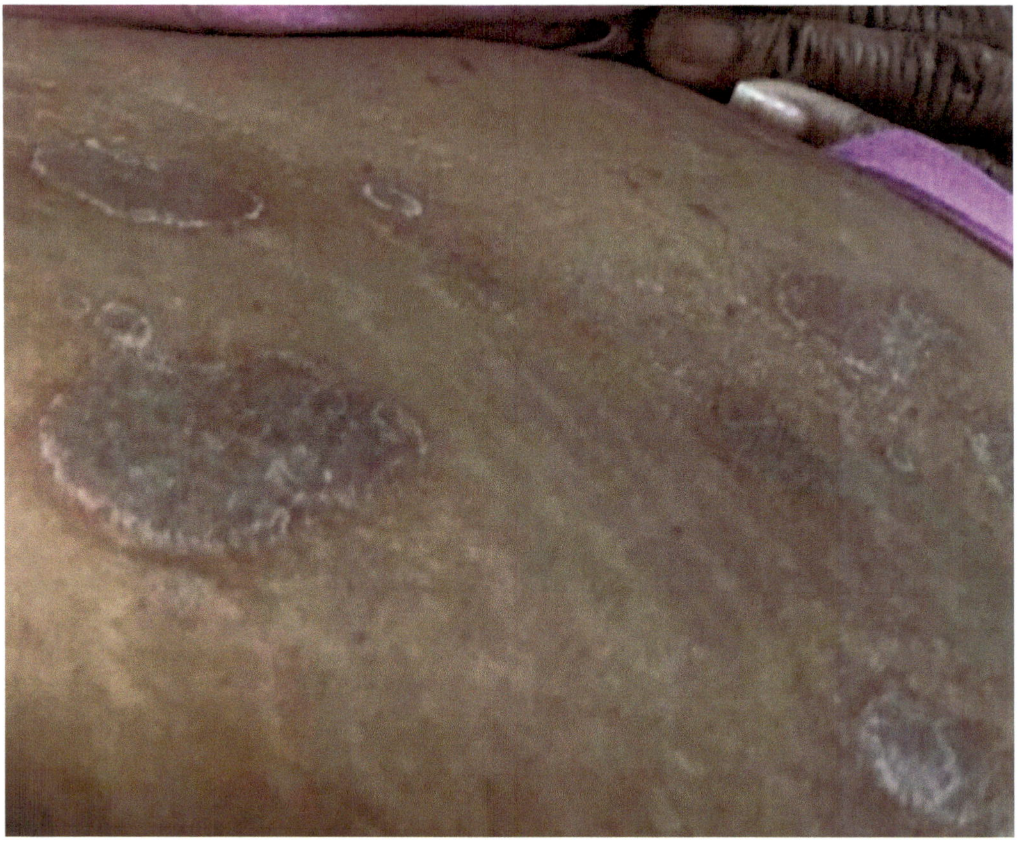

FIGURE 1.82 Erythema annulare centrifugum in skin of color.

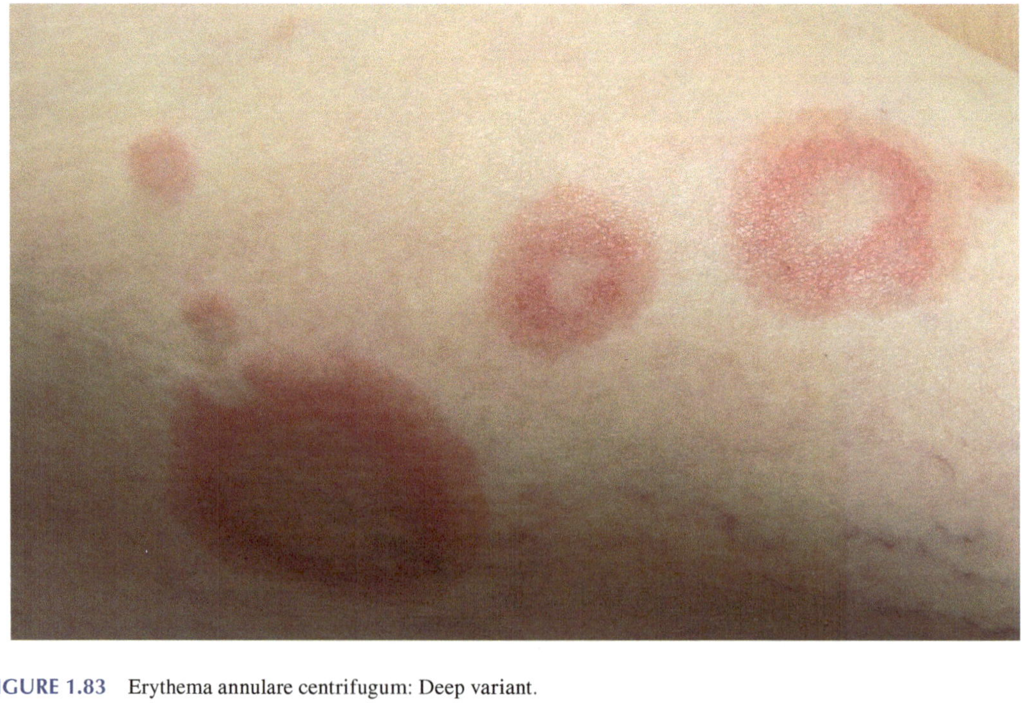

FIGURE 1.83 Erythema annulare centrifugum: Deep variant.

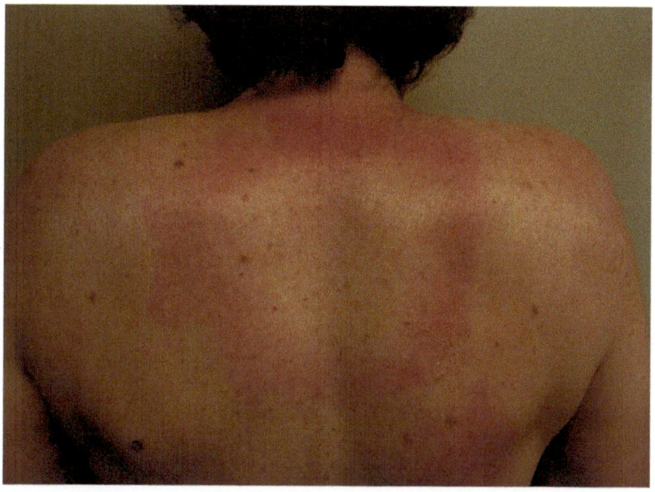

FIGURE 1.84 Erythema migrans.

TABLE 1.9

Gyrate Erythema

Gyrate Erythema	Clinical Findings	Associated Conditions
Erythema annulare centrifugum	Multiple lesions, expanding erythematous macule or slightly raised plaque with trailing scale, central clearing	Superficial fungal or yeast infections, medications
Erythema chronicum migrans	Often single lesion, can be multiple in early systemic disease Erythematous macule, sometimes with targetoid appearance, rarely bullous	Lyme disease
Erythema gyratum repens	Multiple lesions, "wood grain" appearance	Internal malignancy
Erythema marginatum	Multiple migratory lesions, annular macules with serpiginous borders, central clearing, asymptomatic Lesions coalesce into polycyclic macules.	Acute rheumatic fever

BIBLIOGRAPHY

Boehner A, Neuhauser R, Zink A, et al. Figurate erythemas – Update and diagnostic approach. J Dtsch Dermatol Ges 2021;19(7):963–972.

Dogan G. Pregnancy as a possible etiologic factor in erythema annulare centrifugum. Am J Clin Dermatol 2009;10(1):33–35.

Kazandjieva J, Bogdanov G, Bogdanov I, et al. Figurate annulare erythemas. Clin Dermatol 2023;41(3):368–375.

Hypertrichosis and Hirsutism

Etiopathogenesis

Hypertrichosis is the growth of hair (lanugo, vellus, terminal) in an excessive amount on any part of the body. Hirsutism, a subset of hypertrichosis, is androgen-dependent terminal hair growth in women in a male distribution. Increased growth of eyelashes is called trichomegaly. The etiology of new growth or transition from vellus to terminal hairs is relatively unknown. The conversion and increase to terminal hairs occur at puberty or exposure to increased androgen production. Additional mechanisms of action are poorly understood changes in hair follicular density and the hair growth cycle.

Clinical Manifestations

Hypertrichosis can be congenital/acquired and localized/generalized. Vellus hairs (short, nonpigmented, variably medullated) differ from terminal hairs (long, pigmented, medullated). Lanugo hairs (long, nonpigmented, unmedullated) grow in utero and are shed at or after birth. With hirsutism, terminal hair growth occurs specifically on the face (chin [**Figure 1.85**], lip), breast (**Figure 1.86**), abdominal, suprapubic, thigh (**Figure 1.87**), and lumbosacral areas. Hirsutism can occur concomitantly with acne, alopecia, breast discharge, clitoromegaly, striae, truncal obesity, enhanced musculature, and deepening of voice.

Systemic Manifestations

Acquired generalized hypertrichosis from systemic diseases include porphyrias (face and extremity), neurologic disorders/injury, malnutrition/anorexia (extremity, trunk, face), hypothyroidism (back, extremities), or HIV/AIDS (torso, occasional eyelash trichomegaly [**Figure 1.88**]). The sudden onset of hypertrichosis lanuginosa (**Figures 1.89** and **1.90**) has been associated with malignancy (GI, genitourinary [GU], breast, and lung cancers and lymphomas). Medication-induced hypertrichosis has been reported (**Table 1.10**, **Figure 1.91**) predominately involving the torso and extremities, but may be seen on the face. Although idiopathic hirsutism (functional ovarian hyperandrogenicity) is most common, polycystic ovarian syndrome, IR syndromes, androgen/ovarian tumors, and endocrinopathies (adult-onset congenital adrenal hyperplasia, Cushing syndrome, hyperprolactinemia, acromegaly, thyroid dysfunction) are secondary causes of hirsutism.

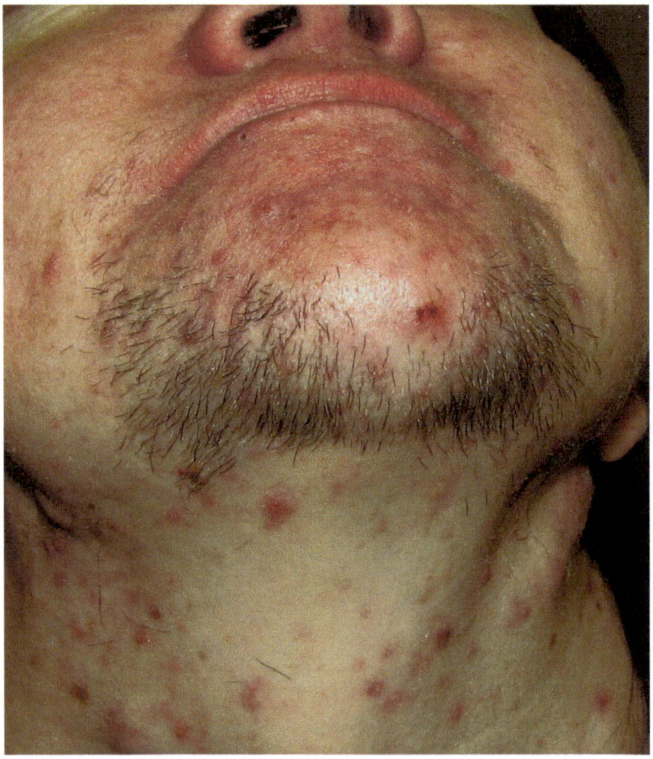

FIGURE 1.85 Hirsutism: Chin.

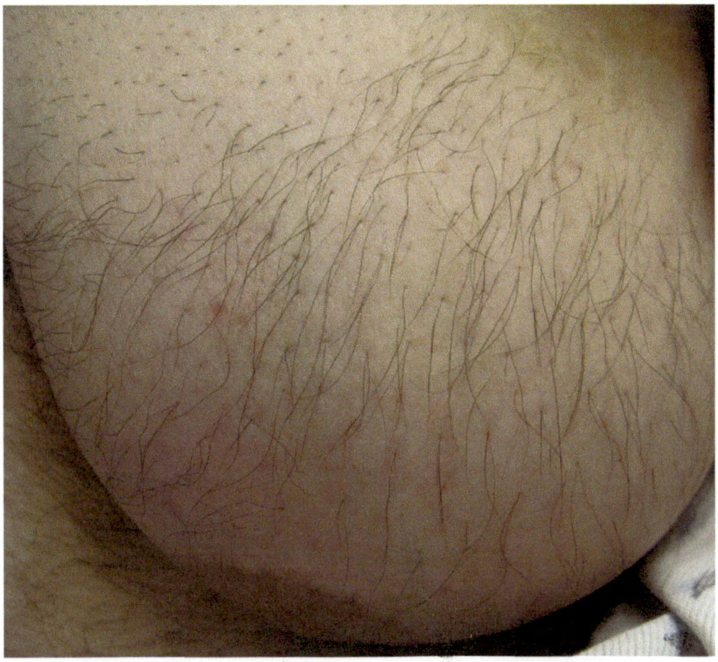

FIGURE 1.86 Hirsutism: Breast.

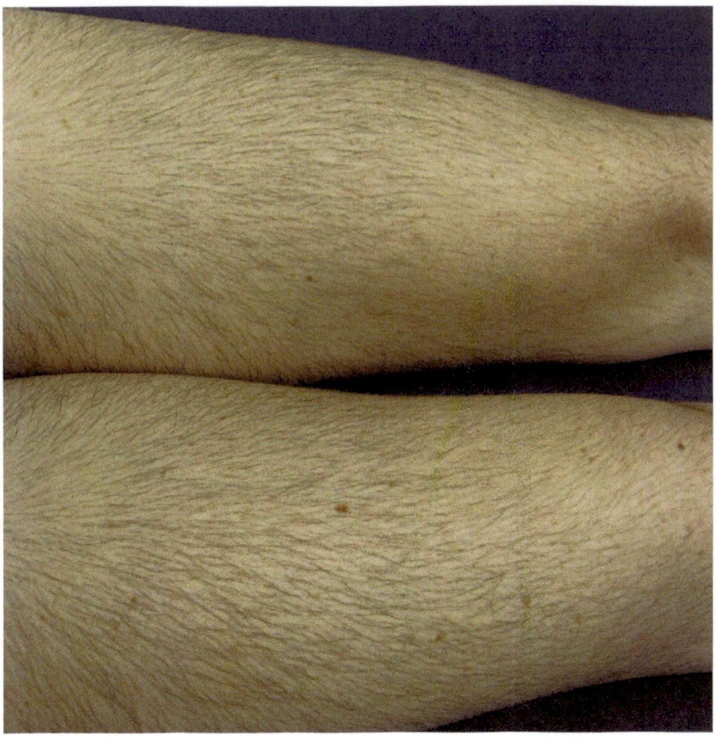

FIGURE 1.87 Hirsutism: Thighs.

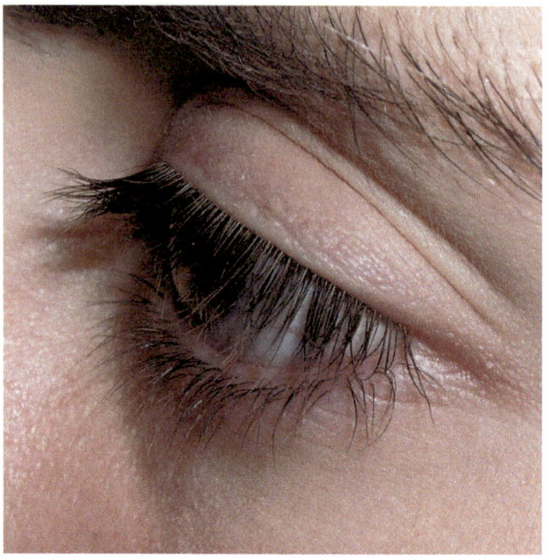

FIGURE 1.88 Trichomegaly: Eyelashes.

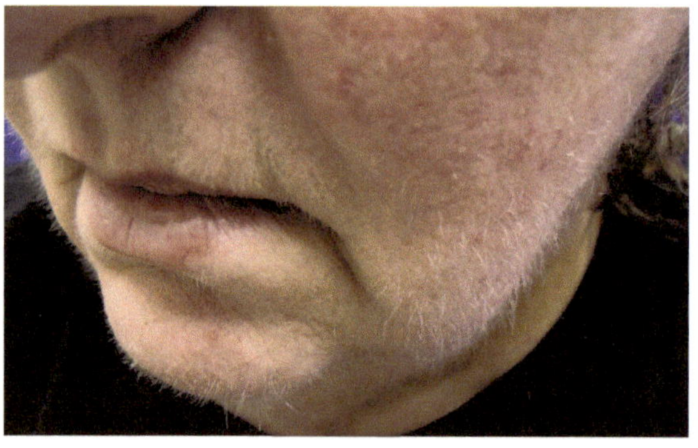

FIGURE 1.89 Hypertrichosis lanuginosa: Pancreatic cancer.

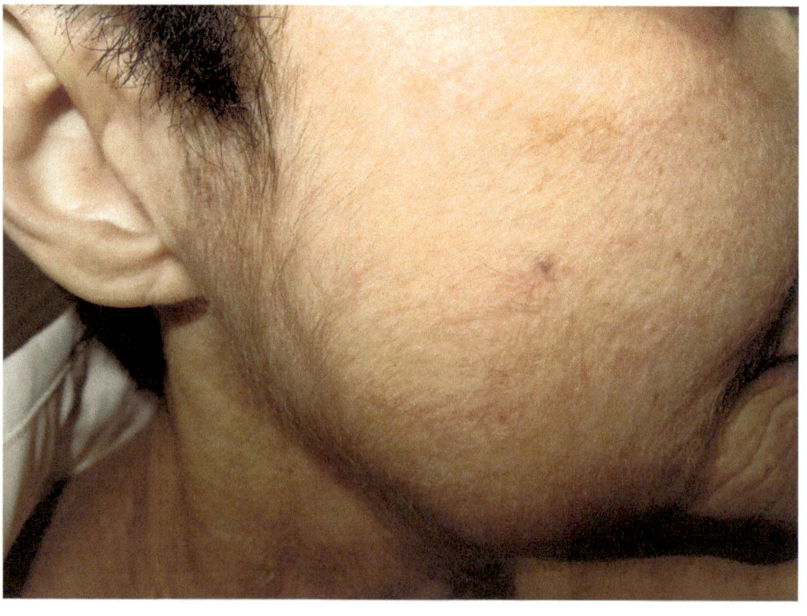

FIGURE 1.90 Hypertrichosis lanuginosa: Lung cancer.

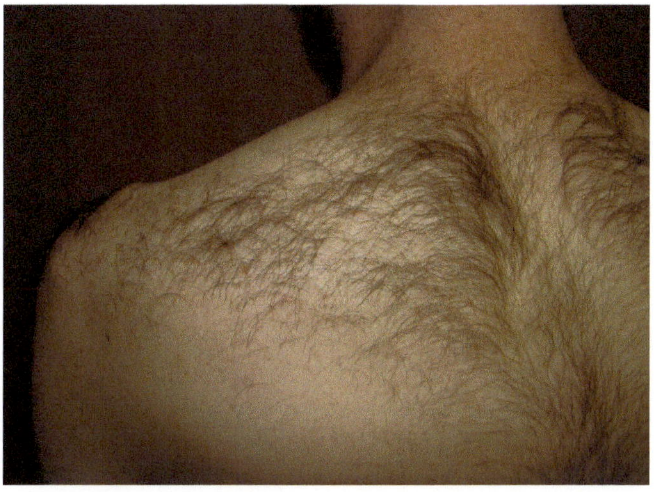

FIGURE 1.91 Hypertrichosis: Cyclosporine.

Medication-induced hirsutism occurs with testosterone, androgenic progestins, anabolic steroid, and corticosteroid use.

TABLE 1.10

Medication 'Induced Hypertrichosis'
Amlodipine
Bimatoporst
Corticosteroids
Cetuximab
Crisaborole
Cyclosporine
Diazoxide
Dopamine
Latanoprost
Minoxidil
Panitumumab
Pemigatinib
Phenytoin
Serotonin reuptake inhibitors
Travoprost

Evaluation and Management

Obtaining an extensive review of systems and medication lists is important. On the basis of findings, testing for hypertrichosis may include serum/urine porphyrins, vitamins, prealbumin, albumin, HIV, and Hep C. Laboratory testing for hirsutism may include testosterone (TEST), sex hormone-binding globulin (SHBG), dehydroepiandrosterone-sulfate (DHEA-s), 17-hydroxyprogesterone (HyPROG), follicle-stimulating hormone (FSH), luteinizing hormone (LH), prolactin (PRL), a.m. cortisol, FBG, TFTs, and growth hormone (GH). Radiographic imaging with CT may be required for malignancy evaluation. Treating underlying disorders is fundamental. Hair removal techniques (shaving, depilatories, electrolysis, and lasers) may be used for both diseases. Antiandrogen therapies of low-androgenic progestin birth control pills and use of oral antiandrogens may prevent hair growth in hirsutism.

BIBLIOGRAPHY

Hasan R, Juma H, Eid FA, et al. Effects of hormones and endocrine disorders on hair growth. Cureus 2022;14(12):e32726.

Sardana K, Muddelbihal A, Sehrawat M, et al. An updated clinic-investigative approach to diagnosis of cutaneous hyperandrogenism in relation to adult female acne, female pattern alopecia & hirsutism a primer for dermatologists. Expert Rev Endocrinolo Metab 2024;19(2):111–128.

Vedak P. Hair and nail conditions: Hypertrichosis and hirsutism. FP Essent 2022;517:22–26.

Ichthyosis and Spicules

Etiopathogenesis

Acquired ichthyosis (AI), hyperkeratotic spicules (HSs), and trichodysplasia spinulosa (TS) represent disorders of keratinization associated with systemic disease. *Ichthyosis* refers to dry fish-like scale changes of the integument. Although most congenital forms are associated with a mutation in keratinization (Ichthyosis vulgaris-filaggrin) the exact etiology of the acquired disease is unknown. HSs are digitate keratoses predominately located on the face. The deposition of monoclonal immunoglobulins has been postulated to be the initiating factor, altering keratinization in some cases. Trichodysplasia spinulosa (TS) are folliculocentric keratin spines most common in immunosuppressed solid-organ transplant patients caused by a polyomavirus.

Clinical Manifestations

AI presents with the symmetrical development of 1 mm to 1 cm plate-like white to gray-brown colored scales. It affects the torso and lower (greater than upper) extremities, with sparing of the flexures. Most congenital forms present before puberty, but xerosis, late-onset ichthyosis vulgaris, and Refsum disease may appear similar. HSs may be non-follicular or follicular-based lesions that predominately occur on the face, particularly the nose. However, lesions may develop on the scalp, trunk, and extremities. Lesions are usually white, spiny, and 1–2 mm in height. TS presents as papular flesh colored, erythematous, or hyperpigmented follicular spicules on the central face, ears, and trunk. Lesions may be pruritic.

Systemic Manifestations

Systemic diseases associated with AI include malignancy (lymphoma, myeloma, solid tumors, and cutaneous T-cell lymphoma), autoimmunity (lupus, dermatomyositis, sarcoidosis [**Figure 1.92**]), nutritional disease (malnutrition, celiac disease), metabolic disease (hepatic/renal failure, hypothyroidism/hypopituitarism, hyperparathyroidism, diabetes), infection (HIV [**Figure 1.93**]), human T-lymphotrophic virus (HTLV-I/II), and medications (cholesterol-lowering agents, cimetidine, clofazimine, hydroxyurea). HSs may be idiopathic but are concerning for associated paraproteinemia or monoclonal gammopathy of undetermined significance (**Figure 1.94**), multiple myeloma (**Figure 1.95**), monoclonal cryoglobulinemia, and follicular mucinosis-associated cutaneous T-cell lymphoma (**Figure 1.96**). TS occurs with immunosuppression from medications, organ transplants, cancer, or HIV (**Figure 1.97**).

Evaluation and Management

A detailed history, review of systems, medications, and physical examination (especially skin and lymph node evaluation) is warranted. Additional evaluation for AI is reviewed in **Table 1.11**). TS requires medication review, screening for malignancy, and HIV testing. Hyperkeratotic spicules require laboratory tests for SPEP/SIFE, UPEP/UIFE, and CRYO. Treating the underlying disease state is vital, and skin treatments include topical retinoids and keratolytics.

TABLE 1.11

Evaluation of Acquired Ichthyosis

Laboratory tests
• Complete blood count with platelets and differential
• Comprehensive metabolic panel
• Anti-nuclear antibodies
• Prealbumin
• Vitamin and Mineral levels
• Thyroid function tests
• Parathyroid hormone
• HIV
• HTLV I/II
• ACTH
• Prolactin
• Growth Hormone
• Anti-gliadin/Endomysial/Transglutaminase antibodies
Radiographic imaging
• Chest X-ray
• Pan-computed tomography scan
Procedures
• Skin biopsy

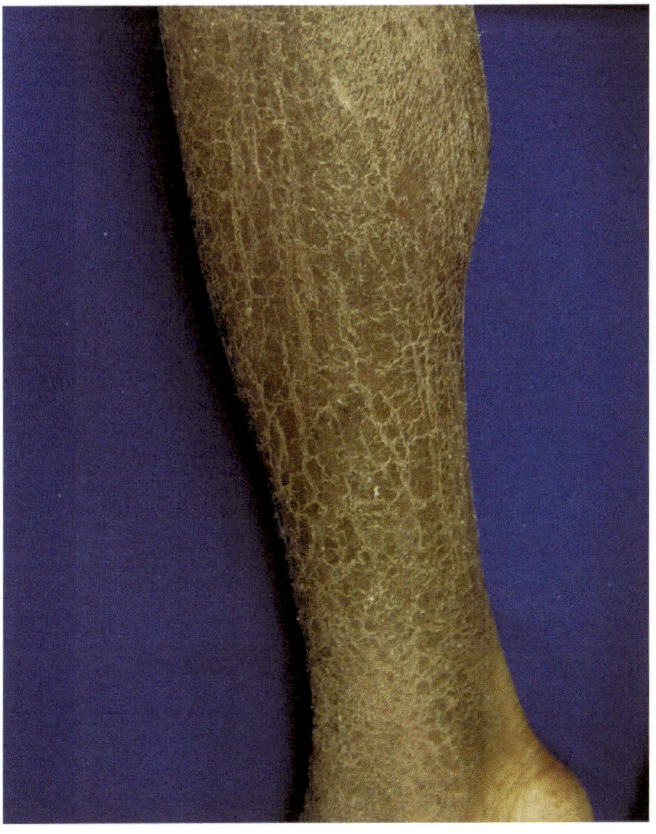

FIGURE 1.92 Acquired ichthyosis: Sarcoidosis.

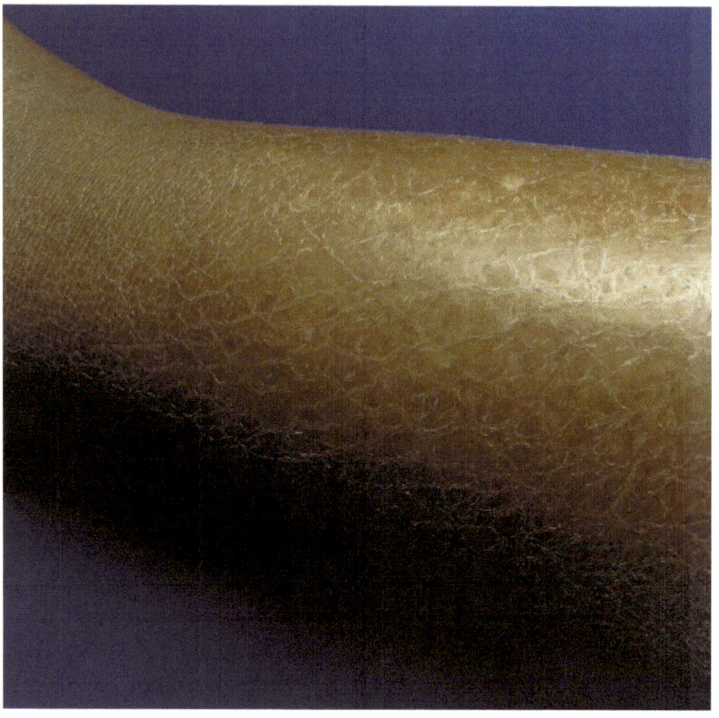

FIGURE 1.93 Acquired ichthyosis: HIV.

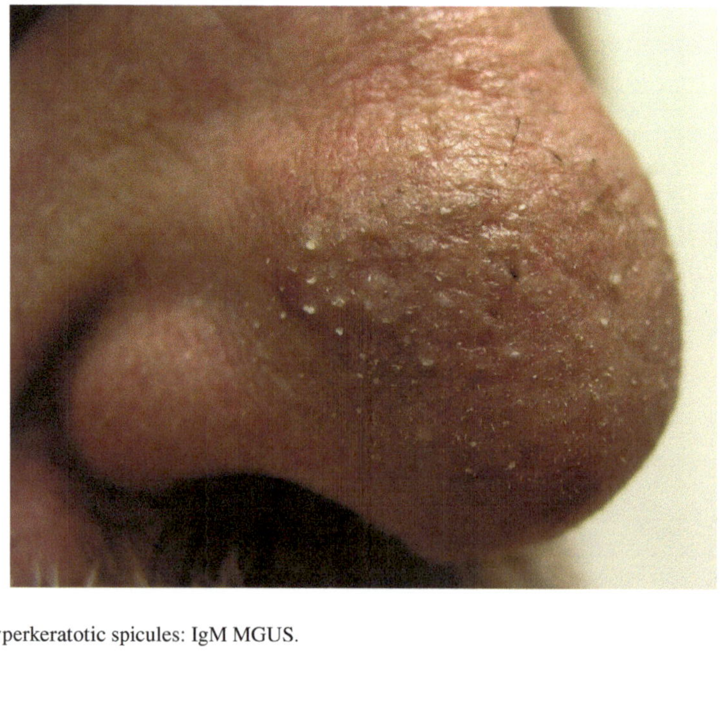

FIGURE 1.94 Hyperkeratotic spicules: IgM MGUS.

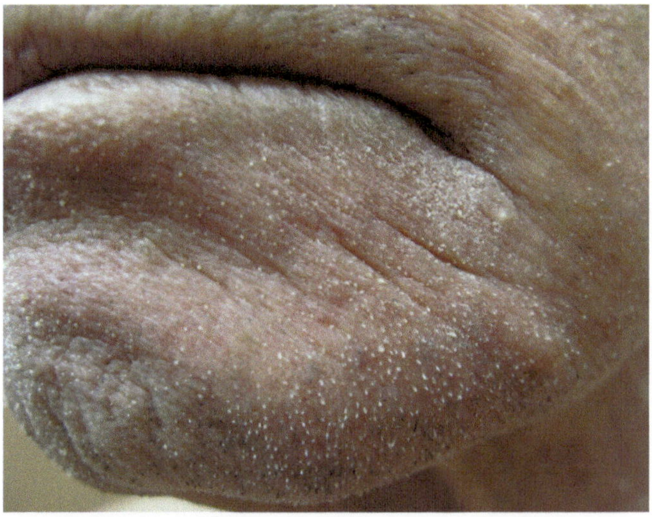

FIGURE 1.95 Hyperkeratotic spicules: IgG multiple myeloma.

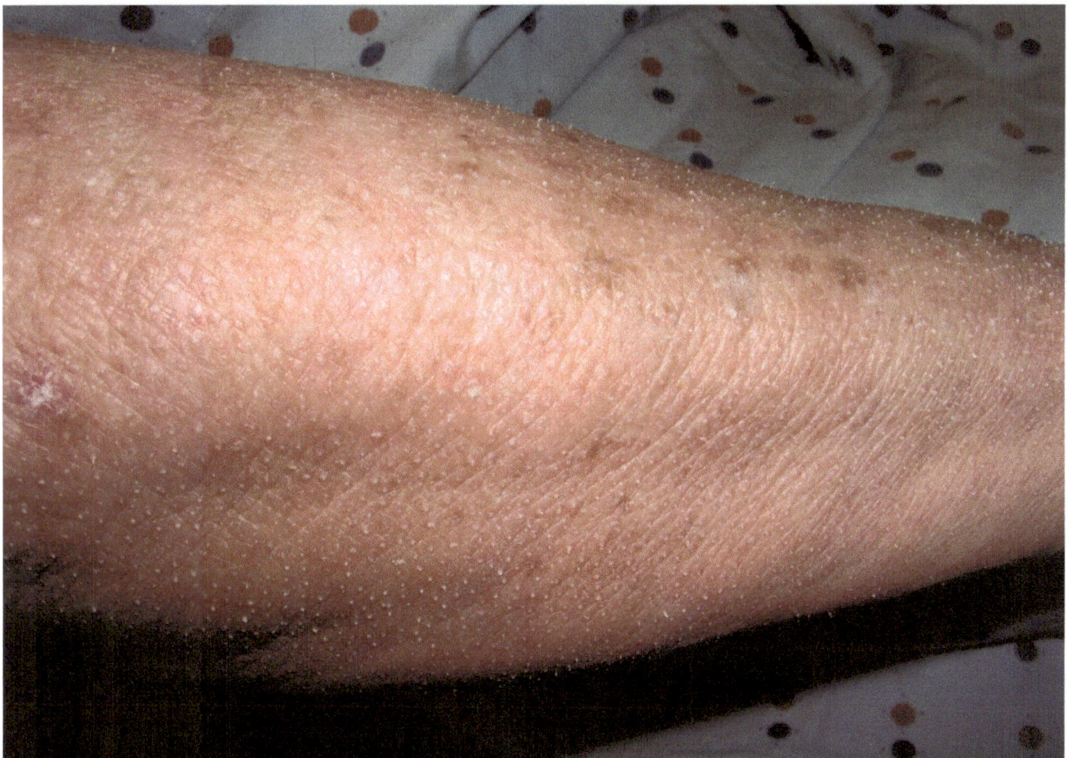

FIGURE 1.96 Hyperkeratotic spicules: Follicular mucinosis-associated cutaneous T-cell lymphoma.

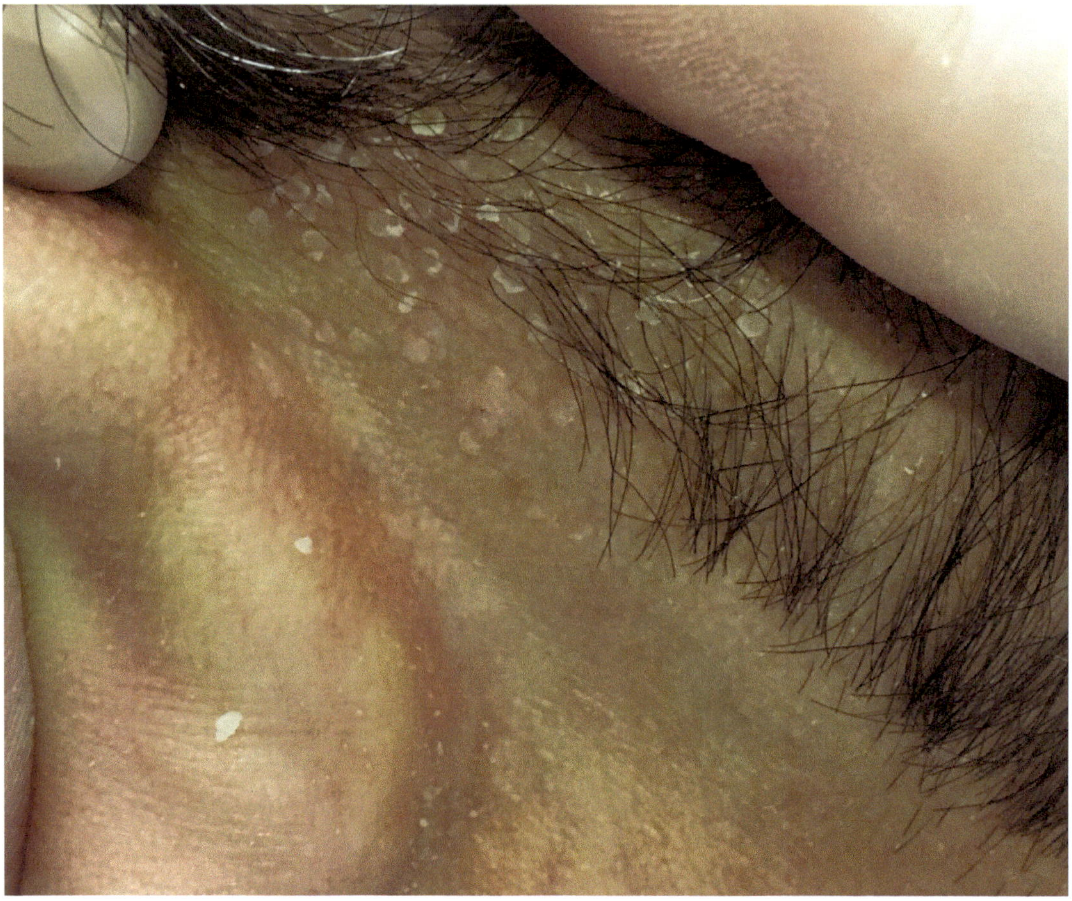

FIGURE 1.97 Trichodysplasia spinulosa.

BIBLIOGRAPHY

Haber R, Feghali J, Nadir U, et al. Acquired ichthyosis: A clinical review. Arch Dermatol Res 2023;315(9):2529–2543.

Jose A, Dad T, Strand A, et al. Trichodysplasia spinulosa: Case reports and review of the literature. Transpl Infect Dis 2020;22(5):e133342.

Patel N, Spencer LA, English JC III, et al. Acquired ichthyosis. J Am Acad Dermatol 2006;55(4):647–656.

Smith MP, Manabat-Hidalgo C. Follicular spicules of multiple myeloma. Dermatol Online J 2019;25(10):13030/qt5bp8s5nn.

Tomasini C, Kempf W, Novelli M, et al. Spiky follicular mycosis fungoides: A clinicopathologic study of 8 cases. J Cutan Path 2015;42 (3):164–172.

Keratodermas

Etiopathogenesis

The term *hyperkeratosis* typically describes thickened skin; however, *keratodermas* refers to thickened skin of the hands and feet. Keratodermas are divided into congenital or acquired etiologies. Congenital causes include a large range of gene defects affecting proteins involved in cellular adhesion and the formation of cytoskeletal proteins. Acquired causes are from inflammatory dermatoses, infections, drug reactions, systemic diseases, and malignancies.

Clinical Manifestations

Acquired keratoderma can present as >50% diffuse thickening or hardening of the skin on the palmar and/or plantar surfaces. It can also present with punctuate lesions and focal thickening of the skin over pressure points or along skin tension lines. Lesions may appear with or without peripheral erythema.

Systemic Manifestations

Systemic diseases associated with acquired keratoderma are predominately endocrinopathies and malignancies. When occurring in the context of menopause, it has been termed keratoderma climacterium (**Figure 1.98**). Hypothyroidism (**Figure 1.99**) with and without myxedema has been associated with acquired keratoderma. In a setting of liver disease, biliary acute cholangitis can present with acquired keratoderma. Morbid obesity may induce predominately plantar keratoderma, which is more from the pressure of excess weight than a metabolic issue. Most concerning are malignancies associated with keratoderma (esophageal, gastric, colon, breast, lung, bladder, peripheral T-cell lymphoma, cutaneous T-cell lymphoma, Sezary syndrome). In addition, protein/vitamin malnutrition and reactive arthritis may lead to keratoderma (keratoderma blenorrhagicum [**Figure 1.100**]). The differential diagnoses include arsenic exposure, allergic/irritant dermatitis, psoriasis, pityriasis rubra pilaris, syphilis, tinea pedis, encrusted scabies, leprosy, and drug-induced keratoderma (lithium, quinacrine, bleomycin, hydroxyurea, verapamil, glucan, or venlafaxine). Notably, a rare condition causing keratoderma after water exposure (aquagenic pseudokeratoderma [**Figure 1.101**]) has also been described, which may have concomitant hyperhidrosis and has been reported at a higher frequency in patients with cystic fibrosis.

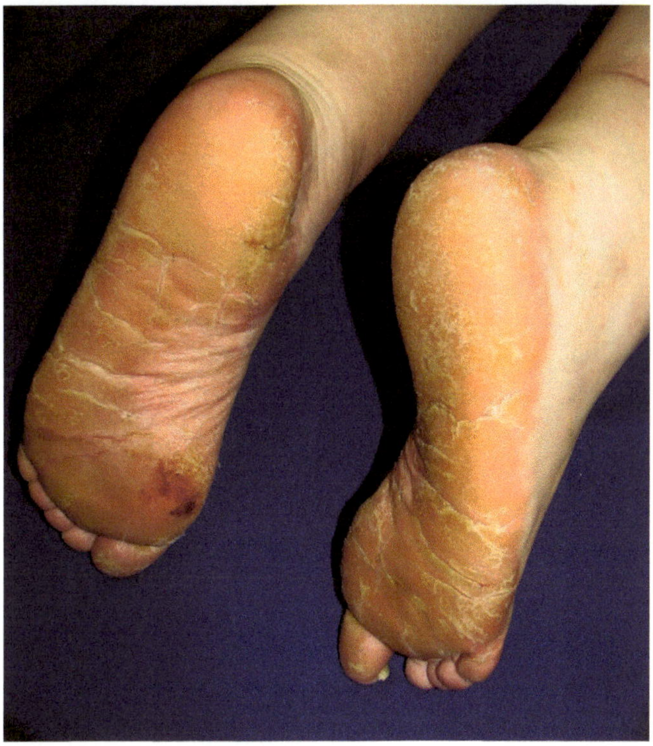

FIGURE 1.98 Acquired keratoderma: Keratoderma climacterium.

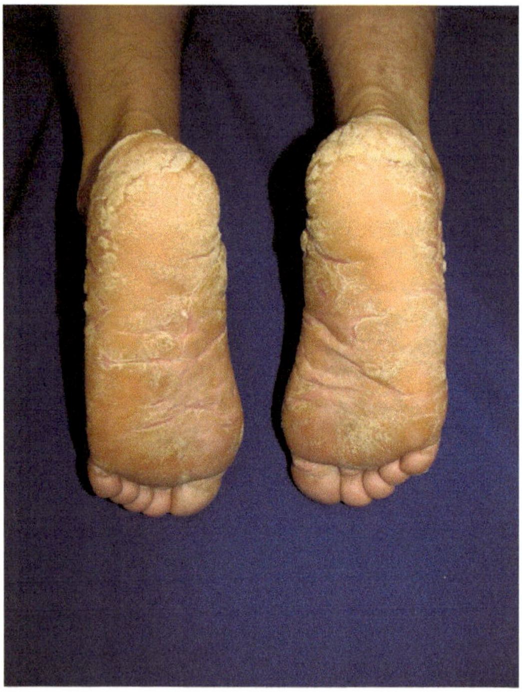

FIGURE 1.99 Acquired keratoderma: Hypothyroidism.

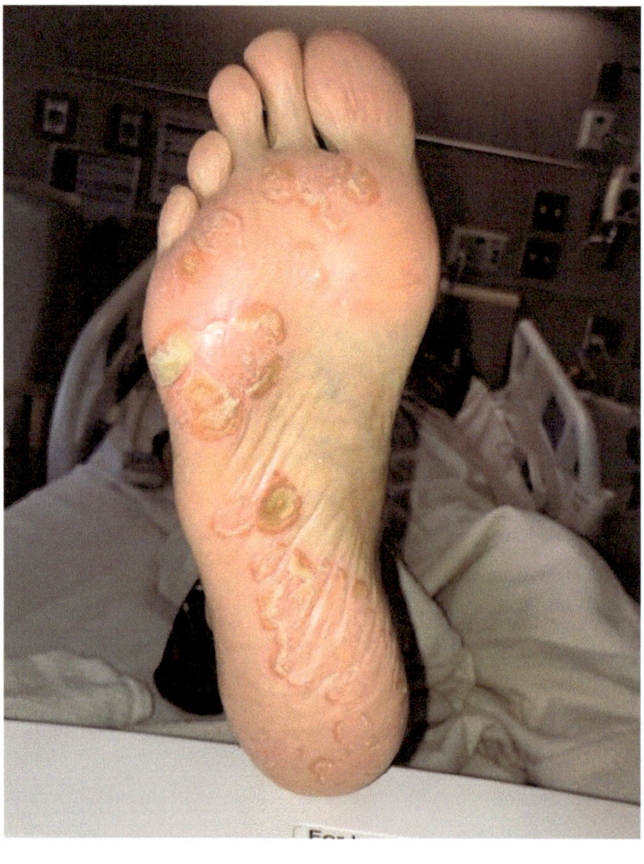

FIGURE 1.100 Acquired keratoderma: Keratoderma blenorrhagicum.

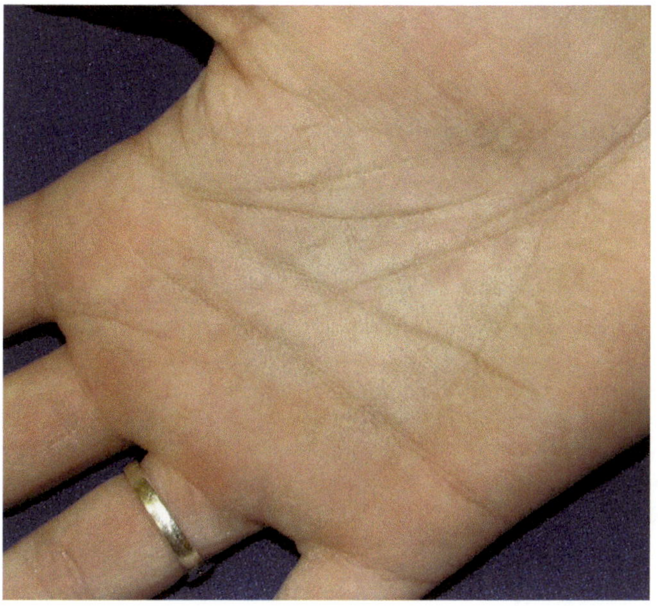

FIGURE 1.101 Acquired keratoderma: Aquagenic pseudokeratoderma.

Evaluation and Management

A thorough history, medication list, physical exam, and review of systems to help guide further testing is warranted. Consider skin biopsy to help differentiate among inflammatory and infectious skin disorders. Laboratory testing may include TFTs, triglycerides (TGs), thyroid peroxidase enzymes (TPOs), erythrocyte sedimentation rate (ESR), C-reactive protein (CRP), hemoccult stool testing, prealbumin, vitamin, and mineral levels. Age/gender-appropriate cancer screening should be brought up to date. Further consideration of a pan CT scan and EGD/CS is based on clinical findings. Diagnosing aquagenic pseudokeratoderma should warrant CXR and pulmonary function testing (PFT). The gene mutation deltaF508 of the *CFTR* gene can be tested because up to 84% of cystic fibrosis patients and up to 25% of cystic fibrosis carriers can develop aquagenic pseudokeratoderma. Treating the underlying etiology may resolve the keratoderma (e.g., thyroid hormone replacement, surgery/chemotherapy). The use of topical keratolytics (e.g., ammonium lactate, urea) or topical/systemic retinoids may be used as needed.

BIBLIOGRAPHY

Atzori L, Ferreli C, Rongioletti F. Aquagenic (pseudo)keratoderma (aquagenic palmoplantar keratoderma, aquagenic wrinkling to the palms). Clin Dermatol 2021;39(2):256–260.

March-Rodriguez A, Marcantonio O, Olmos-Alpiste F, et al. Complete and persistent resolution after ursodeoxycholic acid treatment. Australas J Dermatol 2022;63(1):e49–e51.

Mizutani Y, Ito M, Takahashi T, et al. Acquired palmoplantar keratoderma associated with hypothyroidism. J Dermaol 2016;43(10):1246–1247.

Patel S, Zirwas M, English JC III. Acquired palmoplantar keratoderma. Am J Clin Dermatol 2007;8(1):1–11.

Leonine Facies

Etiopathogenesis

Leonine facies is best described as thickening of the skin, most often the forehead, cheeks, and upper lip due to coalescing, indurated, or granulomatous plaques causing accentuated skin lines that give a lion-like appearance, often with decreased range of motion. The causes are various; however, one consistent feature is the presence of a dense dermal infiltrate of inflammatory cells or granuloma formation.

Clinical Manifestations

Exaggerated skin grooves are formed by the presence of firm, coalescing nodules and plaques. These lines frequently include transverse furrows of the forehead. Infiltration of the skin of the periorbital area frequently results in furrowing of the glabellar area, as well as exaggerated infraorbital lines. Involvement of the cheeks gives exaggerated nasolabial and mesolabial folds. Once lesions become coalescent, the overlying skin can attain a pebbly or cobblestone-like appearance.

Systemic Manifestations

Systemic manifestations are dependent on the underlying etiology (**Table 1.12**). Symptoms of dysphagia, obstructive or restrictive pulmonary disease, myopathy, or arthralgia could suggest scleromyxedema. With pulmonary symptoms, sarcoidosis should also be considered. A history of steroid-resistant skin eruption could suggest lymphocytoma cutis, mycosis fungoides (**Figure 1.102**), systemic mastocytosis, chronic actinic dermatitis (**Figure 1.103**), or recalcitrant atopic dermatitis (**Figure 1.104**). A corroborating travel or exposure history could suggest infectious etiology, including lepromatous leprosy, leishmaniasis, and syphilis.

Evaluation and Management

Given the classical association of leonine facies with leprosy, skin biopsy should be obtained to assess for acid-fast bacilli. Touch prep of the skin biopsy specimen can also be processed with Giemsa stain for rapid screening. Sarcoidosis can be distinguished due to its granulomatous inflammatory pattern on histology. Cutaneous T-cell lymphoma and leukemia cutis can also be considered if abnormal dense dermal inflammatory infiltrates with corroborating immunohistochemical markers are identified on pathology specimens. Scleromyxedema (**Figure 1.105**) is suggested if there is evidence of dermal fibrosis, mucin deposition, and fibroblast proliferation on histology. SPEP/SIFE and UPEP/UIFE will help identify associated paraproteinemia. The presence of excessive numbers of mast cells should prompt consideration for serum tryptase testing and a possible bone marrow biopsy to evaluate for mastocytosis. Multiple enlarged sebaceous glands are seen histologically in patients with presenile diffuse familial gland hyperplasia. A rapid plasma reagin (RPR) should be considered to screen and rule out secondary syphilis. Patch testing may be performed if chronic actinic or atopic dermatitis is considered.

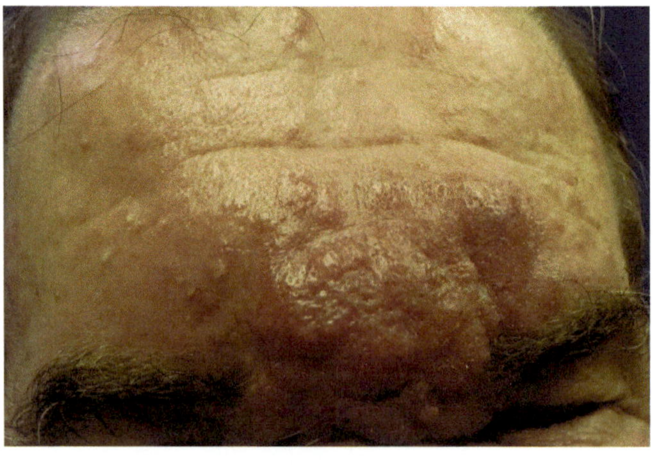

FIGURE 1.102 Leonine facies: Cutaneous T-cell lymphoma.

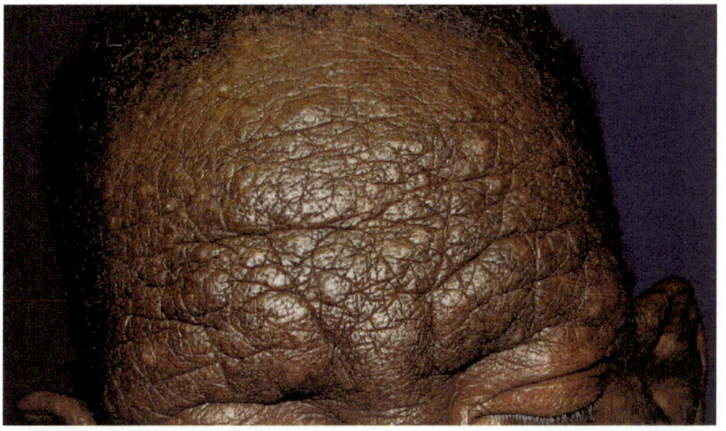

FIGURE 1.103 Leonine facies: Chronic actinic dermatitis.

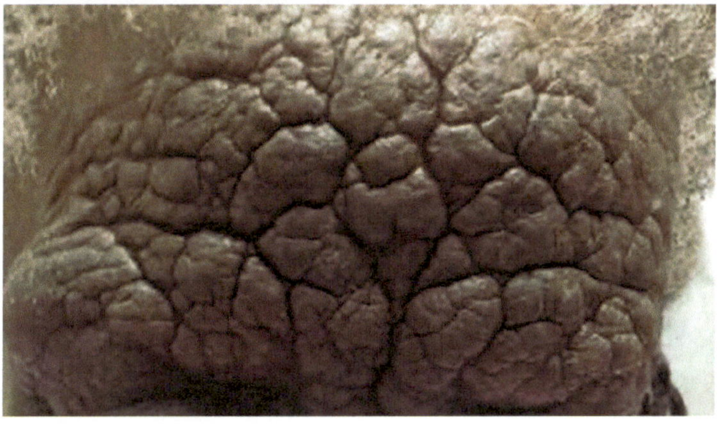

FIGURE 1.104 Leonine facies: Recalcitrant atopic dermatitis.

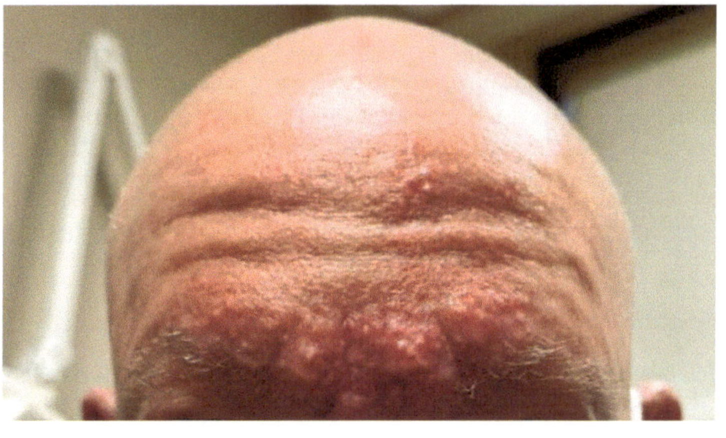

FIGURE 1.105 Leonine facies: Scleromyxedema.

TABLE 1.12

Differential Diagnosis of Lenonine Facies

Cause	Cutaneous Features	Associated Systemic Findings	Diagnosis
Scleromyxedema	Furrowed brow, coalescing "waxy" papules into larger plaques	Pulmonary symptoms, myopathy, arthralgia	Skin biopsy, SPEP, UPEP
Sarcoidosis	Reddish-brown papules and nodules, involvement of tattoos/scars	Pulmonary symptoms, arthralgia	Skin biopsy
Chronic actinic dermatitis	Sharp demarcation between sun-exposed and sun-protected skin	None	Skin biopsy, phototesting
Lepromatous leprosy	Hypoesthesia in some of the lesions	Fevers	Skin biopsy
Cutaneous T-cell lymphoma	Alopecia, palmar/plantar keratoderma, erythroderma	Sezary cells	Skin biopsy, peripheral blood flow cytometry

BIBLIOGRAPHY

Brown DN, Wieser I, Wang C, et al. Leonine facies (LF) and mycosis fungoides (MF): A single-center study and systematic review of the literature. J Am Acad Dermatol 2105;73(6):976–986.

Lim JH, Lin FL. Unusual leonine facies: A rare presentation. Kaohsiung J Med Sci 2024;40(10):951–952.

Ochi H, Kwong HL, Lim SPR. Leonine facies in a masseuse as a result of allergic contact dermatitis. Contact Dermatitis 2021;84(4):268–270.

Livedo Reticularis

Etiopathogenesis

Livedo reticularis is a skin change that is due to a physiologic response of skin arterial and venous vasculature to temperature or underlying disease. The increased visibility of the vessels is attributed to venodilation and deoxygenated blood from decreased arteriolar inflow or increased resistance to venous outflow. When this violaceous pattern becomes atypical, it is referred to as livedo racemosa, which is due to focal and persistent impairment of blood flow due to underlying disease. Complete vascular occlusion from inflammation or occlusive pathology may produce retiform purpura, which is, by definition, not livedo reticularis/racemosa and will be discussed in the Purpura section.

Clinical Manifestations

Livedo reticularis presents as a violaceous blanchable, net-like, generalized, and symmetrical eruption predominately on the extremities (**Figures 1.106** and **1.107**). The eruption may be physiologic, transient, or persistent in nature. Livedo racemosa presents as a violaceous, partially blanchable, branch-like, localized to segmental to widespread, nonsymmetrical eruption (**Figures 1.108** and **109**). Retiform purpura is differentiated because it is non-blanching and has a greater tendency to ulcerate. Erythema ab igne, a reaction to chronic heat exposure, produces a hyperpigmented net-like pattern often confused with livedo reticularis (**Figure 1.110**).

Systemic Manifestations

Persistent livedo reticularis, although often physiologic or idiopathic in nature, has been associated with multiple systemic diseases. Livedo racemosa is always considered a pathologic state from an underlying disease. The most common associations are reviewed in **Table 1.13**.

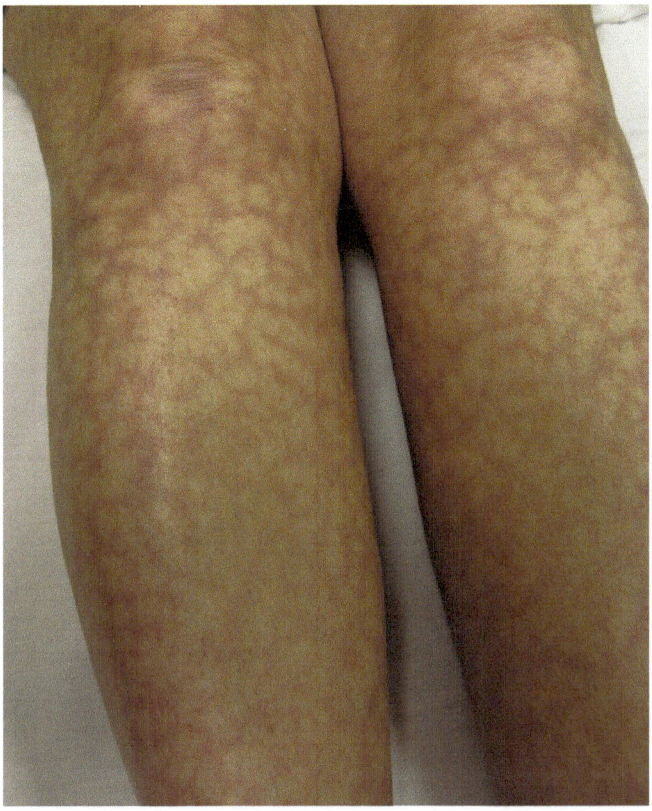

FIGURE 1.106 Livedo reticularis: Antiphospholipid antibody syndrome.

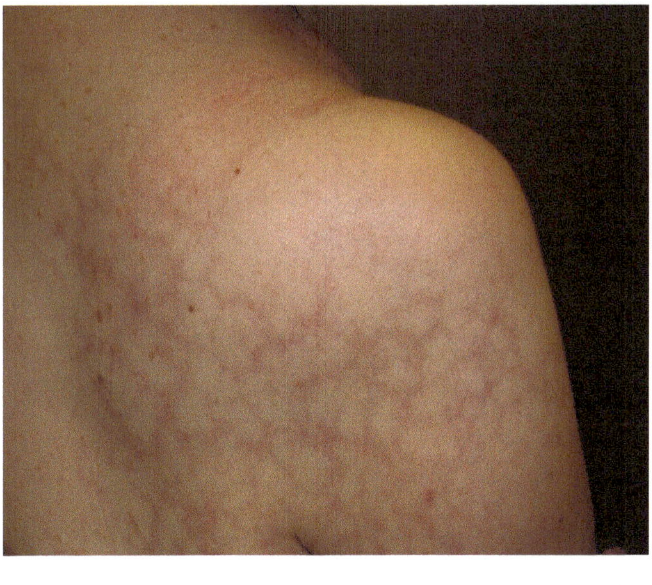

FIGURE 1.107 Livedo reticularis: Systemic lupus erythematosus.

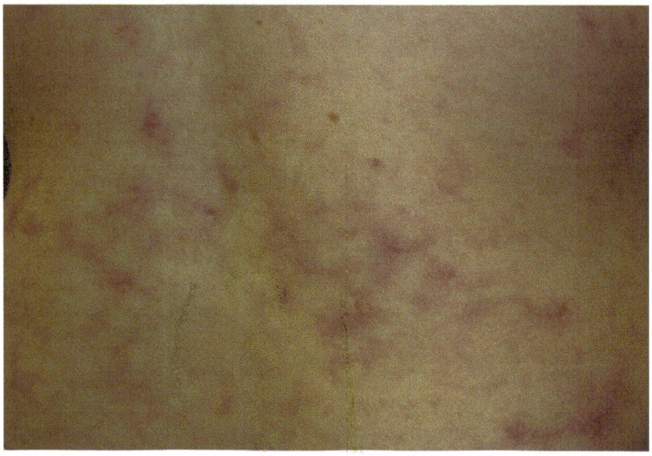

FIGURE 1.108 Livedo racemosa: Systemic lupus erythematosus.

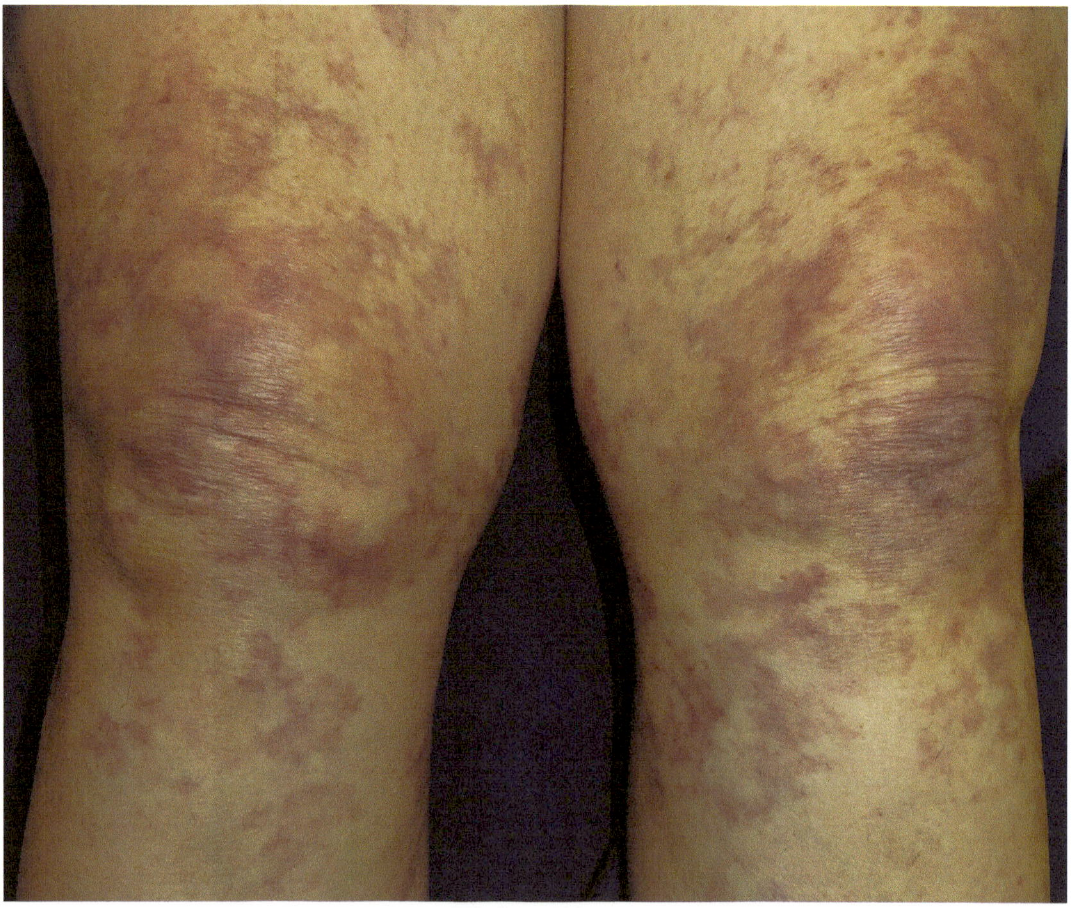

FIGURE 1.109 Livedo racemose: Mixed connective tissue disease.

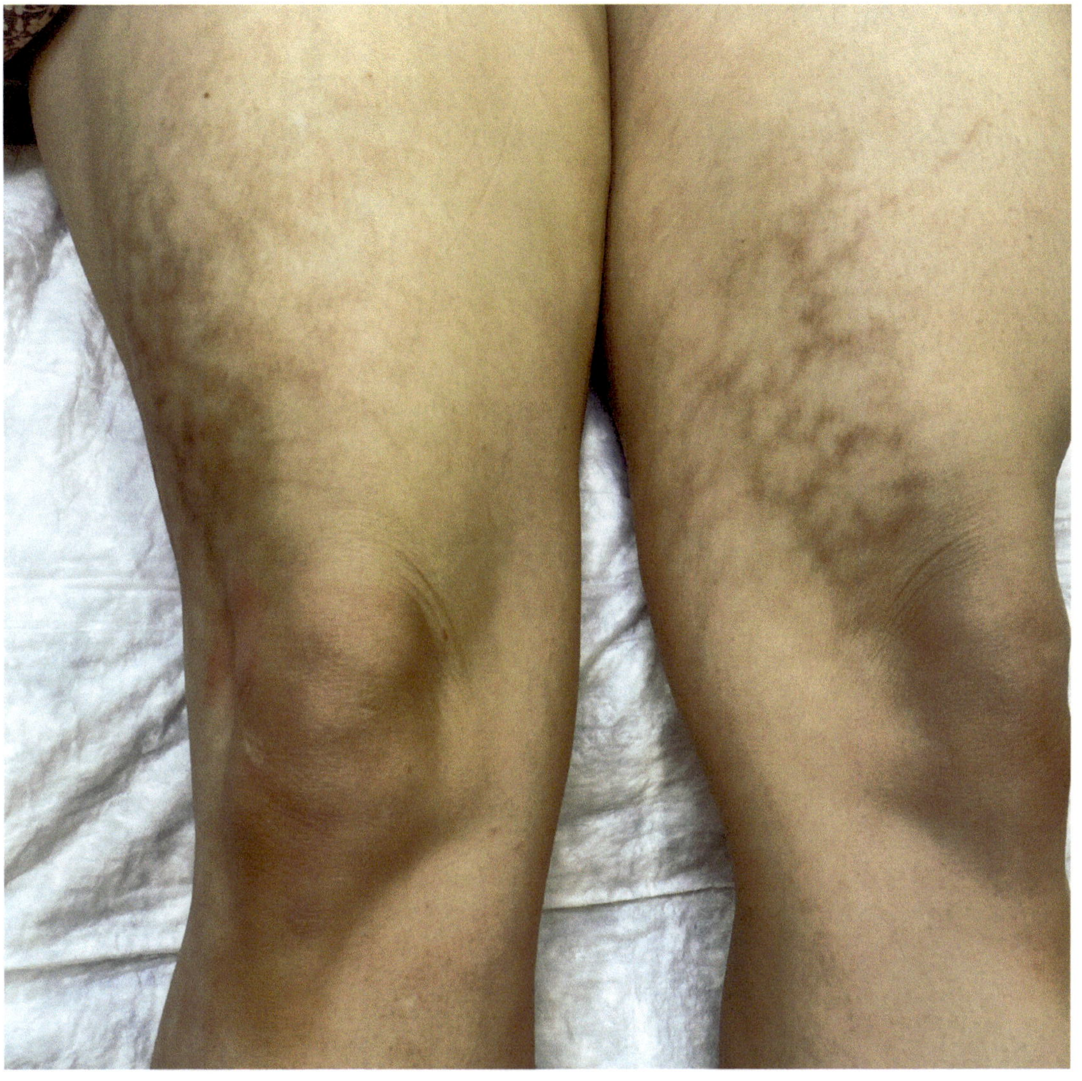

FIGURE 1.110 Erythema Ab Igne mimicking Livedo reticularis.

Evaluation and Management

Identifying the cause of these livedoid patterns is the diagnostician's main concern. An in-depth history, review of systems, and additional physical examination for signs of other associated disease (cutaneous lupus) is beneficial. Additional laboratory testing may include LAC, APLAs, CBC, ESR, CRP, LFTs, renal function tests (RFTs), UA, complement 3 and 4 (C3/4), ANAs, ANCAs, anti-Ro/SSA and anti-La/SSB antibodies (Ro/La), Scl70, ACA, Hep C, CRYO, and RPR. Unfortunately, no treatment is available. The cutaneous manifestations will persist unless treatment of the underlying disease eliminates the mechanism of action producing this pattern.

TABLE 1.13

Causes Associated with Livedo Reticularis/Racemosa

Hematologic/Hypercoagulable states
- Antiphospholipid antibody syndrome
- Cryoglobulinemia
- Polycythemia vera

Systemic vasculitis
- Granulomatosis with polyangiitis
- Polyarteritis nodosa

Connective tissue disease
- SLE
- Dermatomyositis
- Scleroderma
- Sjögren syndrome

Infections
- Hepatitis C
- *Mycoplasma pneumoniae*
- Parvovirus B19
- Syphilis
- COVID-19

Embolic phenomenon
- Cholesterol emboli syndrome
- Septic emboli
- Calciphylaxis

Neurologic
- Sneddon syndrome
- Autonomic nervous systemic dysfunction

Medications
- Amantadine
- Gemcitabine
- Rasagiline
- Norepinephrine
- Dapsone
- Gefitinib
- Minocycline

BIBLIOGRAPHY

Gibbs MB, English JC III, Zirwas MJ. Livedo reticularis: An update. J Am Acad Dermatol 2005;52:1009–1019.

Gomez-Flores M, Herrera-Argaez G, Vazquez-Martinez O, et al. Cutaneous manifestations of antiphospholipid antibody syndrome. Lupus 2021;30(4):541–548.

Mitri F, Enk A, Bersano A, et al. Livedo racemosa in neurologic diseases: An update on the differential diagnosis. Eur J Neurol 2020;27(10):1832–1843.

Nakashima C, Kato M, Otuska A. Cutaneous manifestations of COVID-19 and COVID-19 vaccination. J Dermatol 2023;50(3):280–289.

Pincelli MS, Echavarria AMJ, Criado PR, et al. Livedo racemosa: Clinic. Laboratory and histological findings in 33 patients. Int J Low Extrem Wounds 2021;20(1);22–28.

Metastases and Paraneoplasia

Etiopathogenesis

The skin manifestations of internal malignancy can include the presence of cutaneous metastases or the presence of a cutaneous paraneoplastic syndrome. Cutaneous metastases occur in approximately 1%–9% of individuals with internal malignancy and represent approximately 2% of all skin tumors. Melanoma has the highest propensity to metastasize to the skin, but it is a less common malignancy overall, so it occurs as cutaneous metastases less frequently than breast cancer or colon cancer in women, and less frequently than lung cancer or colon cancer in men.

Clinical Manifestations

Lesions of cutaneous metastases (**Figures 1.111–1.118**) can present as subcutaneous indurated nodules, plaques, or exophytic nodules with ulcerations on the skin. Location of the metastases will often correspond to the organ of origin (anterior chest wall for breast cancer, umbilicus for colon cancer), although lesions can also occur at a site on the skin that is not contiguous with the underlying cancer, with the scalp being an area of skin that is frequently involved. In addition to nodules and tumors, there are other presentations of cutaneous metastases, such as a cellulitis-like presentation that can occur in breast cancer (carcinoma erysipeloides), or alopecia that can occur in the setting of scalp lesions (alopecia neoplastica). Another cutaneous sign of internal malignancy is the presence of paraneoplastic phenomena (**Figures 1.119–1.127**) with relatively specific skin findings. **Table 1.14** is a partial list of skin changes that can occur in the setting of some internal malignancies.

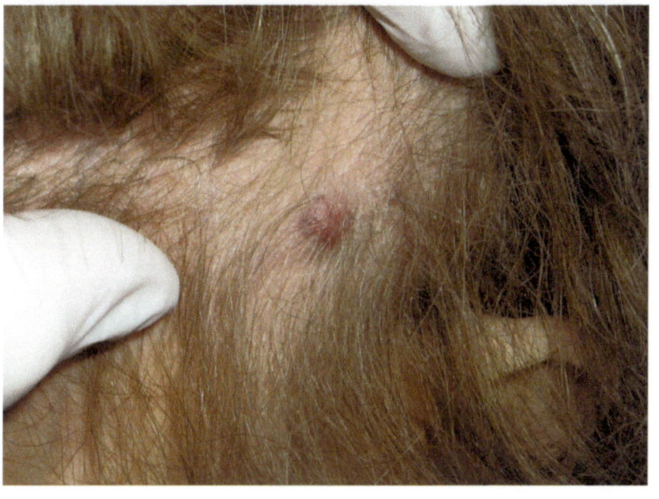

FIGURE 1.111 Skin metastasis: Lung.

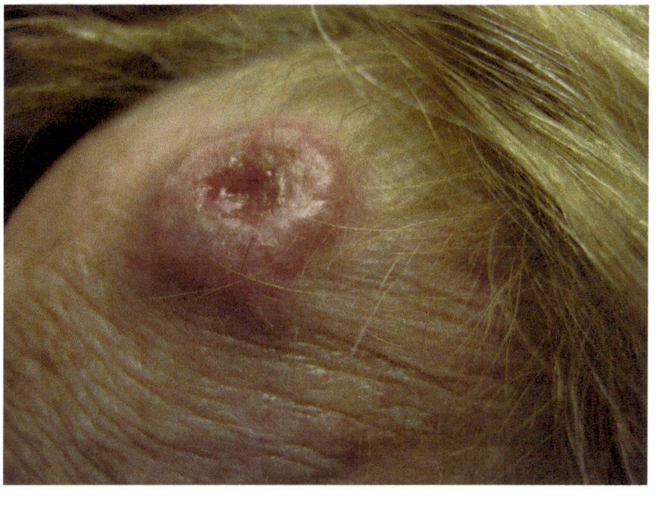

FIGURE 1.112 Skin metastasis: Lung.

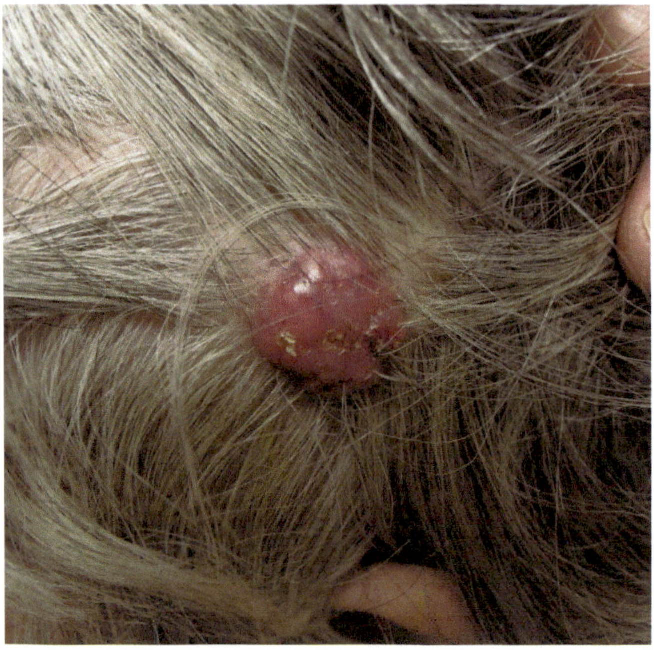

FIGURE 1.113 Skin metastasis: Colon.

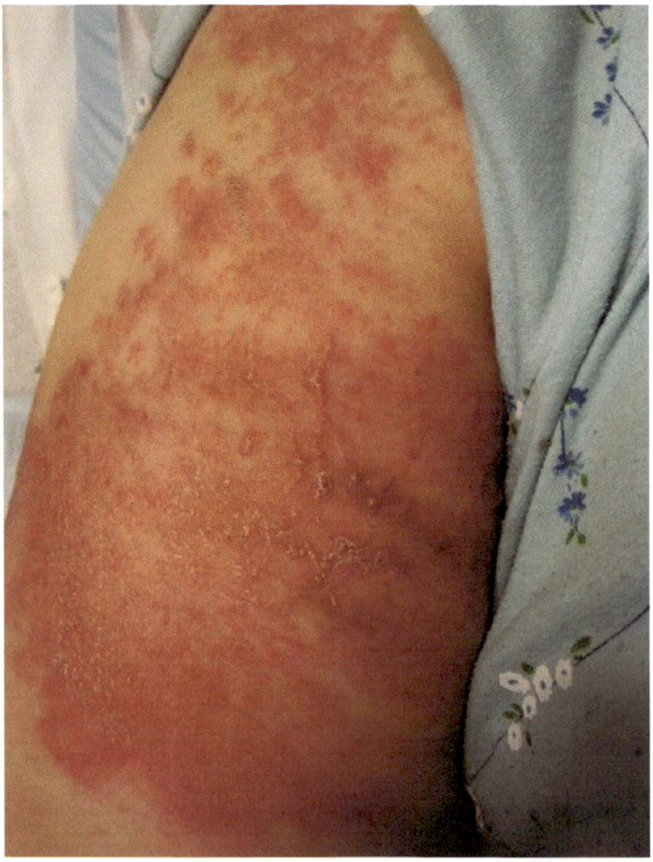

FIGURE 1.114 Skin metastasis: Breast.

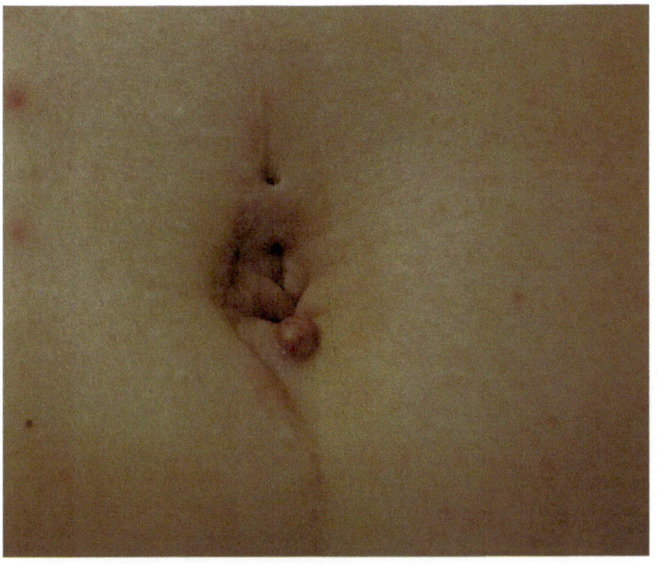

FIGURE 1.115 Skin metastasis: Peritoneal adenocarcinoma.

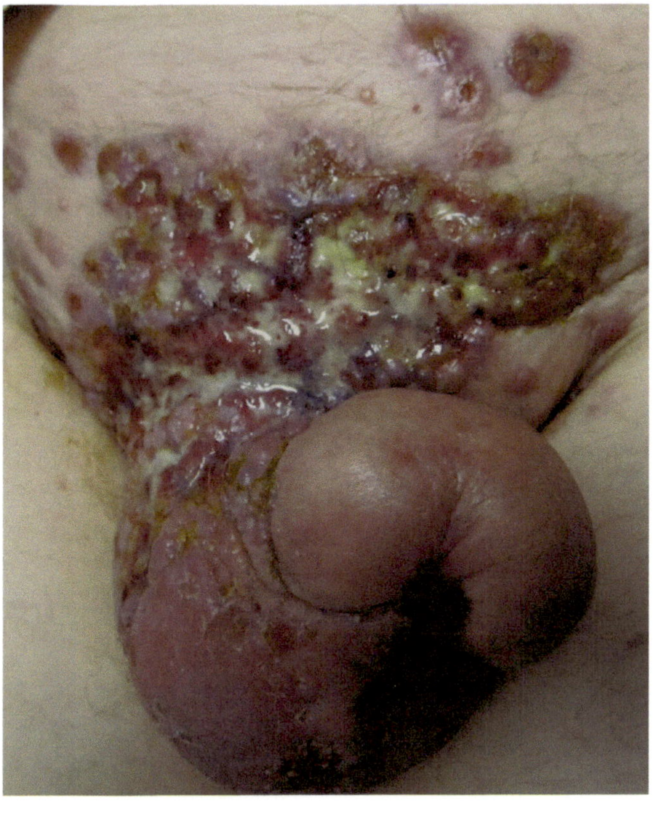

FIGURE 1.116 Skin metastasis: Rectal adenocarcinoma.

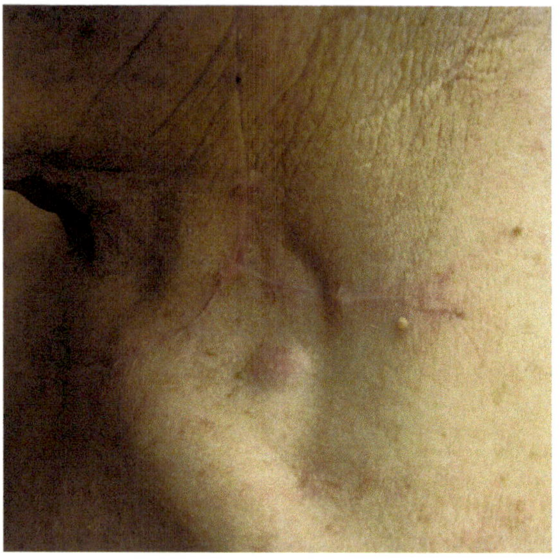

FIGURE 1.117 Skin metastasis: Malignant melanoma.

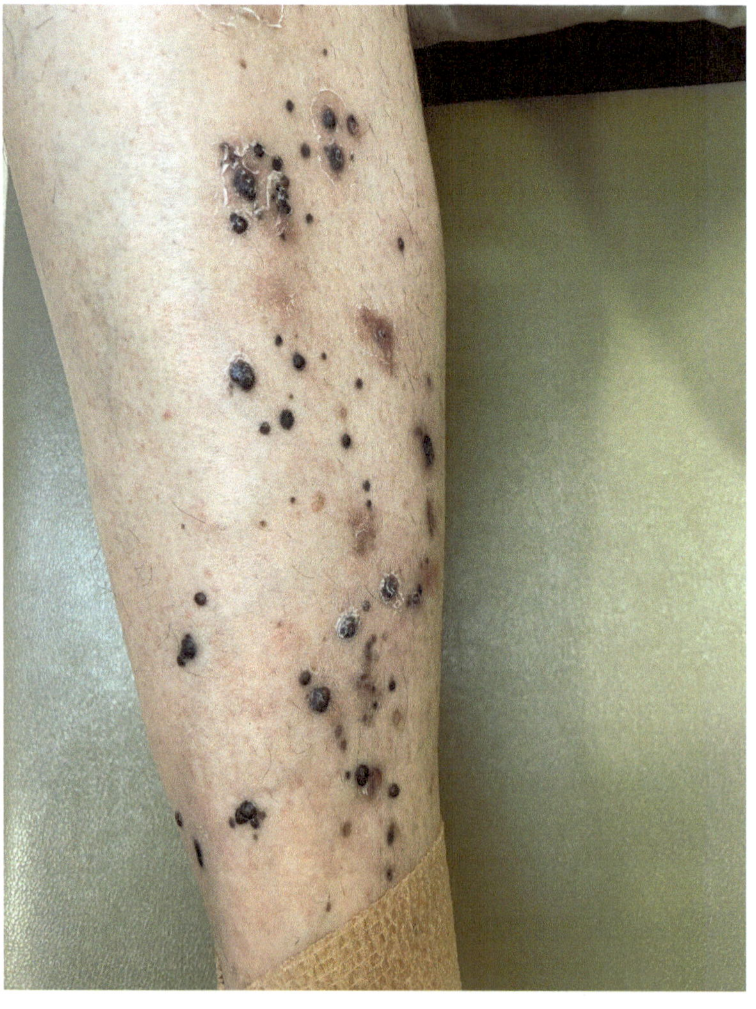

FIGURE 1.118 Skin metastasis: Malignant melanoma.

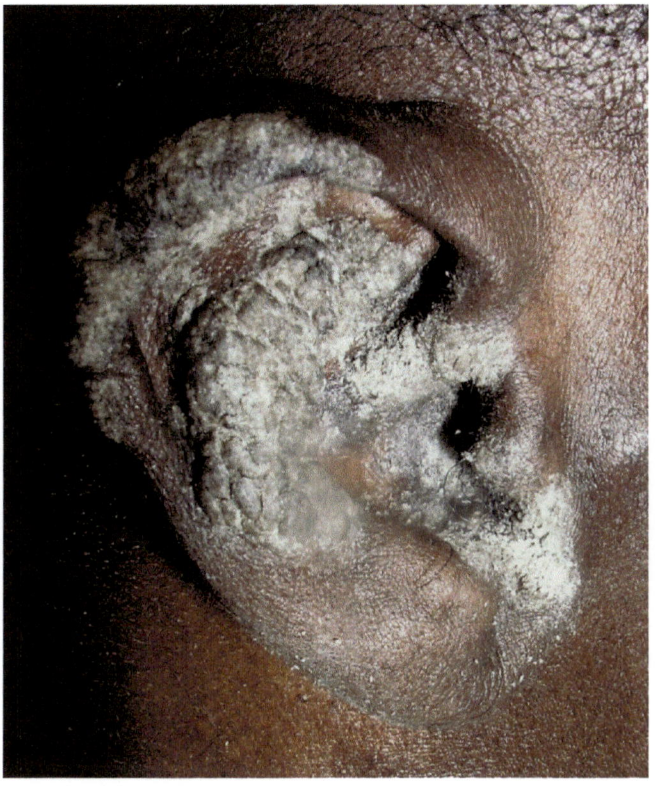

FIGURE 1.119 Acrokeratosis neoplastica.

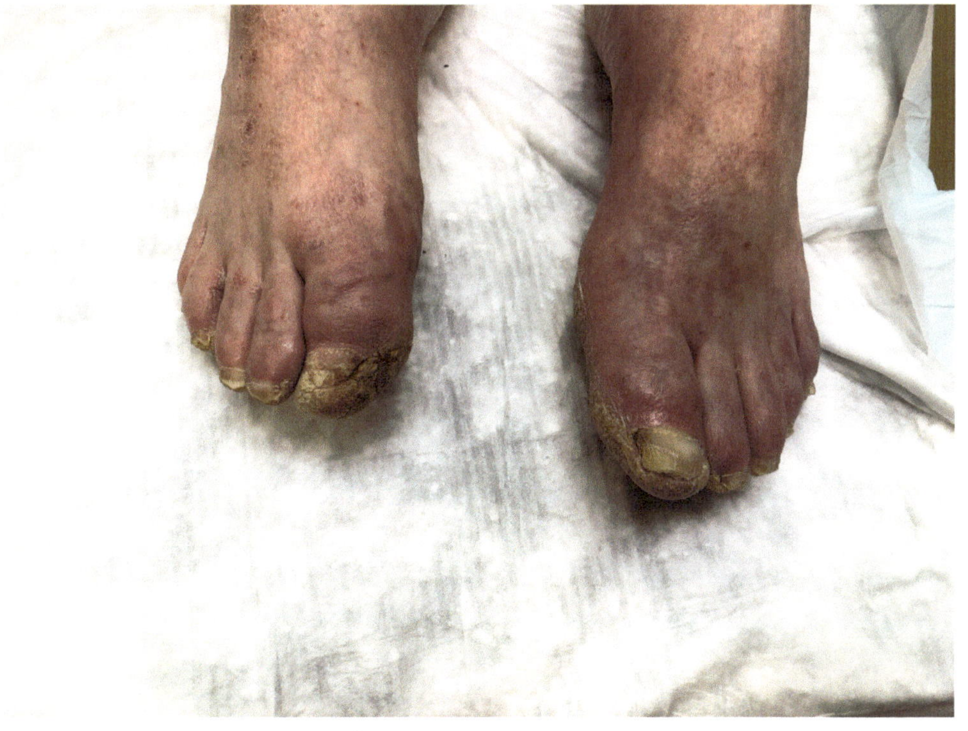

FIGURE 1.120 Acrokeratosis neoplastica.

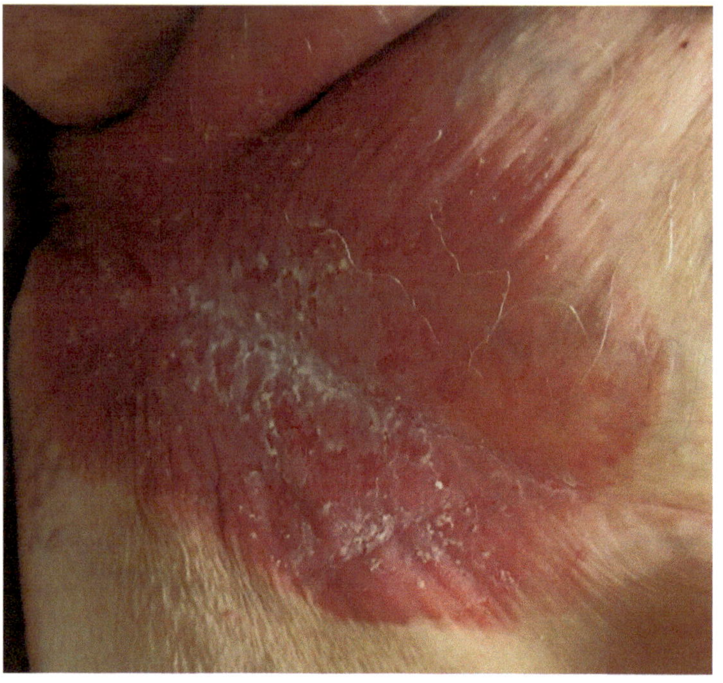

FIGURE 1.121 Extramammary Paget disease.

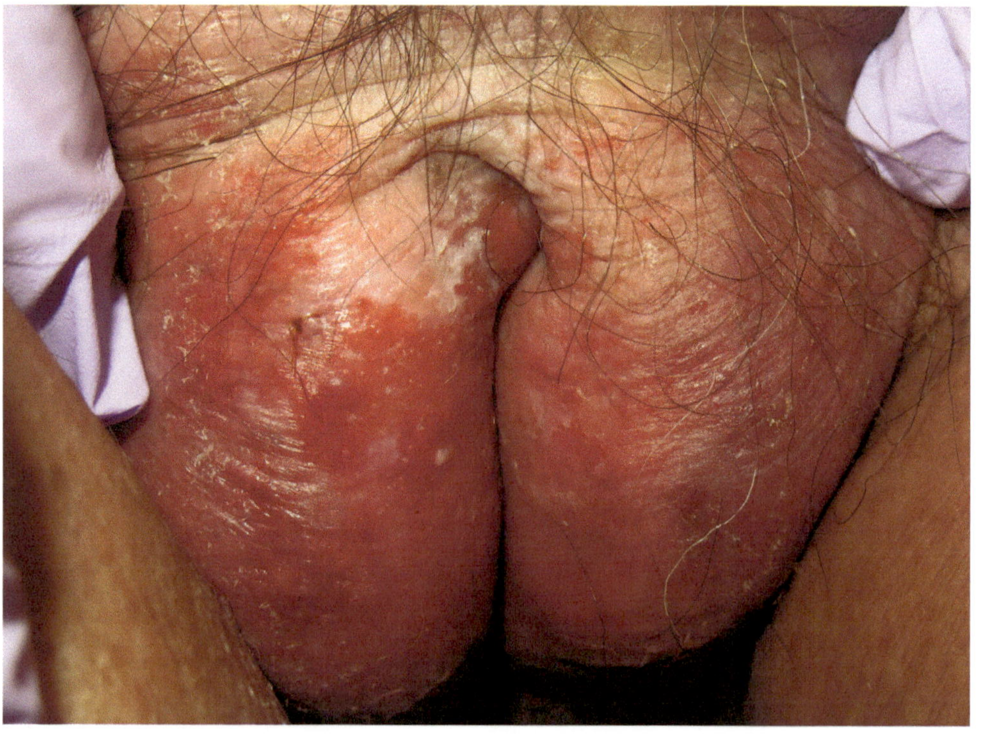

FIGURE 1.122 Extramammary Paget disease.

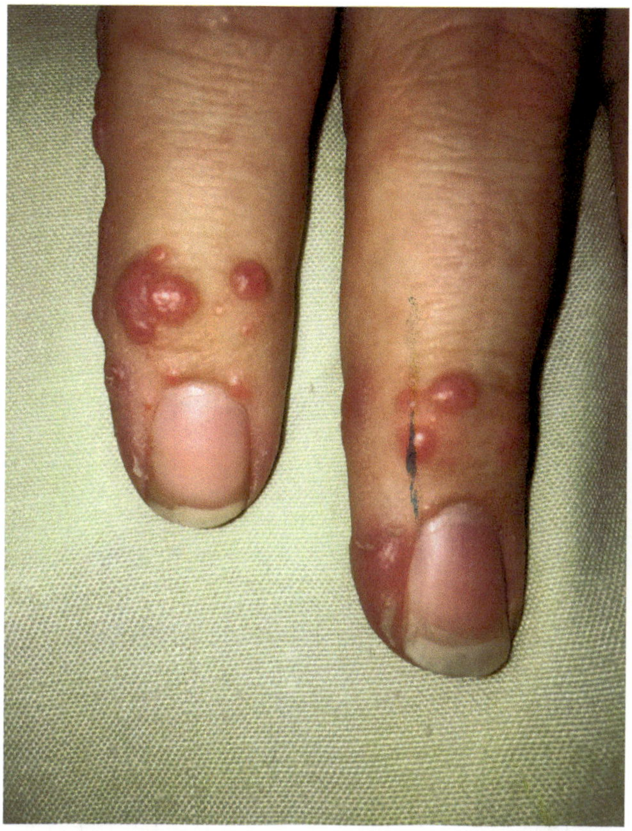

FIGURE 1.123 Multicentric reticulohistiocytosis.

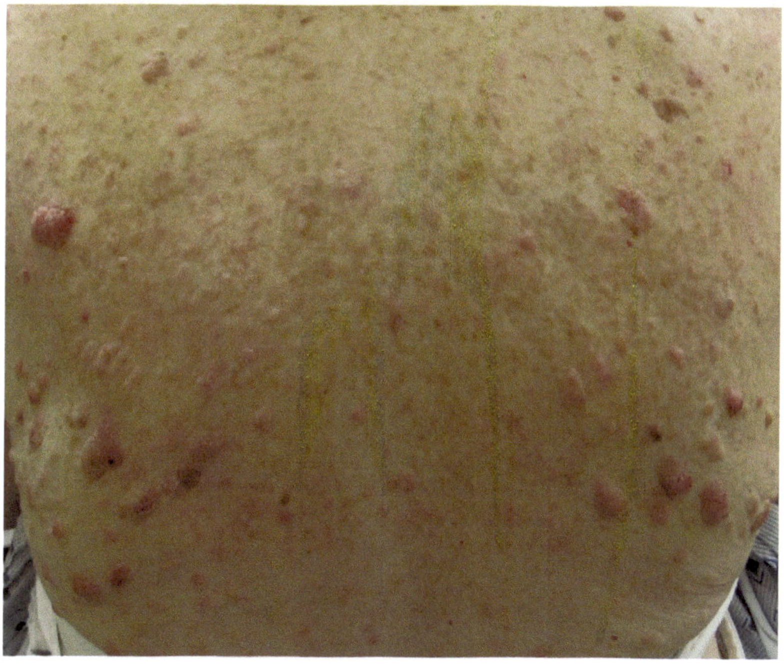

FIGURE 1.124 Sign of Leser–Trelat.

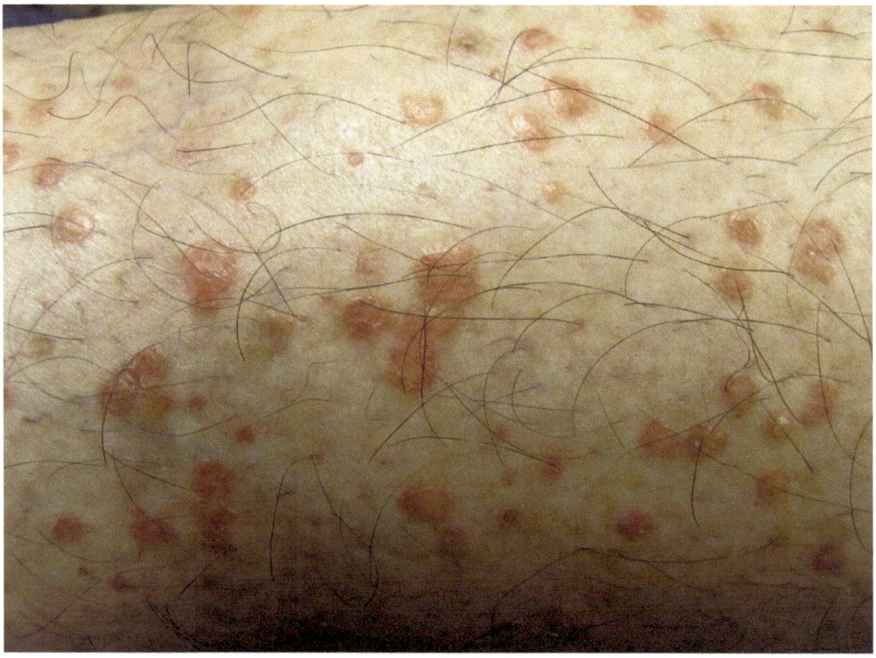

FIGURE 1.125 Disseminated superficial porokeratosis.

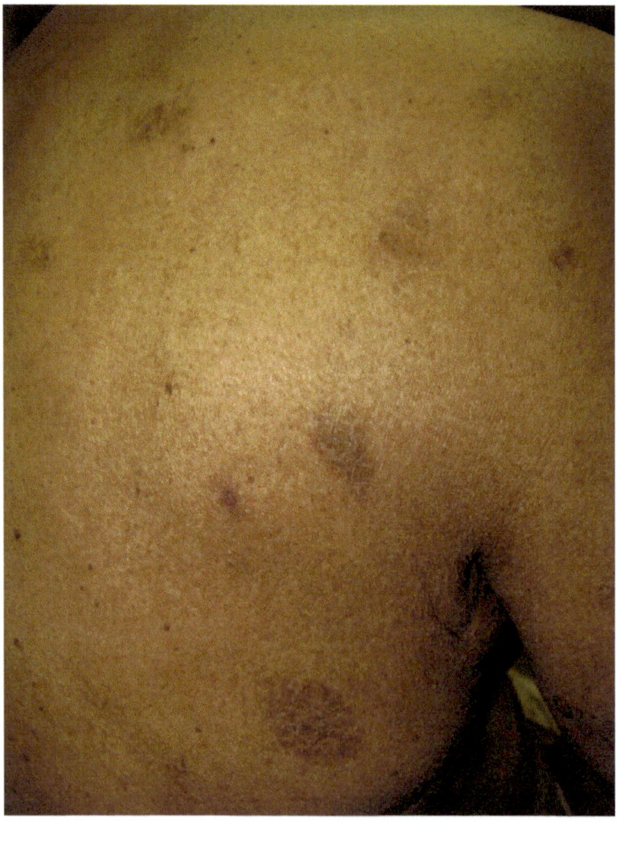

FIGURE 1.126 Pityriasis rotunda.

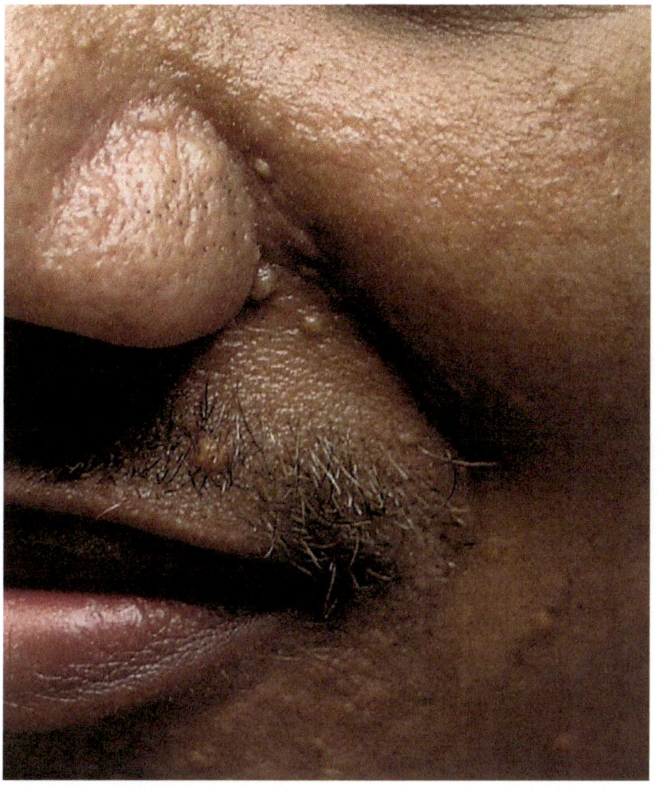

FIGURE 1.127 Adult multiple xanthogranulomas.

TABLE 1.14

Cutaneous Paraneoplastic Disorders

Disease	Clinical Findings	Associated Malignancies	Percentage of Patients with Malignancy
Necrolytic migratory erythema	Erosive scaling plaques in periorificial and genital locations	Pancreatic glucagonoma	Almost 100%
Bazex syndrome (acrokeratosis neoplastica)	Psoriasiform lesions on the distal fingers and toes, ears, and nose	Upper aerodigestive tract malignancies	Almost 100%
Hypertrichosis lanuginosa	The sudden presence of widespread, downy lanugo hairs	Lung, colon	Almost 100%
Tripe palms	Thickened, rugated hyperkeratosis of the palms ± acanthosis nigricans	Lung and GI malignancies	>90%
Erythema gyratum repens	"Wood grain" appearing annular and polycyclic rings	Lung, breast, colon	~80%
Mammary Paget's disease	Erythema with erosions on breast	Breast	~80%–90%
Extramammary Paget's disease	Erythema with erosions on anogenital areas	GU, GI, skin	50%
Multicentric reticulohistiocytosis	Periungual and facial red to orange papules/ nodules with associated polyarthritis	Ovary, breast, colon, lung	~20%
Sign of Leser–Trelat	Eruptive seborrheic keratoses or inflammation of all current seborrheic keratoses ± acanthosis nigricans	Stomach, colon, breast	Low
Disseminate porokeratosis	Erythematous papule with coronoid lamellae	Cholangiocarcinoma Prostate	Low
Pityriasis rotunda	Tan to brown oval patches	Hepatocellular	Low
Adult xanthogranulomas	Red to orange-yellow papules, widespread	Lymphoma	Low

Systemic Manifestations

The systemic manifestations of an internal malignancy will largely reflect the organ involved. In general, patients may also report a history of night sweats, unintended weight loss, fevers, or lymphadenopathy.

Evaluation and Management

In the setting of an undiagnosed primary malignancy, a biopsy of the skin lesion with histopathologic evaluation can lead to appropriate workup, staging, and treatment of the underlying malignancy.

BIBLIOGRAPHY

Fernández-Antón Martínez MC, Parra-Blanco V, Avilés Izquierdo JA, et al. Cutaneous metastases of internal tumors. Actas Dermosifiliogr 2013;104(10):841–853.

Habermehl G, Ko J. Cutaneous metastases: A review and diagnostic approach to tumors of unknown origin. Arch Pathol Lab Med 2019;143(8):943–957.

Turner N, Ware O, Bosenberg M. Genetics of metastasis: Melanoma and other cancers. Clin Exp Metastasis 2018;35(5–6):379–391.

Mucinoses

Etiopathogenesis

Cutaneous mucinoses are the result of increased production/deposition of dermal mucopolysaccharides from reactive fibroblast production. The exact etiology of focal, follicular, and diffuse cutaneous mucinoses is unknown; however, immunologic disturbances may be underlying. Newer cutaneous mucinosis includes obesity-associated, pretibial stasis mucinosis, and toxic dermal mucinoses from medications (tumor necrosis factor [TNF] alpha inhibitors, Type 1 interferon, colony stimulating factor 1, tocilizumab, ustekinumab). Several entities have established associations with systemic disease. Scleredema, reticular erythematous mucinosis (REM), follicular mucinosis, and scleromyxedema will be further elaborated.

Clinical Manifestations

Scleredema presents as indurated, thickened, painless skin, predominately on the upper back, that is associated with significant restriction in mobility of the upper extremities (**Figures 1.128–1.131**), head, and neck. The skin may have a blanchable erythema present. REM presents as asymptomatic erythematous macular, papular, or plaque lesions that have a reticular pattern (**Figure 1.132**). Lesions favor the chest and back, more commonly in women. Lesions may demonstrate photosensitivity, which may produce pruritus. Follicular mucinosis (**Figures 1.133** and **1.134**) may cause follicular erythematous papules to nodules on the face, torso, extremities, and scalp (alopecia mucinosa). Scleromyxedema presents usually with generalized waxy papules with sclerodermoid indurations (**Figure 1.135**).

Systemic Manifestations

Scleredema is associated with viral/bacterial infections in younger patients, whereas in the adult population it is associated with diabetes mellitus and plasma cell dyscrasia (IgGκ monoclonal gammopathy to myeloma). REM has been seen more often in cigarette smokers and patients with autoimmune thyroiditis, psoriatic/rheumatoid arthritis, hypertension, and malignancy (breast, rectal, lymphoma). Some feel it is related to tumid lupus, a form of chronic cutaneous lupus erythematosus. Both have a low association with developing systemic lupus. Follicular mucinosis may be found in reactive inflammatory conditions as an incidental finding, a primary condition, or due to follicular mycosis fungoides (cutaneous T-cell lymphoma). Scleromyxedema is associated with monoclonal gammopathy.

Evaluation and Management

Skin biopsy is helpful in diagnosing these cutaneous mucinoses. Scleredema will reveal a nonfibroplastic, noninflammatory dermal thickened collagen fibers separated by mucin. REM has superficial and deep perivascular lymphocytic infiltrate with dermal mucin deposition. Follicular mucinosis associated with lymphoma presents with perifollicular neoplastic infiltrates with follicular mucin. Scleromyxedema demonstrates mucin deposition, fibroblastic proliferation, and fibrosis. Investigative testing for FBS, HAIc, SPEP/SIFE, and UPEP/UIFE (scleredema and scleromyxedema); TFTs, TGs, TPOs, ANA, mammography (MMGX), and CT (REM); and CBC (follicular mucinosis) is recommended. Scleredema, REM, and primary follicular mucinosis may respond to hydroxychloroquine. Scleredema may also be treated with phototherapy (ultraviolet A-1) and superficial electron beam radiation. Scleromyxedema is treated with intravenous immunoglobulin (IVIG). Treating the underlying systemic associations may not alter the course of skin disease, except for follicular mycosis fungoides.

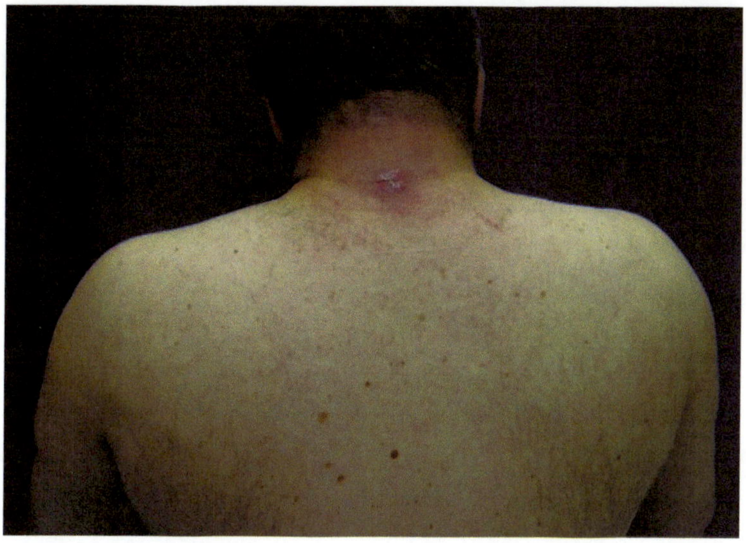

FIGURE 1.128 Scleredema: Baseline (diabetic).

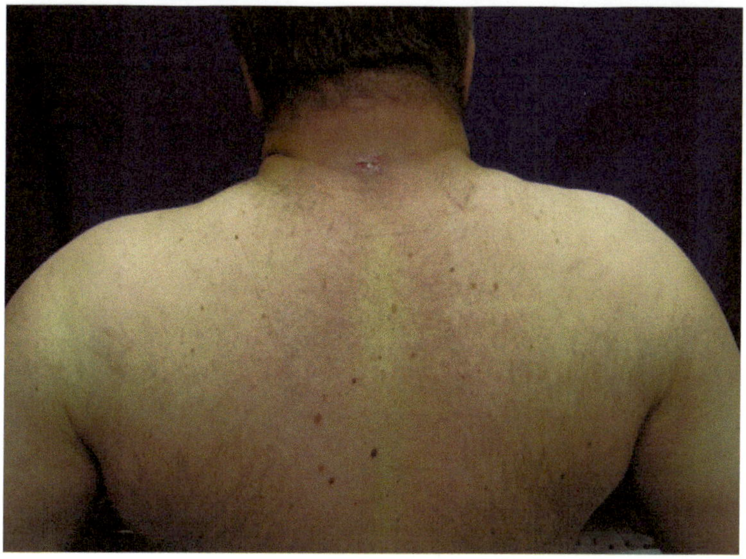

FIGURE 1.129 Scleredema: Shoulder adduction.

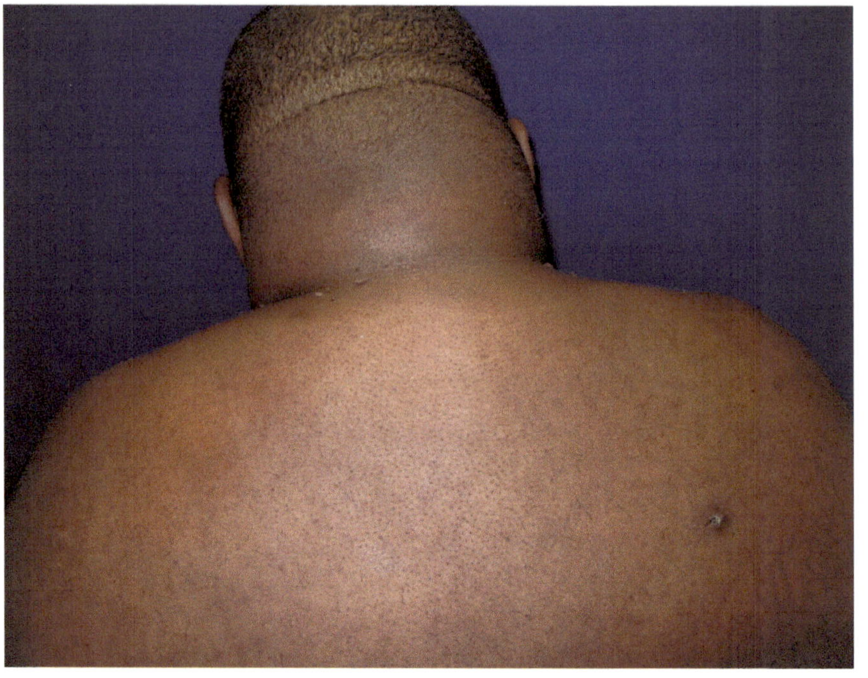

FIGURE 1.130 Scleredema: Baseline (diabetic).

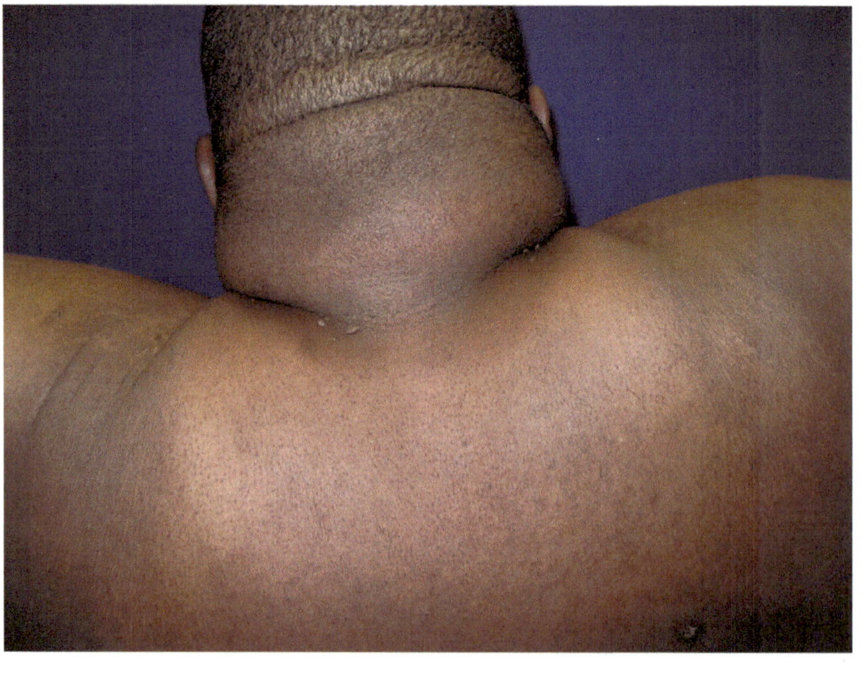

FIGURE 1.131 Scleredema: Maximum shoulder elevation.

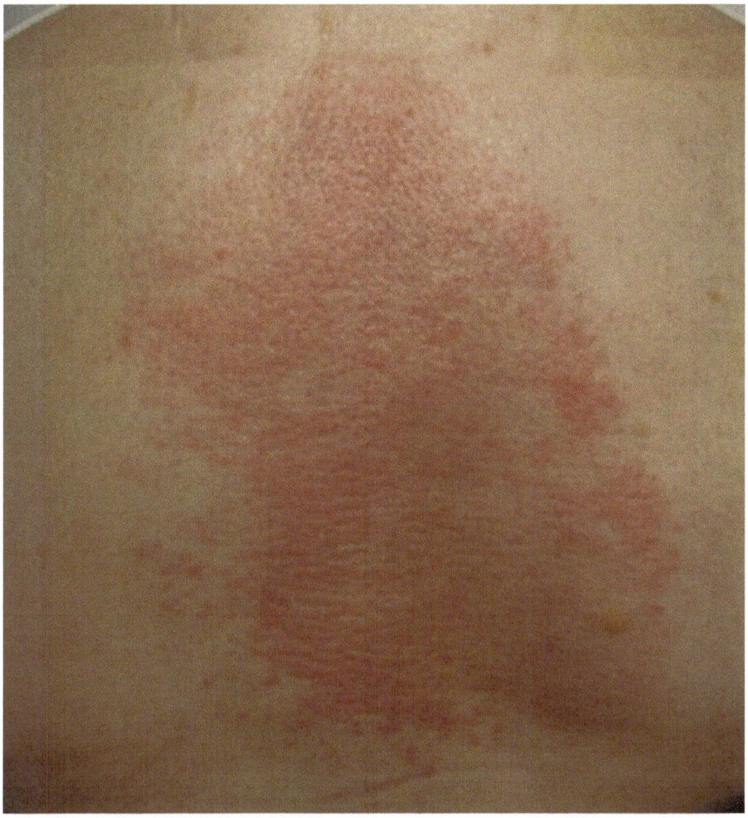

FIGURE 1.132 Reticular erythematous mucinosis.

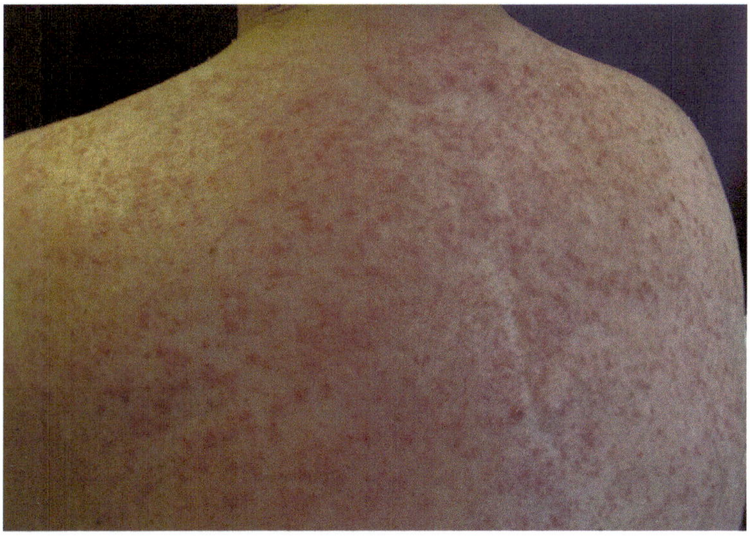

FIGURE 1.133 Follicular mucinosis: Cutaneous T-cell lymphoma.

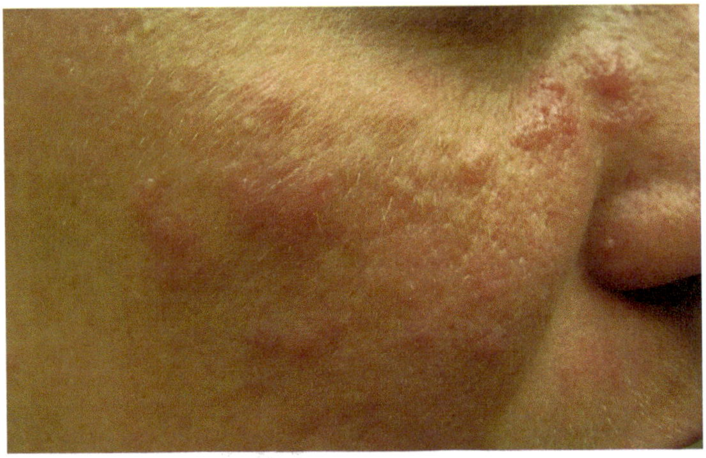

FIGURE 1.134 Follicular mucinosis: Primary.

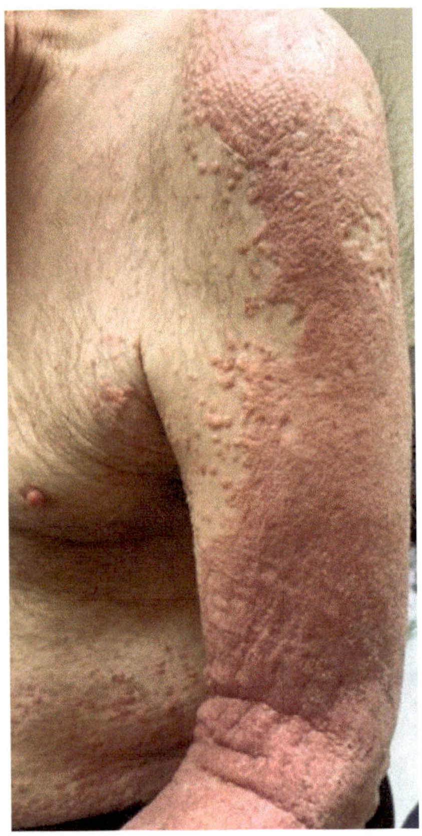

FIGURE 1.135 Scleromyxedema.

BIBLIOGRAPHY

Hoffman JHO, Enk AH. Scleromyxedema. J Dstch Dermatol Ges 2020;18(12):1449–1467.

Khalil J, Kurban M, Abbas O. Follicular mucinosis: A review. Int J Dermatol 2021;60(2):159–165.

Ocanha-Xavier JP, Cola-Senra CO, Xavier-Junior JCC. Reticular erythematous mucinosis: Literature review and case report of 24-year-old patient with systemic erythematosus lupus. Lupus 2021;30(2):325–335.

Pereira M, Pinheiro RR, Lencastre A, et al. Scleredema diabeticorum. Dermatol Rep 2022;14(4):9477.
Rongioletti F. New and emerging conditions of acquired cutaneous mucinoses in adults. J Eur Acad Dermatol Venereol 2022;36(7):1016–1024.

Onychodystrophy

Etiopathogenesis

Onychodystrophy (abnormal nail) manifesting from a systemic disease is due to matrix disruption, matrix keratinization, matrix melanin production, matrix pigment deposition, separation of the plate from the bed, bed vascularization, or unknown growth disturbances.

Clinical Manifestations

Transverse depression of the nail plate that will grow out with the nail is called a Beau line (**Figures 1.136 and 1.137**). Mees' lines (**Figure 1.138**) are transverse white lines in the plate (true leukonychia) that do not fade with compression and changes with nail growth. Bissell's lines (**Figure 1.139**) are longitudinal melanonychia in multiple nails. Onycholysis (**Figure 1.140**) is the separation of the nail plate from the bed, whereas spooning of the plate is referred to as koilonychia (**Figure 1.141**). Transverse apparent leukonychia fades with compression and does not change with growth (**Table 1.15**). When extending to half the nail plate, it is referred to as half-and-half or Lindsay nails (**Figure 1.142**), whereas extension to the distal end is called Crescent or Terry's nails (**Figure 1.143**). Muehrcke's nails present as two reddish lines with an edematous-appearing nail bed (**Figure 1.144**). Thickened and hard yellow nail changes of all digits is referred to as yellow-nail syndrome (**Figure 1.145** Blue lunulae can be seen during states of hypoxia but when persistent consider drug induced discoloration (Minocycline, Silver ingestion [argyria, **Figure 1.145**]). Greyish lunula can be seen with hydroxychloroquine use. Red lunulae are also a sign of systemic disease (**Figure 1.147**). Vascular dilation of proximal nail fold vessels can cause hairpin or globular telangiectasia (**Figures 1.148** and **1.149**). Hemorrhage in the nail bed produces splinter hemorrhages (**Figure 1.150**), and microthrombi at the nail fold produce Bywaters lesion (**Figure 1.151**).

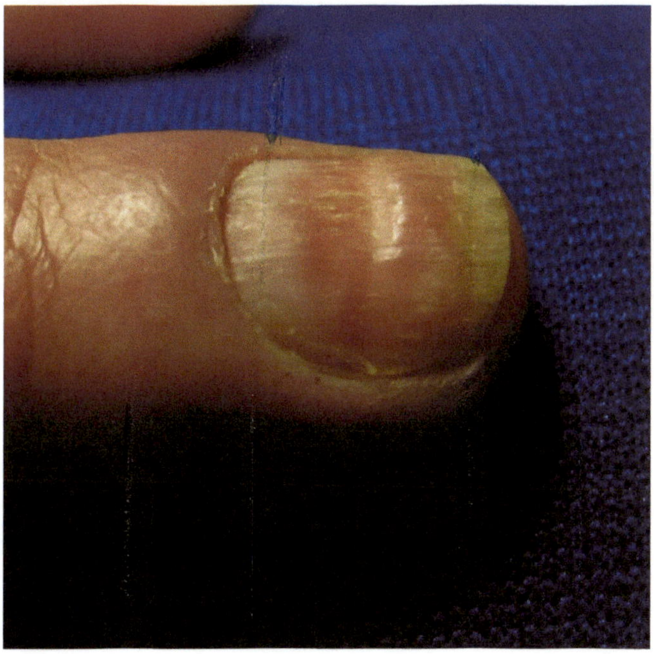

FIGURE 1.136 Beau lines.

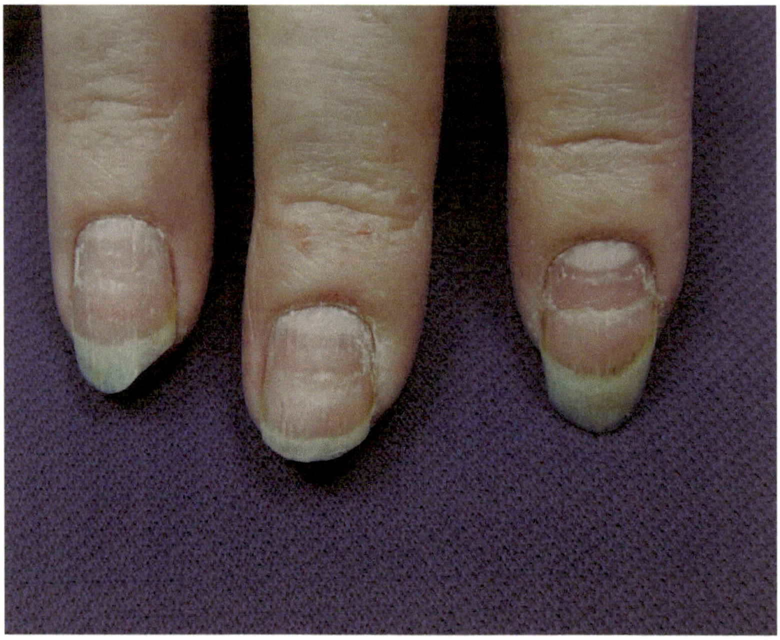

FIGURE 1.137 Beau lines.

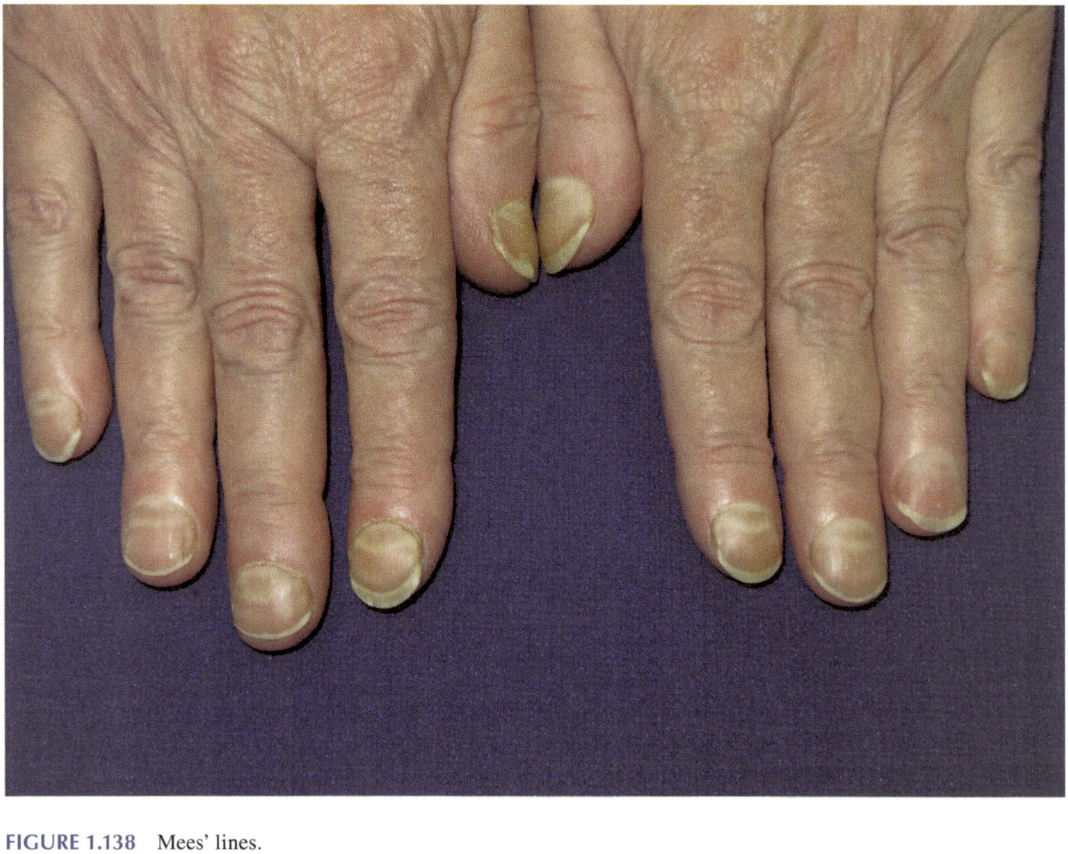

FIGURE 1.138 Mees' lines.

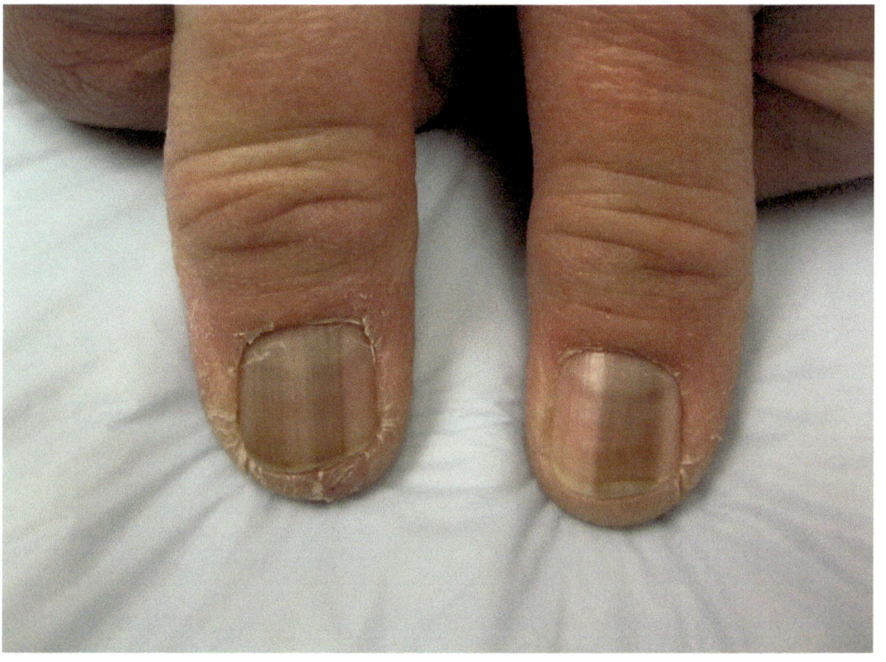

FIGURE 1.139 Bissell's lines.

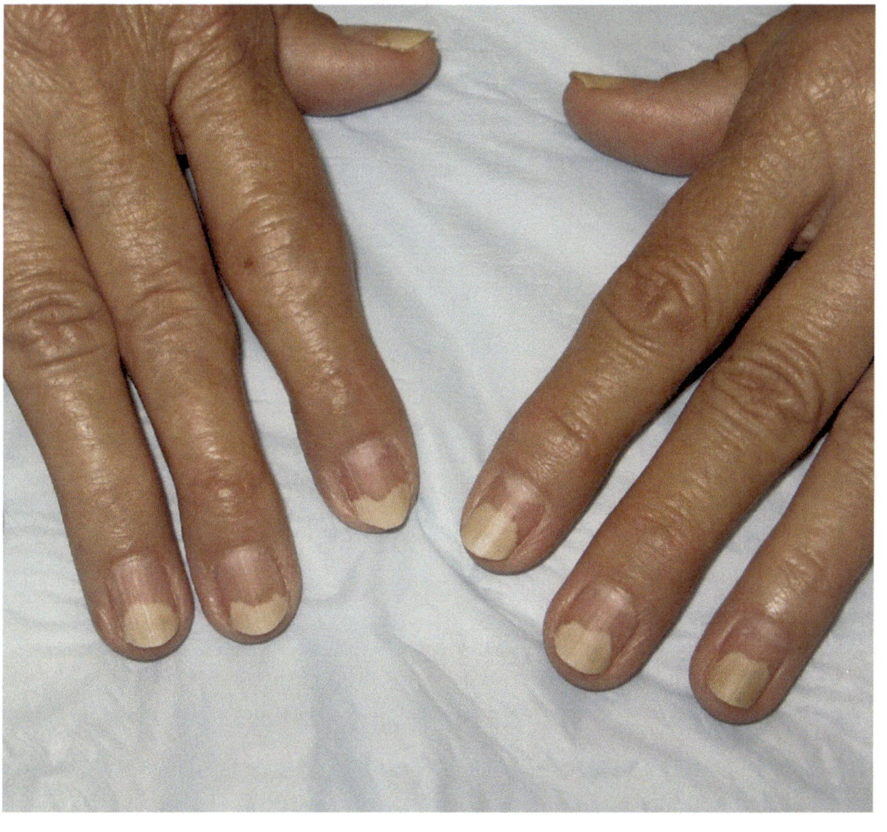

FIGURE 1.140 Onycholysis.

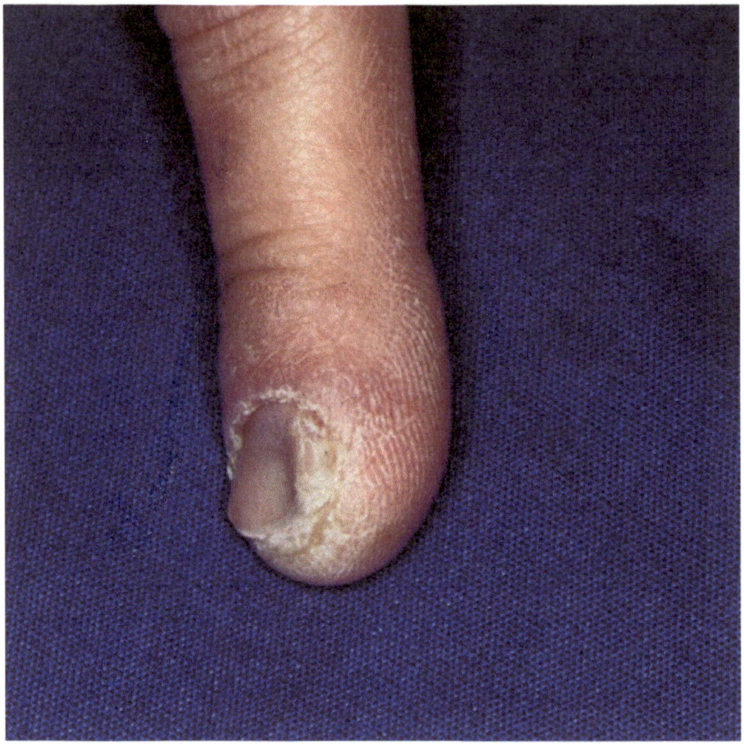

FIGURE 1.141 Koilonychia.

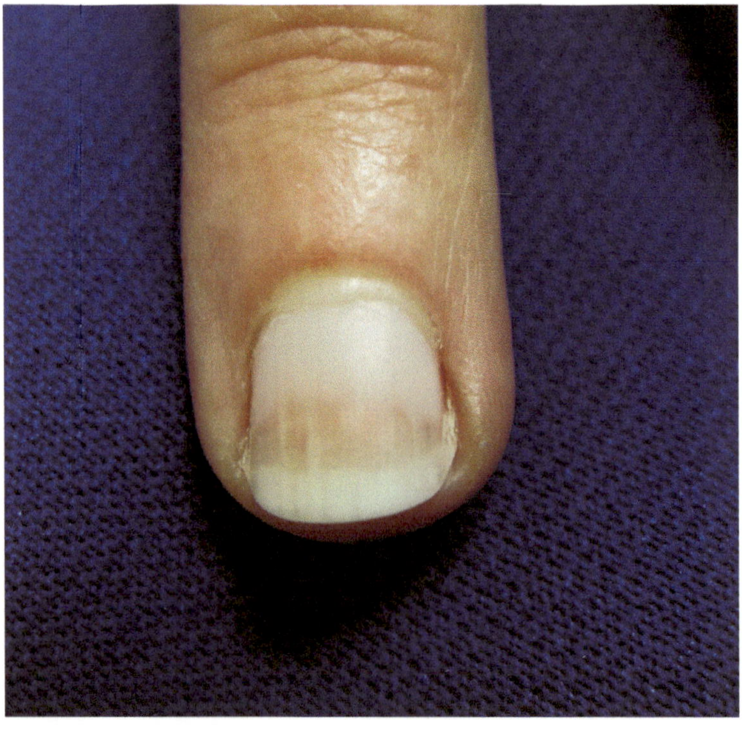

FIGURE 1.142 Half-and-half nail (Lindsay nails).

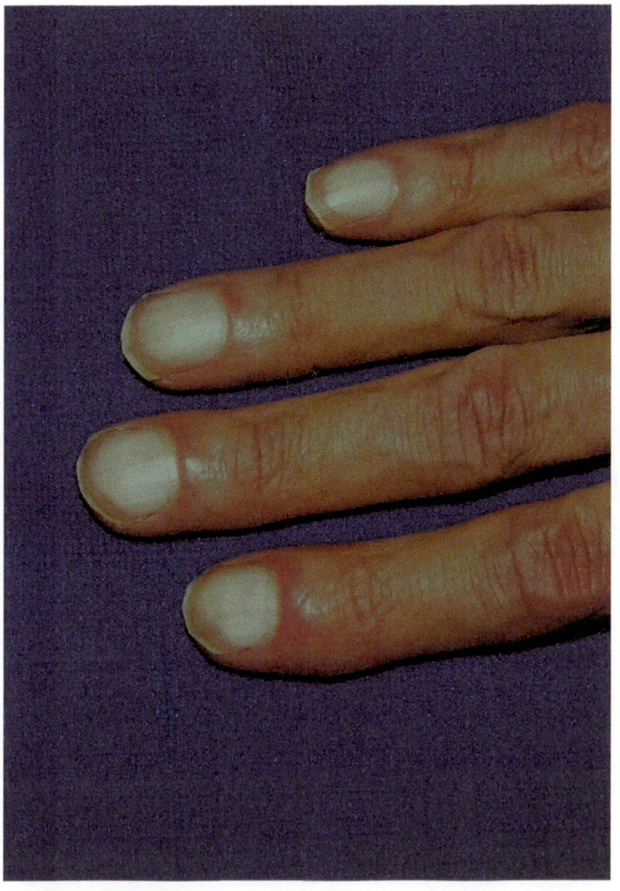

FIGURE 1.143 Crescent nails (Terry nails).

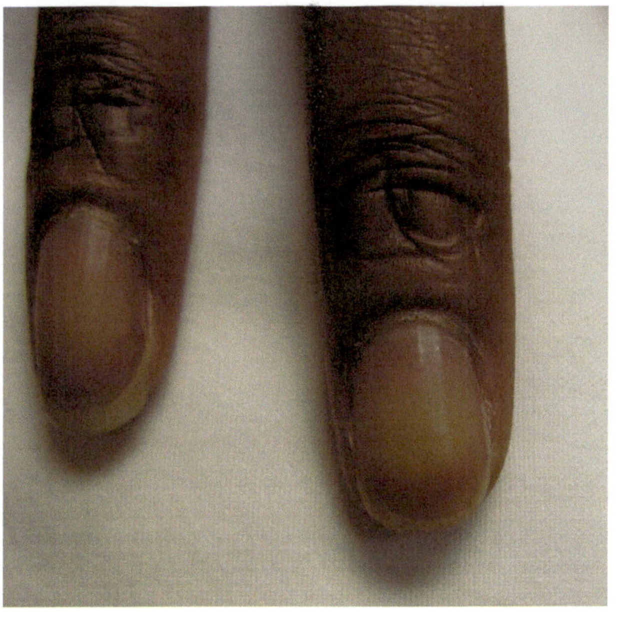

FIGURE 1.144 Muehrcke's nails.

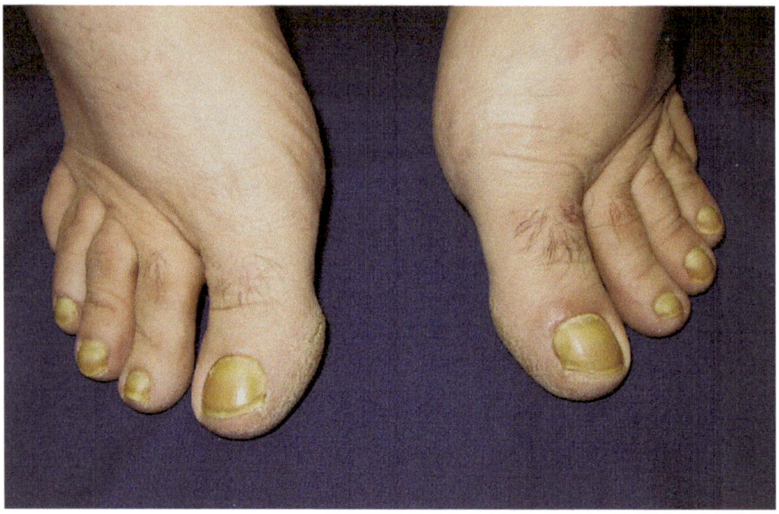

FIGURE 1.145 Yellow-nail syndrome.

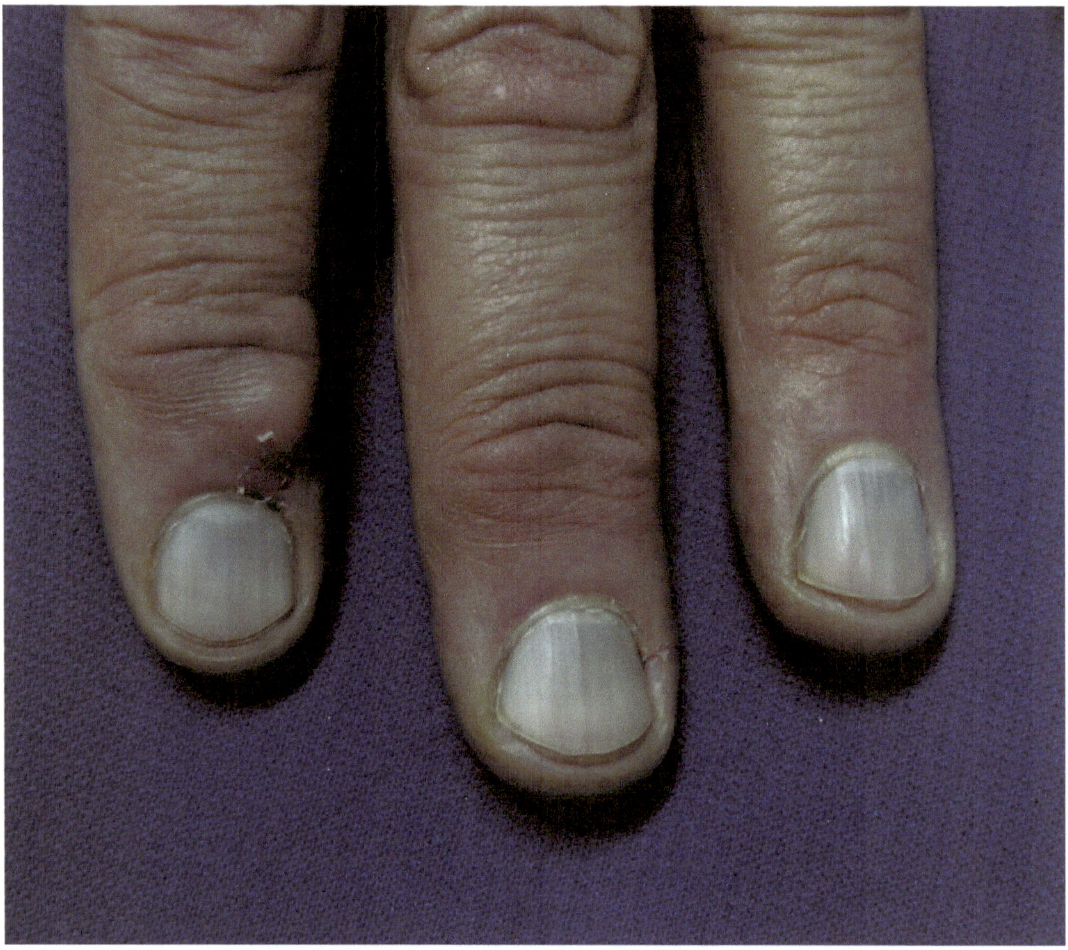

FIGURE 1.146 Argyria.

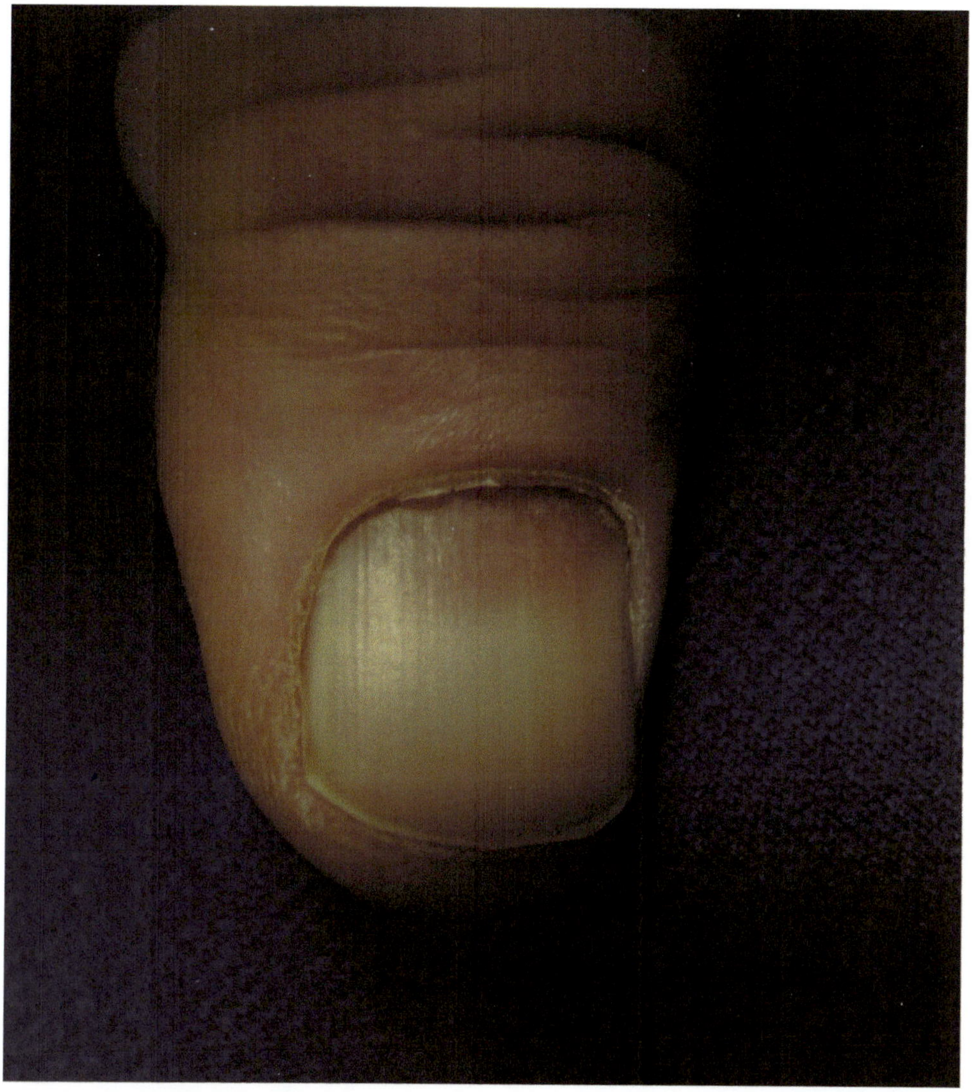

FIGURE 1.147 Alopecia areata.

Systemic Manifestations

Beau lines occur with any significant stressors to the body. Mees' lines are historically associated with arsenic and thallium exposure but may occur in systemic infections to malignancy. Although common in patients with skin of color, multiple longitudinal melanonychia associated with mucosal and palmar crease pigmentation due to Addison's disease constitute Bissell's lines. Onycholysis can be induced by hyperthyroidism, autoimmune disorders, and amyloidosis. Koilonychia can be seen in iron deficiency anemia and hemochromatosis. Muehrcke's nails represent hypoalbuminemia (malnutrition, renal and liver diseases). Half-and-half nails (Lindsay's nails) have been seen in patients with chronic renal disease and renal transplant. Crescent nails (Terry's nails) may be seen with renal disease, cirrhosis, diabetes, and chronic congestive heart failure. Yellow-nail syndrome is associated with lymphedema and pulmonary disease. Lupus produces nail fold hairpin telangiectasia, whereas dermatomyositis and scleroderma cause globular vessels with skip spaces. Splinter hemorrhages when extensive with a heart murmur should raise suspicion for bacterial endocarditis but can be seen with autoimmune diseases. Red lunulae can be seen in alopecia areata, carbon dioxide poisoning, and connective tissue disease.

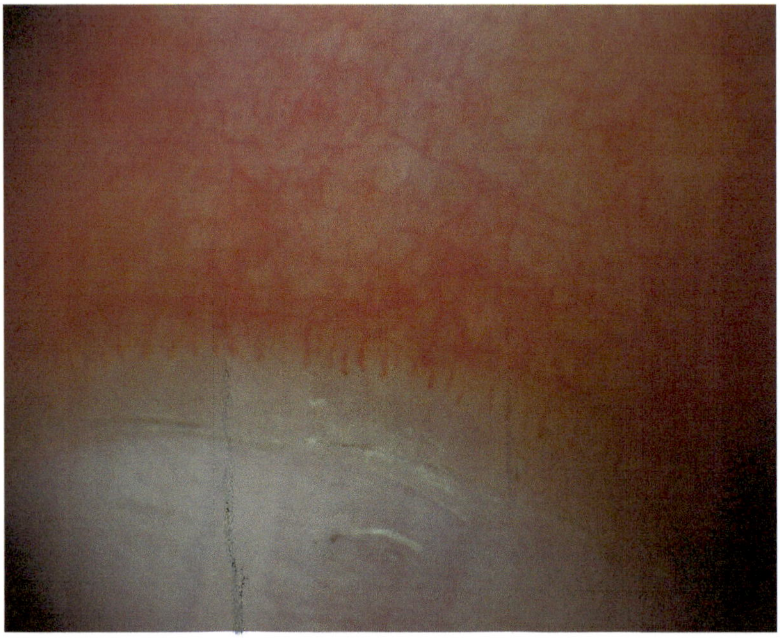

FIGURE 1.148 Nail fold telangiectasia: Lupus.

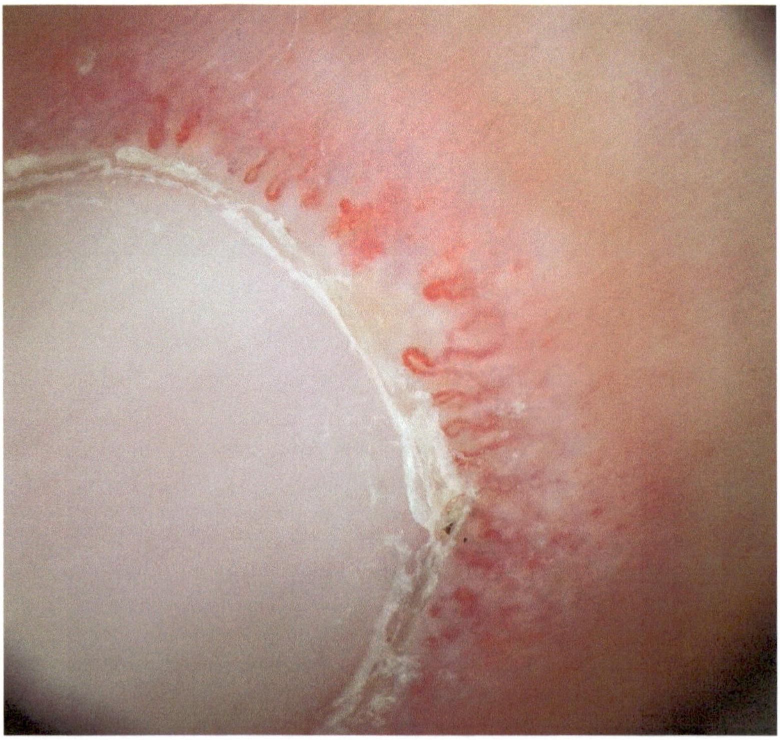

FIGURE 1.149 Nail fold telangiectasia: Dermatomyositis or scleroderma.

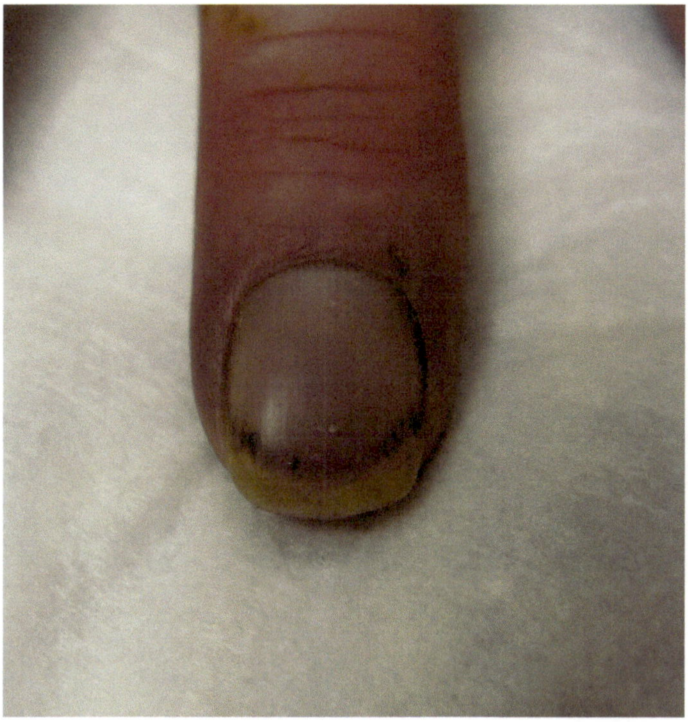

FIGURE 1.150 Splinter hemorrhages and acrocyanosis.

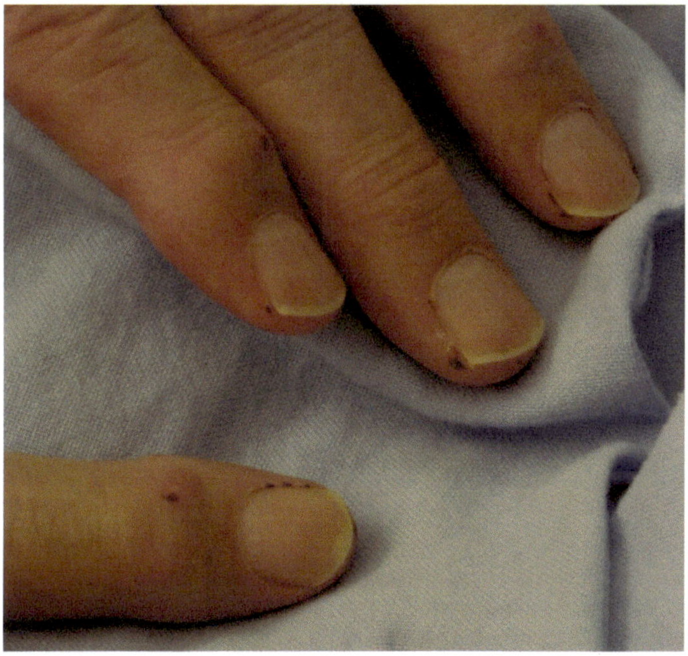

FIGURE 1.151 Bywaters lesions: Rheumatoid arthritis.

TABLE 1.15

Lines vs. Nails

"… Lines" are a plate phenomenon

- Beau's lines
  - Nail plate transverse groove
  - Growth arrest due to systemic illness/drug
- Mee's lines
  - Nail plate transverse leukonychia
  - Arsenic, infections, systemic illness
- Bissel's lines
  - Longitudinal melanonychia (striata)
  - Addison's disease

"… Nails" are a nail bed phenomenon

- Muehrcke's nails
  - Nail bed edema from hypoalbuminemia giving the appearance of two transverse red lines
- Terry's nails
  - Crescent nail in liver disease, CHF, DM, normal aging
- Lindsay's nails
  - Half-and-half nail in renal disease, normal aging

Evaluation and Management

After determining the type of onychodystrophy, the systemic evaluation may be limited to the reported associations. In addition to a history and physical exam, laboratory testing may include CBC, IRON, TFTs, a.m. cortisol, LFTs, RFTs, UA, albumin, FBG, HA1c, ANAs, C3/4, RF, Scl70, ACAs, creatinine phosphokinase (CPK), and aldolase. Additional studies may include a CXR, echocardiogram, and blood cultures. Treating the underlying disease may return nails to normal and can be enhanced with the use of acetyl mandelic acid solution, nail supplements (non-biotin), and moisturization.

BIBLIOGRAPHY

Gollins CE, deBerker D. Nails in systemic disease. Clin Med (Lond) 2021;21(3):166–169.

Iorizzo M, Starace M, Pasch MC. Leukonychia: What can white nails tell us? Am J Clini Dermatol 2022;23(2):177–193.

Smith V, Icklinger C, Hysa E, et al. Nailfold capillaroscopy. Best Pract Res Clin Rheumatol 2023;37(1):101849.

Palmar Erythema

Etiopathogenesis

The development of palmar erythema is not completely understood in all instances. However, circulating factors may be playing a role. Elevated free estrogen can promote increased capillary density; impaired metabolism of vasoactive factors can alter vascular tone; and in the case of malignancy, the generation of proangiogenic factors could promote vascular proliferation.

Clinical Manifestations

Palmar erythema is characterized by nonpainful, nonpruritic redness of the palmar surface of skin and most often affects the hypothenar and thenar eminences (**Figures 1.152–1.154**). Palmar erythema occurs in the absence of other surface findings such as ulceration, hyperkeratosis, and lichenification. Palmar erythema lacks anemic-appearing macules, which distinguishes it from benign physiologic mottling of the palms.

Systemic Manifestations

There are many causes of palmar erythema (**Table 1.16**). The classic association of palmar erythema has been with hepatic disease (cirrhosis, hemochromatosis) secondary to the associated hyperestrogenic state. Endocrinopathies that feature palmar erythema include diabetes and thyrotoxicosis. In the right clinical contexts, autoimmune disorders (lupus, rheumatoid arthritis, Sjögren syndrome, sarcoidosis) can also be considered when confronted with the finding of palmar erythema. Palmar erythema in the oncology patient may be seen with GVHD but must be distinguished from toxic erythema of chemotherapy (TEC) of the palms (also referred to as palmar erythrodysesthesia or chemotherapy acral erythema). TEC initially develops like palmar erythema, but then becomes painful with secondary vesiculobullous changes from chemotherapy: cytarabine, doxorubicin, anthracyclines, and immunotherapies: sunitinib and sorafenib therapies, for example. Various malignancies (brain malignancies, leukemia/lymphoma, gastric adenocarcinoma) can also result in palmar erythema. Infectious etiologies from hepatitis B/C virus, brucellosis, trichinellosis, HIV, and HTLV-1 have been reported with palmar erythema.

TABLE 1.16

Causes of Palmar Erythema

Causes of Palmar Erythema
Physiologic
• Idiopathic
• Hereditary
• Senility
• Pregnancy
Secondary to systemic diseases
• Hepatic
• Endocrinopathies
• Autoimmunity
• Infections
• Malignancy

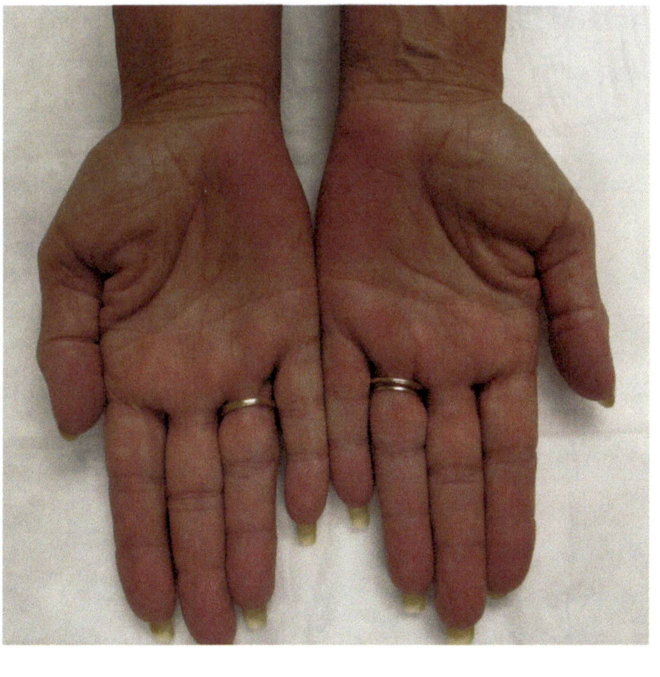

FIGURE 1.152 Palmar erythema: Hepatitis C infection.

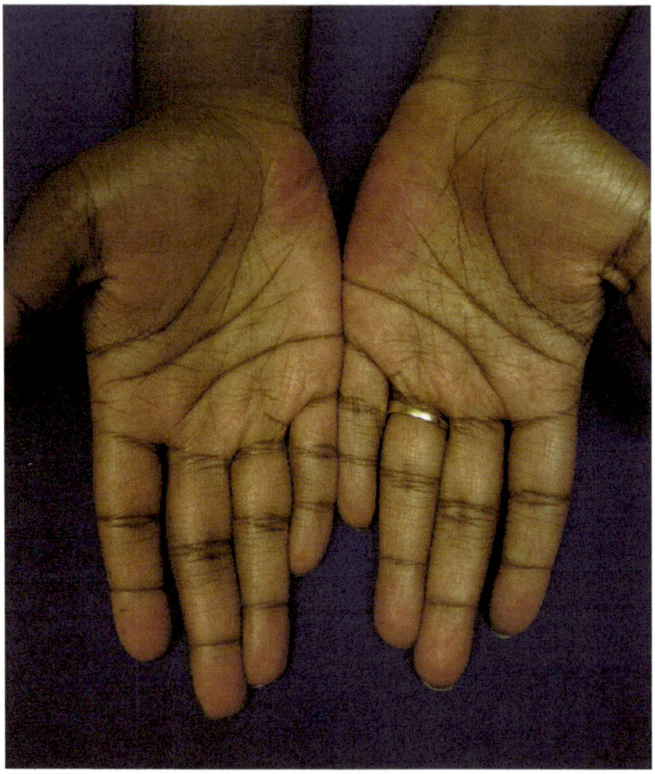

FIGURE 1.153 Palmar erythema: Systemic lupus erythematosus.

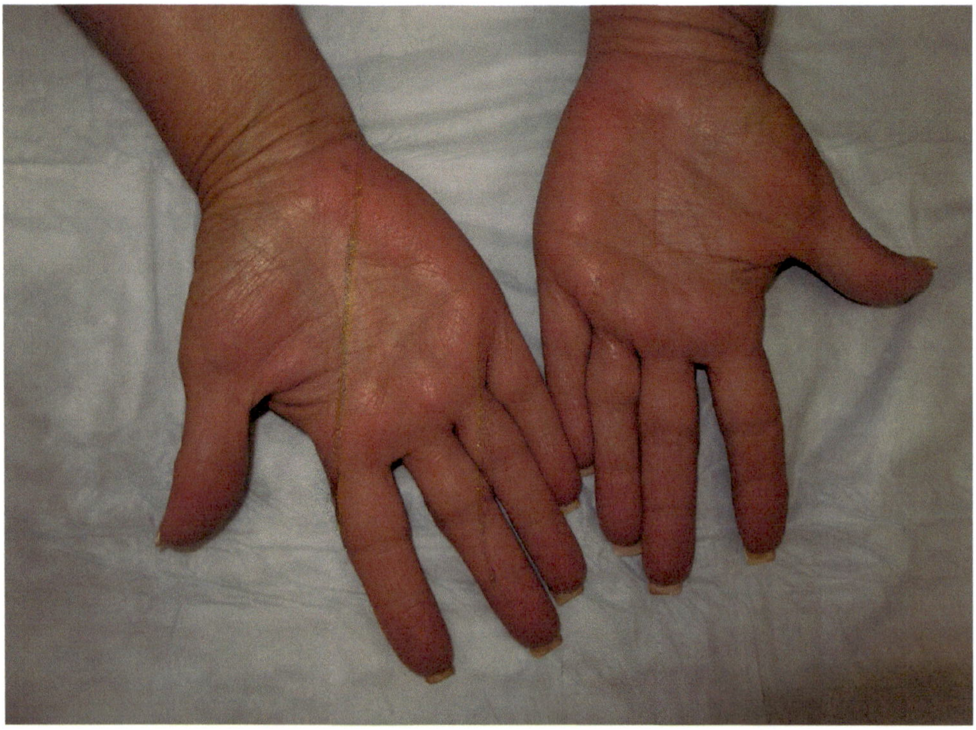

FIGURE 1.154 Palmar erythema: Rheumatoid arthritis.

Evaluation and Management

Given the wide range of differential diagnoses, evaluation should begin with a detailed history and review of systems. Laboratory testing should include CBC, RFTs, LFTs, IRON, Hep B, Hep C serology, FBG, TSH, CBC, and ANAs initially, and consider further testing for hemochromatosis gene mutation, RF, and Ro/La if clinically indicated. CXR screening with additional pan-CT scan and MRI of the brain can be determined on a case-by-case basis. No treatment is required, as the clinical finding is asymptomatic.

BIBLIOGRAPHY

Bhandari A, Mahajan R. Skin changes in cirrhosis. J Clin Exp Hepatol 2022;12(4):1215–1224.
Maekawa M. Palmar erythema as a sign of cancer. Cleve Clin J Med 2017;84(9):666–667.
Serrao R, Zirwas M, English JC. Palmar erythema. Am J Clin Dermatol 2007;8(6):347–356.

Panniculitis

Etiopathogenesis

Panniculitis, or inflammation of the subcutaneous fat, is a nonspecific finding seen in association with a range of conditions. It can be differentiated histologically as septal or lobular, based on the area of inflammation within the fat. Panniculitis can also be differentiated based on underlying pathology (**Table 1.17**) The cause of the inflammation varies based on the underlying etiology. The most common type of panniculitis, erythema nodosum (EN), is considered a delayed-type hypersensitivity reaction to a variety of antigenic stimuli. Other forms of panniculitis, including pancreatic panniculitis and α1-antitrypsin-deficiency panniculitis, occur as a result of direct injury to the adipocytes.

Clinical Manifestations

Panniculitis typically presents as tender, erythematous subcutaneous nodules on the lower extremities. Multiple lesions, ulcerations, indurated atrophy, and involvement of the upper extremities are possible. Given the similarity in clinical presentation of many of the panniculitides, a deep incisional biopsy (through the level of the subcutaneous fat) is often necessary to help delineate the underlying cause if it is not clear based on the patient's history. This will also allow differentiation of secondary "spillover" panniculitis from localized infection, cutaneous vasculitis, thrombophlebitis, lipodermatosclerosis, and granulomatous disorders.

Systemic Manifestations

EN (**Figures 1.155** and **1.156**) has been associated with pregnancy, systemic infection (bacterial, viral, fungal, and protozoal), drugs (sulfonamides, bromides, oral contraceptives, phenytoin), malignancies (Hodgkin disease, non-Hodgkin lymphoma, leukemia, sarcoma, renal carcinoma), and other inflammatory disorders such as sarcoidosis, inflammatory bowel disease, polyarteritis nodosa, Sweet syndrome, and Behcet syndrome. Other systemic conditions that present with panniculitis from systemic disease include pancreatic panniculitis, α-1-antitrypsin-deficiency panniculitis, lupus panniculitis (**Figures 1.157** and **1.158**), subcutaneous panniculitis-like T-cell lymphoma, and lipodermatosclerosis (**Figure 1.159**) from chronic venous insufficiency and early calciphylaxis.

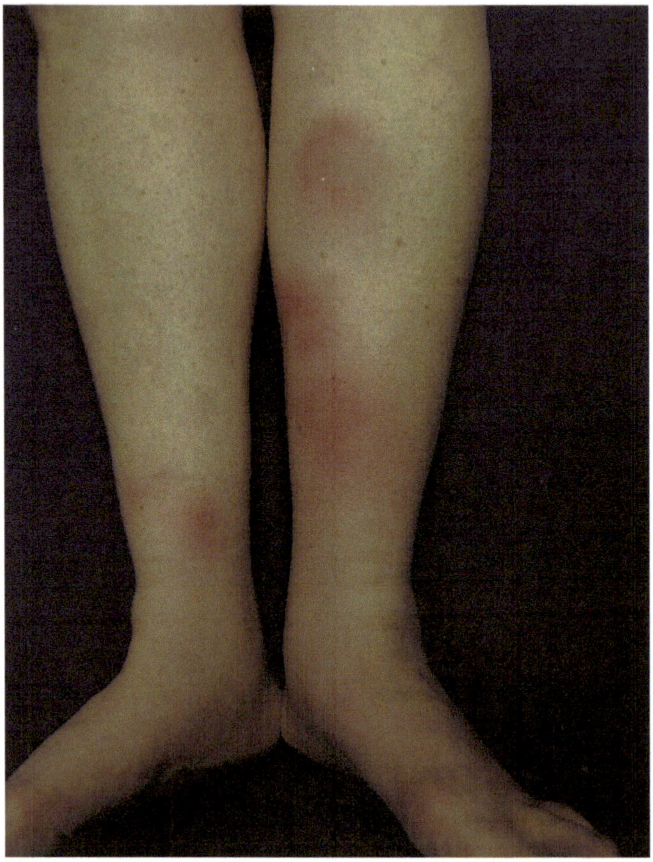

FIGURE 1.155 Panniculitis: Erythema nodosum (sarcoidosis).

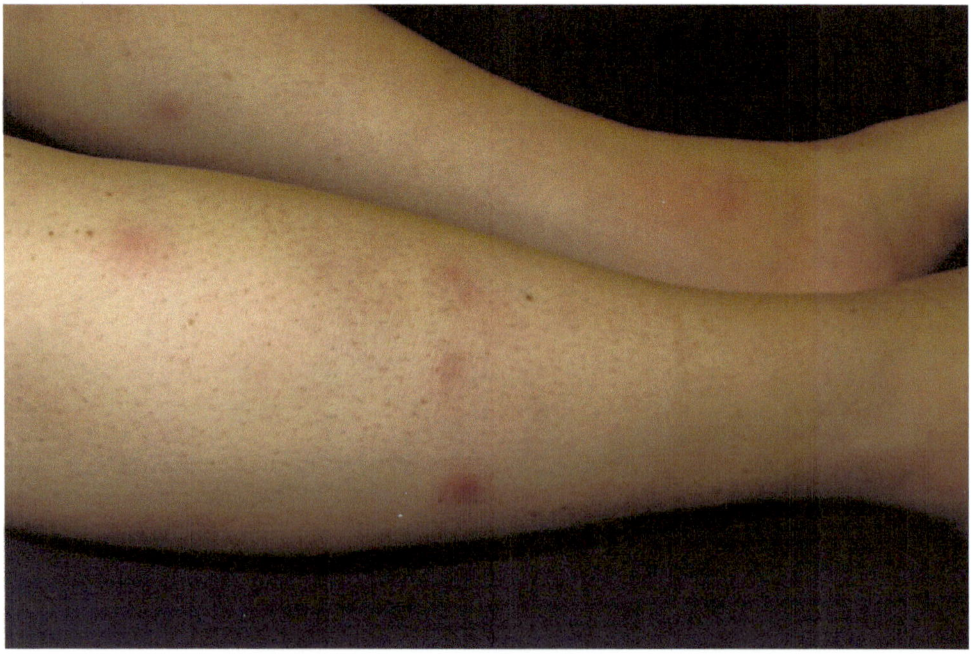

FIGURE 1.156 Panniculitis: Erythema nodosum (Crohn's disease).

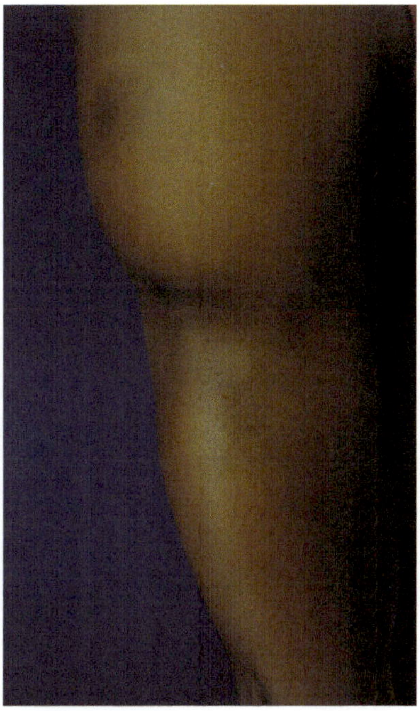

FIGURE 1.157 Panniculitis: Lupus panniculitis.

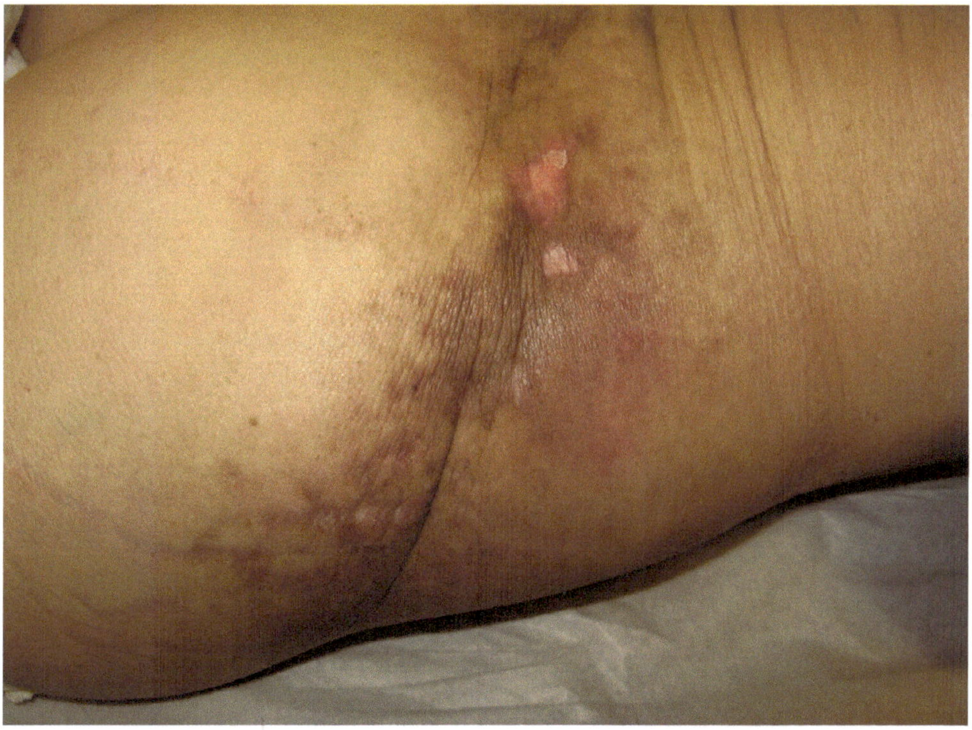

FIGURE 1.158 Panniculitis: Lupus panniculitis (profundus).

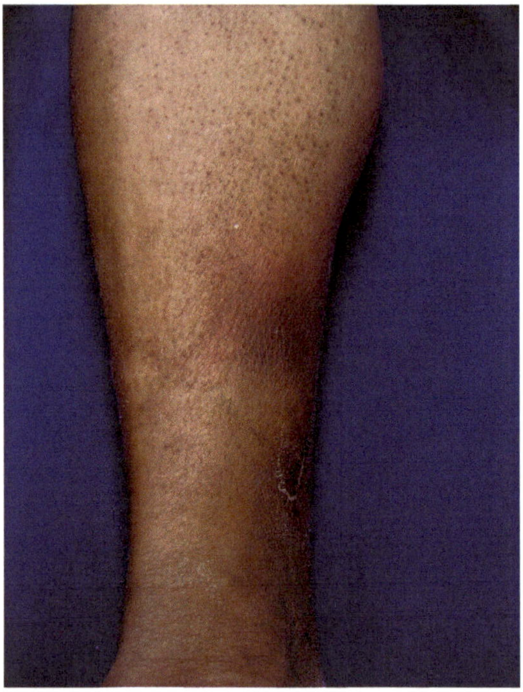

FIGURE 1.159 Panniculitis: Lipodermatosclerosis.

Evaluation and Management

While awaiting histologic confirmation of a primary panniculitis, laboratory testing may include serum or urine HCG, cultures (throat, blood, urine, tissue), CBC, LFTs, RFTs, UA, C3/4, ANAs, ANCAs, and ESR. Radiographic analysis with CXR is indicated. If lesions are ulcerated with oily discharge, testing for pancreatic enzymes (lipase, amylase) and serum α1-antitrypsin would be prudent. Treatment for most panniculitides is aimed at treating the underlying disorder. EN typically regresses spontaneously after several weeks. Supportive care, including NSAIDs, rest, compression garments, and elevation of the legs, is often adequate. Other treatment options include a saturated solution of potassium iodide (SSKI) and systemic corticosteroids when severe, once infection has been ruled out.

TABLE 1.17

Panniculitis by Etiology

	Disease	Histopathologic Features
Inflammatory	Erythema nodosum	Septal panniculitis
	Erythema induratum	Mixed septal/lobular panniculitis with caseous necrosis
	Lupus panniculitis	Lobular panniculitis with hyaline necrosis of fat lobules
	Polyarteritis nodosum	Medium-sized vessel vasculitis
	Lipodermatosclerosis	Lipomembranous change with mid-lobular ischemic necrosis
	subcutaneous panniculitis-like T-cell lymphoma	Mixed septal/lobular panniculitis with bean bag cells and atypical lymphocytes
Enzymatic destruction	Pancreatic panniculitis	Lobular panniculitis with ghost cells (saponification of fat)
	Alpha-1-antitrypsin deficiency panniculitis	Liquefactive necrosis of fat lobules

BIBLIOGRAPHY

Seguí M, Rodríguez-Jiménez P, Fraga J, et al. Pancreatic panniculitis revisited: A series of 34 patients. J Cutan Pathol 2023;50(11):983–990.

Wick MR. Panniculitis: A summary. Semin Diagn Pathol 2017;34(3):261–272.

Pruritus

Etiopathogenesis

Chronic pruritus is defined as pruritus lasting more than 6 weeks and can be caused by several different conditions. Generally speaking, pruritus is grouped into several categories: dermatologic, systemic, neuropathic, psychogenic, medications, and idiopathic, although some overlap exists in many cases. Itch can be localized or widespread and is believed to be transmitted via C nerve fibers that ascend the contralateral spinal cord and end in sensory cortex the brain. The precise stimuli that activate these fibers can be peripherally or centrally located and likely differ depending on the underlying condition. Histamine, substance P, and interleukin 4,13, 31 (among others) have been reported as mediators of pruritus.

Clinical Manifestations

The clinical presentation of the itchy patient varies. Some patients have no skin lesions, even while complaining of severe pruritus. Changes in the skin induced by scratching can include excoriations, prurigo nodules, lichenification, and hyperpigmentation from amyloid deposition. If the pruritus is not due to an underlying skin condition (dermatographism [**Figure 1.160**], scabies, dermatitis), evaluation for systemic associations is needed.

Systemic Manifestations

Pruritus can be the first sign of systemic disease. Systemic causes of pruritus that have been reported in the literature include lymphoproliferative malignancies, liver diseases, renal failure (**Figure 1.161**), iron deficiency anemia (**Figure 1.162**), thyroid disease, and infection (hepatitis C, HIV). Some cases of localized pruritus, such as notalgia paresthetica or brachioradial pruritus, are believed to be caused by nerve compression secondary to spinal disease or muscle fiber compression and are discussed in the Dysesthesia section. Psychologic itch can be caused by depression, anxiety, stress, or delusion of parasitosis (DoP). DoP is when patients believe they have "bugs" in their skin causing the itch. They often present with the matchbox sign (**Figure 1.163**) of bits of dried-blood-crusted skin that the patient believes are the insects they have removed from their skin.

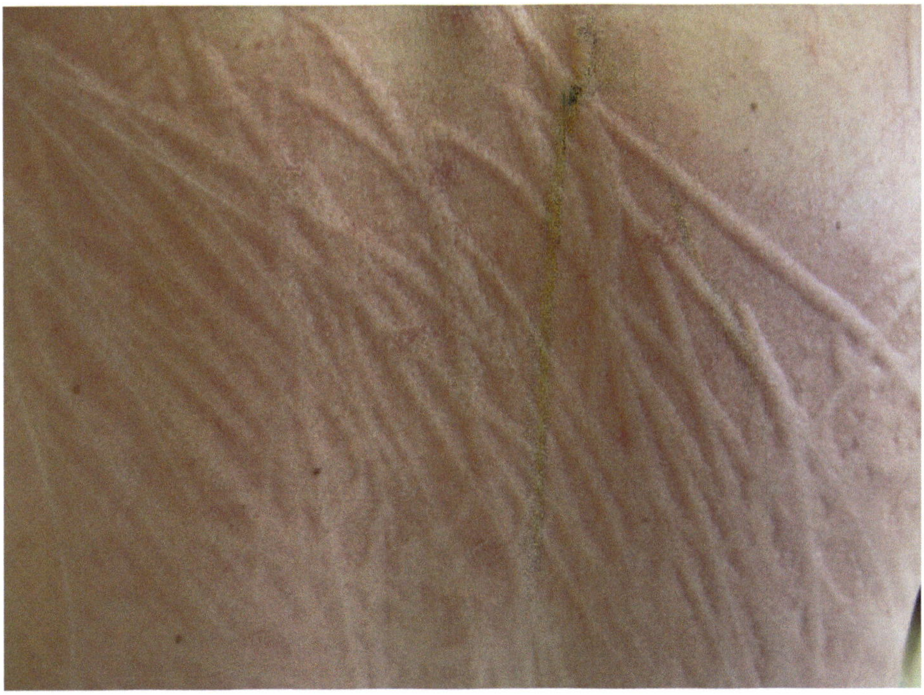

FIGURE 1.160 Pruritus: Dermatographism.

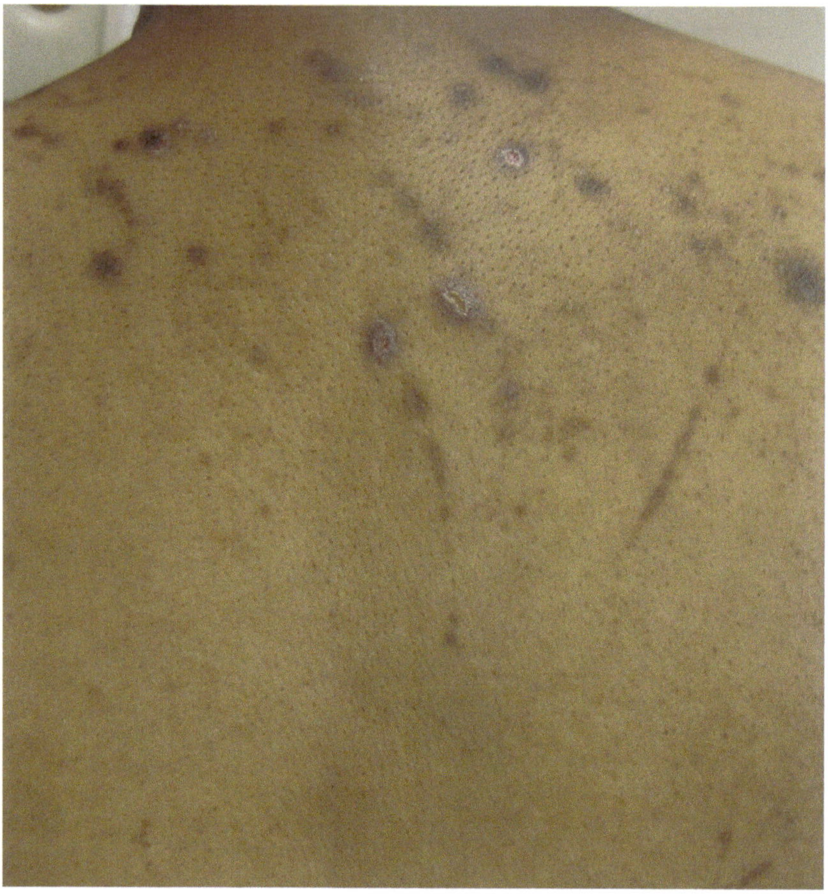

FIGURE 1.161 Pruritus: Renal insufficiency (with prurigo nodules).

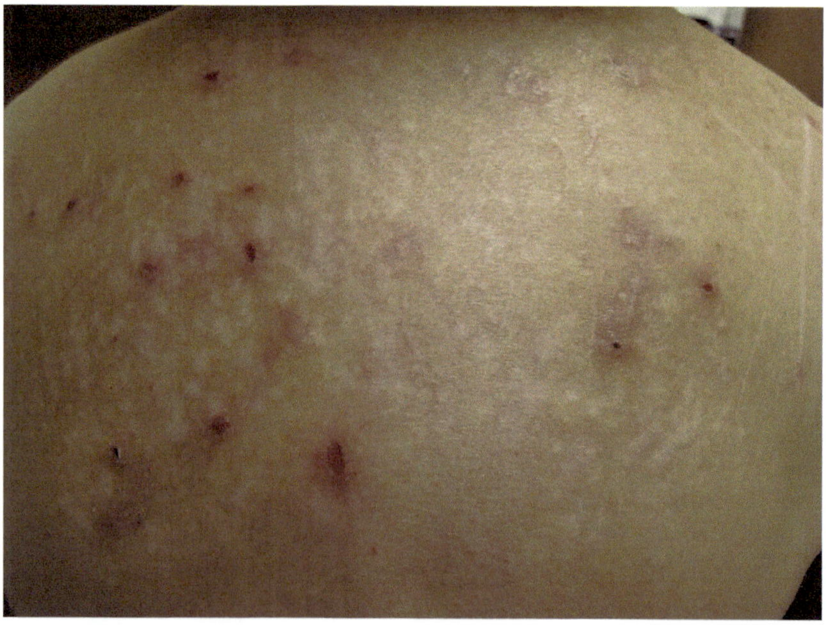

FIGURE 1.162 Pruritus: Iron deficiency anemia.

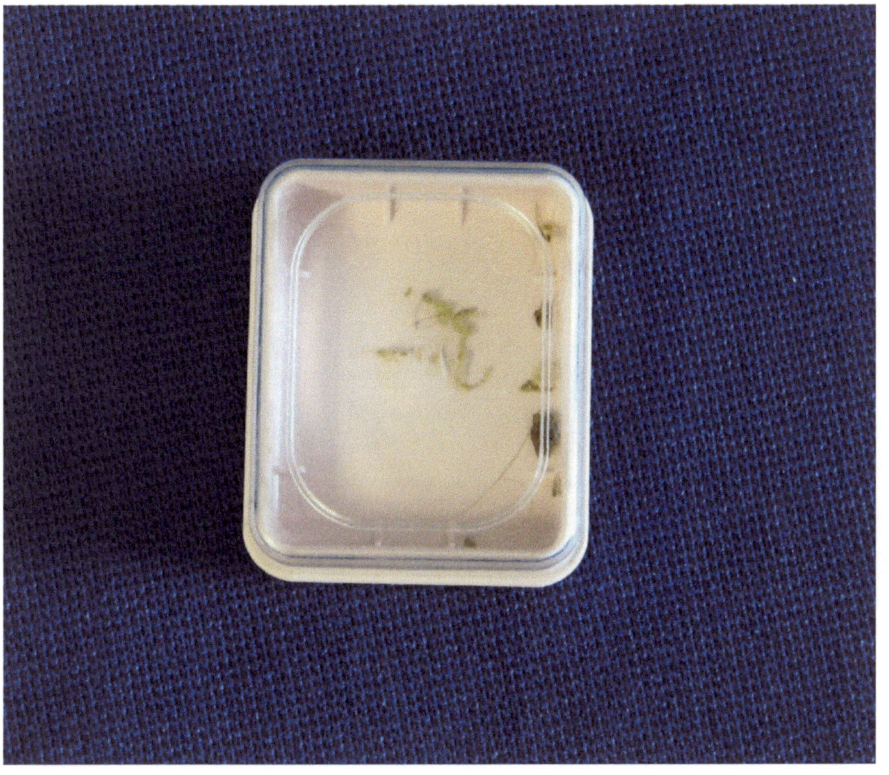

FIGURE 1.163 Pruritus: Matchbox sign (delusions of parasitosis).

Evaluation and Management

The management of the itchy patient is challenging (**Table 1.18**). History should focus on any symptoms (weight loss, night sweats) that may be related to an underlying condition or recent medication use (e.g., opiates for pain). A physical exam should be performed, looking for signs of underlying diseases (e.g., jaundice in liver disease). Evaluation for scabies and dermatographism should be performed in all patients. A reasonable initial workup is summarized in **Table 1.19**. In many instances, no systemic disease is present, and patients benefit from conservative therapies such as aggressive moisturization, minimizing irritants such as hot water and harsh soaps, and humidification of the environment. Topical therapies such as pramoxine, capsaicin, and menthol can be recommended. If inflammation is present, topical corticosteroids can be beneficial. Systemic therapies for treatment-resistant itch include antihistamines, gabapentin, opioid antagonists, ondansetron, and aprepitant. Biologic medications targeting particular cytokines have proven to be effective therapies for patients with prurigo nodularis. These include dupilumab (anti-IL-4/13) and nemolizumab (anti-IL 31); antipsychotic agents risperidone, olanzapine, and pimozide are treatments for DoP.

TABLE 1.18

Differential Diagnosis of Pruritus

Pruritus Subtype	Associated Conditions
Dermatologic	Atopic dermatitis, psoriasis, urticaria, dermatitis herpetiformis, xerosis, scabies, dermatographism
Systemic	Renal disease, liver disease, lymphoproliferative disease, diabetes, thyroid and parathyroid disease, iron deficiency anemia, HIV, viral hepatitis.
Neuropathic	Notalgia paresthetica, brachioradial pruritus, multiple sclerosis, brain tumors
Psychogenic	Stress, anxiety, delusional and eating disorders
Medications	Opioids, heparin, calcium channel blockers, ACE inhibitors
Idiopathic	Itch without any associated systemic, dermatologic, psychogenic factors

TABLE 1.19

Evaluation of Pruritus

Labs
• Complete blood count with platelets and differential
• Iron panel with ferritin
• Thyroid function tests
• Liver function tests
• Renal function tests
• Hepatitis B&C
• HIV
• Serum protein electrophoresis/Serum immunofixation/Serum free light chains and 24-h urine protein electrophoresis/Urine immunofixation (if >60 years).
Imaging
• CXR
• Pan-CT scans

BIBLIOGRAPHY

Butler D, Berger T, Elmariah S, et al. Chronic pruritus: A review. JAMA 2024;331(24):2114–2124.

Ständer S, Yosipovitch G, Legat FJ, et al. Trial of nemolizumab in moderate-to-severe prurigo nodularis. N Engl J Med 2020;382(8):706–716.

Stander S, Zeidler C, Augustin M, et al. S2k guideline: Diagnosis and treatment of chronic pruritus. J Dtsch Dermatol Ges 2022;20(10):1387–1402.

Yosipovitch G, Mollanazar N, Ständer S, et al. Dupilumab in patients with prurigo nodularis: Two randomized, double-blind, placebo-controlled phase 3 trials. Nat Med 2023;29(5):1180–1190.

Purpura

Etiopathogenesis

Purpura is the extravasation of red blood cells into the skin. The etiology is based on histologic findings: noninflammatory purpura without microvascular occlusion, noninflammatory purpura with microvascular occlusion, and inflammatory purpura (neutrophilic, lymphocytic, or necrotizing granulomatous infiltrates).

Clinical Manifestations

Purpura (**Figure 1.164**) presents as 5- to 20-mm, non-blanchable, violaceous to purple lesions. Depending on the underlying cause, lesions can be macular or papular with linear, circular, annular, or retiform patterns and may cause vesiculation or necrosis. If purpuric lesions are less than 5 mm, it is referred to as petechiae, and if greater than 20 mm, the term *ecchymosis* may be applied. Lesions may be localized to extremities, but based on underlying disease, may affect any part of the body (ears, face, abdomen). Branching (retiform) can correlate with microvascular occlusion and medium-sized vessel vasculitis. Non-branching dependent purpura favors small vessel vasculitis. Skin biopsy is required to distinguish.

Systemic Manifestations

Systemic diseases associated with cutaneous purpura range from benign to life-threatening. Clinical pathologic correlation includes noninflammatory purpura without microvascular occlusion (scurvy, amyloidosis [**Figure 1.165**], thrombocytopenia); noninflammatory purpura with microvascular occlusion (disseminate intravascular coagulation [**Figure 1.166**] **Table 1.20**, thrombotic thrombocytopenic purpura, type I cryoglobulinemia [**Figure 1.167**], antiphospholipid antibody syndrome [**Figures 1.168** and **1.169**], calciphylaxis, bacterial endocarditis, cholesterol emboli [**Figure 1.170**], and drugs such as coumadin necrosis, and heparin-induced thrombotic thrombocytopenia, and cocaine-induced),; neutrophilic inflammatory purpura (autoimmune disorders such as lupus, Sjögren syndrome, rheumatoid arthritis, scleroderma, IgA vasculitis [**Figure 1.171**], infection from hepatitis C-induced type II cryoglobulinemia, malignancy [lymphoproliferative types but solid malignancies for IgA vasculitis if >60 years]); lymphocytic inflammatory purpura (viral or drug-induced), necrotizing granulomatous purpura or ANCA-associated (polyarteritis nodosa, microscopic polyangiitis, GPA, eosinophilic GPA), and drugs.

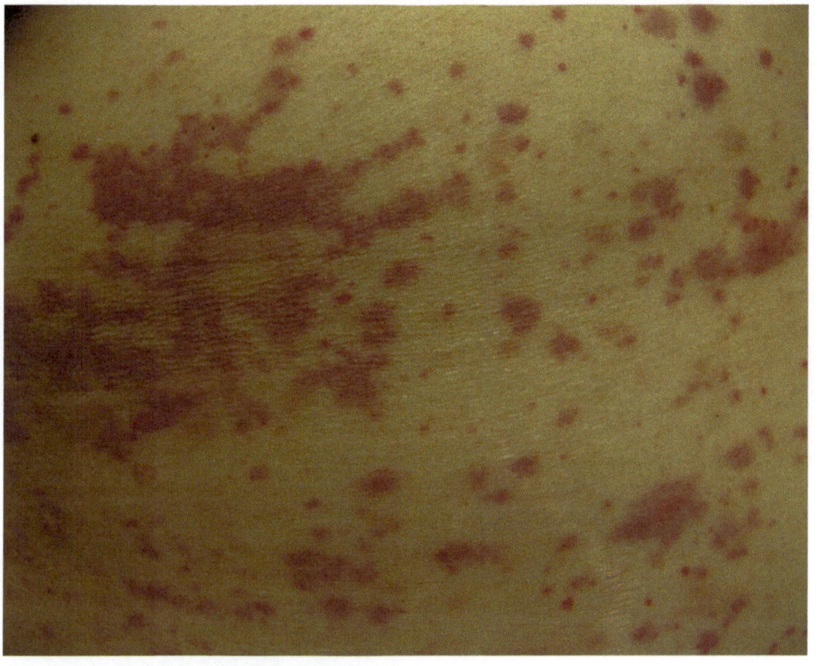

FIGURE 1.164 Purpura.

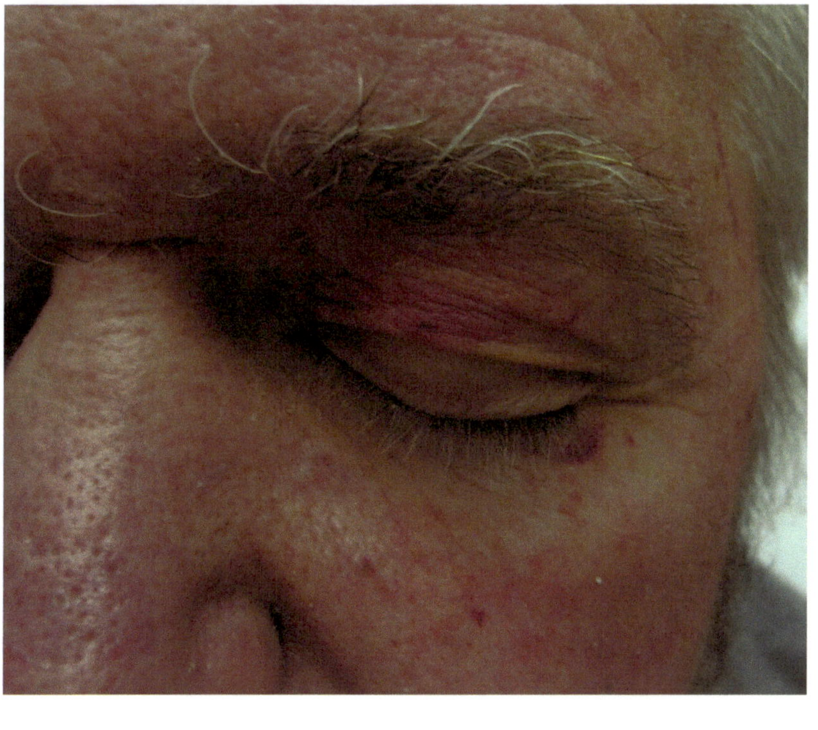

FIGURE 1.165 Noninflammatory purpura without vascular occlusion: Amyloidosis.

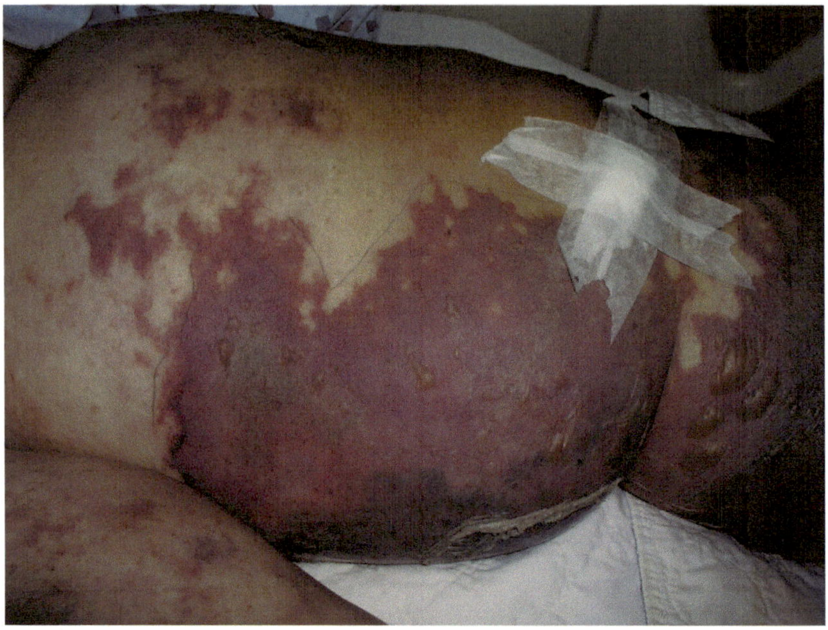

FIGURE 1.166 Noninflammatory purpura with microvascular occlusion: Infectious purpura fulminans.

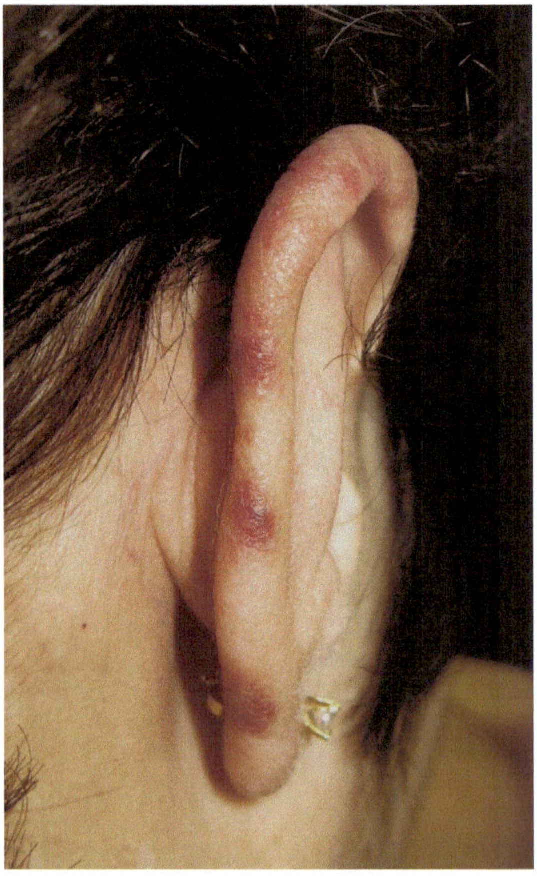

FIGURE 1.167 Noninflammatory purpura with microvascular occlusion: Type I monoclonal cryoglobulinemia.

TABLE 1.20

Laboratory Evaluation for Disseminated Intravascular Coagulation

Labs	Results
• Platelets	Decreased
• PT/PTT	Increased
• Fibrin D-Dimer	Increased*
• Protein C	Decreased
• Protein S	Decreased
• Anti-thrombin III	Decreased
• Fibrinogen	Decreased

Note: *Normal Fibrin D-Dimer levels have a high negative predictive value.

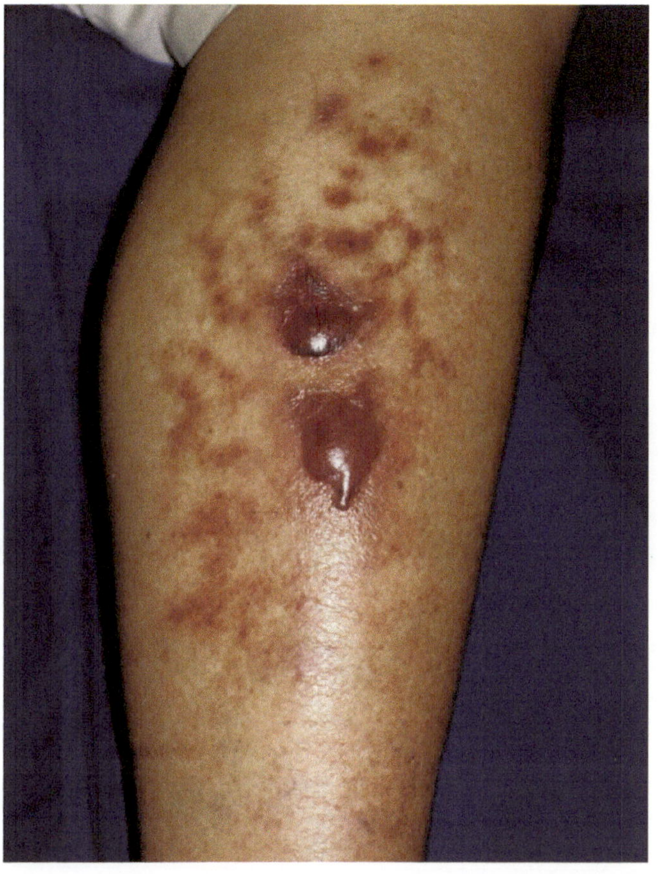

FIGURE 1.168 Noninflammatory purpura with microvascular occlusion: Antiphospholipid antibody syndrome.

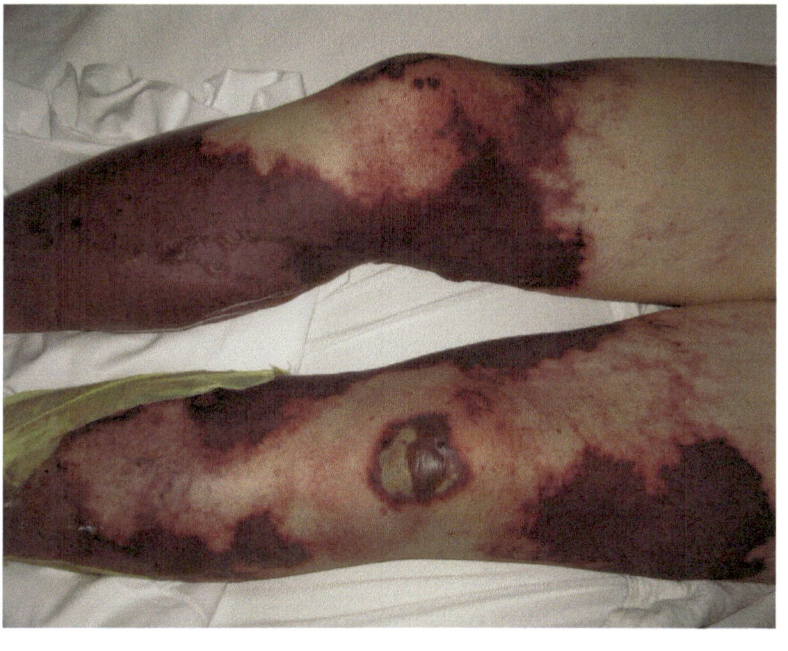

FIGURE 1.169 Noninflammatory purpura with microvascular occlusion: Catastrophic antiphospholipid antibody syndrome.

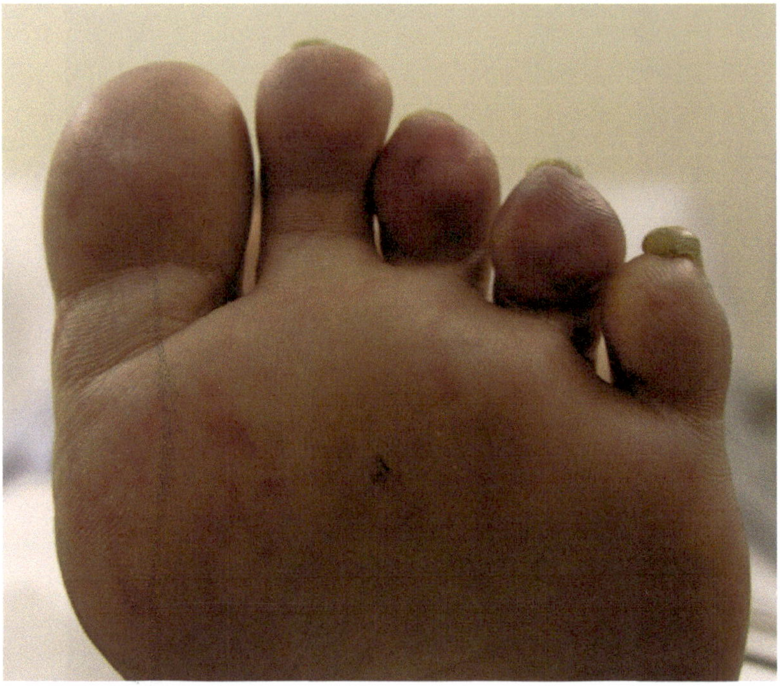

FIGURE 1.170 Noninflammatory purpura with microvascular occlusion: Cholesterol emboli.

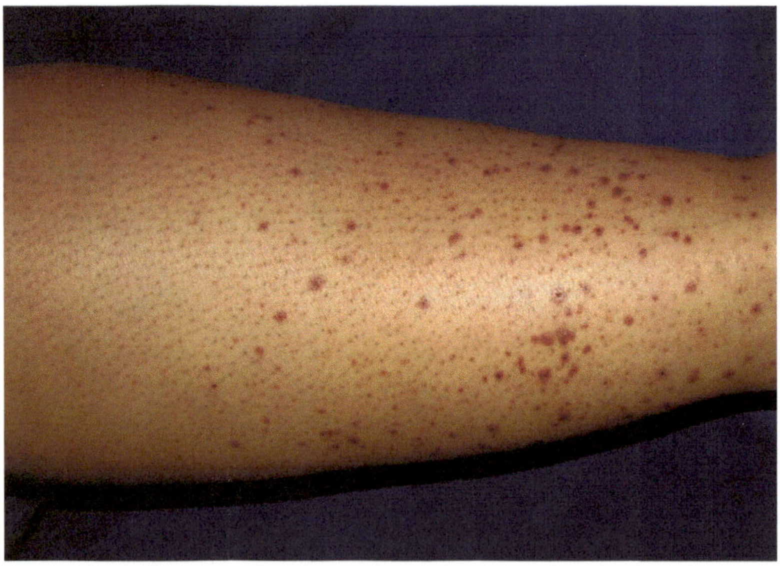

FIGURE 1.171 Inflammatory purpura: IgA vasculitis.

Evaluation and Management

An in-depth history, review of systems, and physical exam are prudent to look for coexisting signs/symptoms in the lung, heart, kidneys, and GI tract as well as the nervous system and musculoskeletal systems. Once again, the first essential diagnostic step is performing a biopsy of active lesions for histology as well as direct immunofluorescence. Investigative tests may include CBC, LFTs, RFTs, UA, PT/PTT, LAC, APLAs, Proteins C and S, antithrombin III, gene mutations (factor V, prothrombin, methylenetetrahydrofolate reductase [MTHFR]), platelet factor 4, ADAMTS13 d-Dimer, fibrinogen, ANAs, Ro/LA, rheumatoid factor (RF), Scl-70, ACAs, SPEP/SIFE, UPEP/UIFE, ANCAs, ESR, CRP, CPK, C3/4, vitamin C, Hep B, Hep C, CRYO, CXR, and CT. Treatment depends on the underlying etiology and may range from oral glucocorticoids to plasmapheresis.

BIBLIOGRAPHY

Gelhausen JR, Wetter DA, Nelson C, et al. A detailed analysis of the distribution, morphology and histopathology of complex purpura in hospitalized patients: A case series of 68 patients. J Am Acad Dermatol 2021;84(4):1188–1196.

Georgesen C, Fox LP, Harp J. Retiform purpura: A diagnostic approach. J Am Acad Dermatol 2020a;82(4):783–796.

Georgesen C, Fox LP, Harp J. Retiform purpura: Work-up and therapeutic considerations in select conditions. J Am Acad Dermatol 2020b;82(4):799–816.

Thornsberry LA, Losicco KI, English JC III. The skin and hypercoagulable state. J Am Acad Dermatol 2013;69:450–462.

Telangiectasia

Etiopathogenesis

Telangiectasias are abnormal, enlarged, dilated superficial cutaneous postcapillary venules. The etiology of these aberrant blood vessels is largely unknown. Because of their association with inflammatory diseases, they may be by-products of various produced growth factors. A genetic defect in genes encoding the receptor ligands of the TGF-β/bone morphogenic protein superfamily has been associated with vascular malformations in hereditary hemorrhagic telangiectasia.

Clinical Manifestations

Telangiectasias may present as individual lesions or mats. Lesions may present unilaterally or in a generalized distribution. Telangiectasias associated with atrophy, scarring, and varied macular pigmentation are referred to as poikiloderma.

Systemic Manifestations

Primary generalized essential telangiectasia (GET) may be idiopathic or familial (**Figure 1.172**). Secondary GET may be due to underlying autoimmunity (dermatomyositis [**Figure 1.173**]) or liver disease. Poikilodermatous GET is concerning for dermatomyositis (**Figure 1.174**) and poikiloderma vasculare atrophicans can be seen due to cutaneous T-cell lymphoma (**Figure 1.175**). Unilateral nevoid telangiectasias are idiopathic, but may develop in increased estrogen states (pregnancy, liver disease). Telangiectatic mats of the face, chest, and palms have been associated with scleroderma (**Figure 1.176**), whereas isolated telangiectasia within skin lesions and nail fold capillaries (see the Onychodystrophy section) can be seen in lupus erythematosus, dermatomyositis, and scleroderma. A macular distribution of lesions associated with GI and bone symptoms may represent a form of systemic mastocytosis historically referred to as telangiectasia macularis eruptiva perstans (**Figures 1.177**). When telangiectasias are noticeable on the oral mucosa (lips, tongue, hard palate) in patients with epistaxis and pulmonary/liver vascular malformations, hereditary hemorrhagic telangiectasia should be considered (**Figure 1.178**).

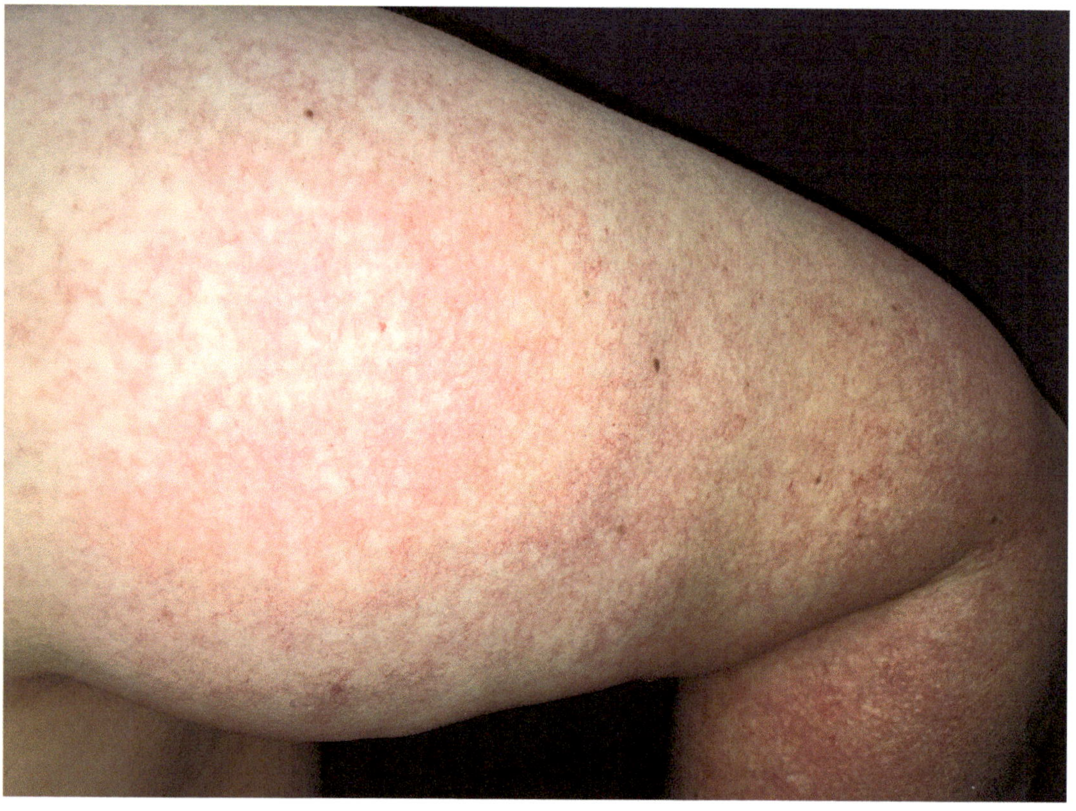

FIGURE 1.172 Primary generalized essential telangiectasias.

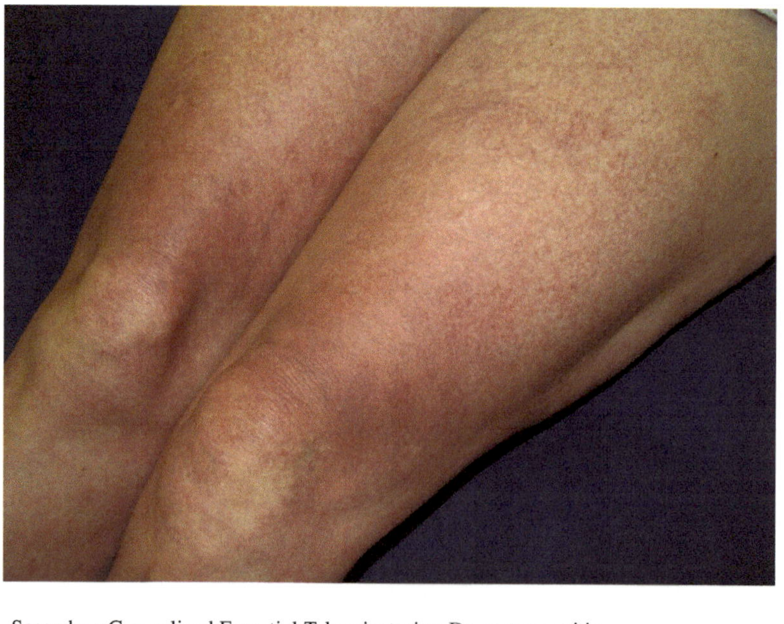

FIGURE 1.173 Secondary Generalized Essential Telangiectasias: Dermatomyositis.

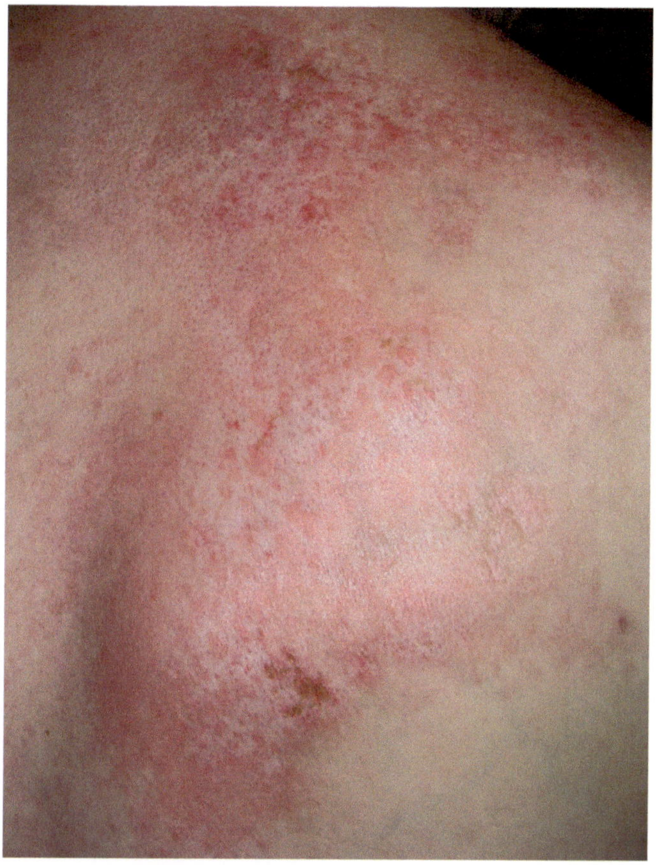

FIGURE 1.174 Poikiloderma: Dermatomyositis.

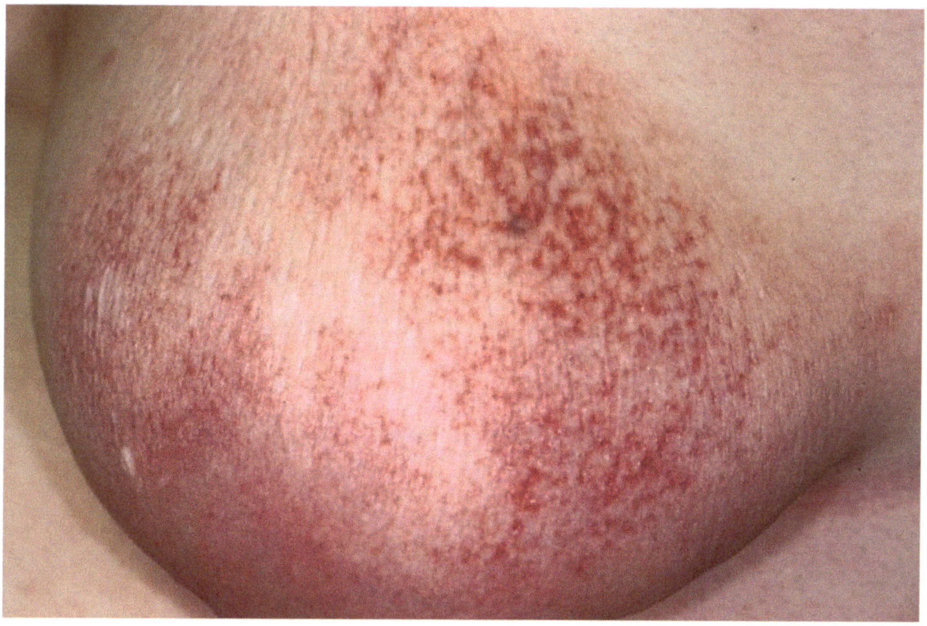

FIGURE 1.175 Poikiloderma atrophicans vasculare: Cutaneous T-cell lymphoma.

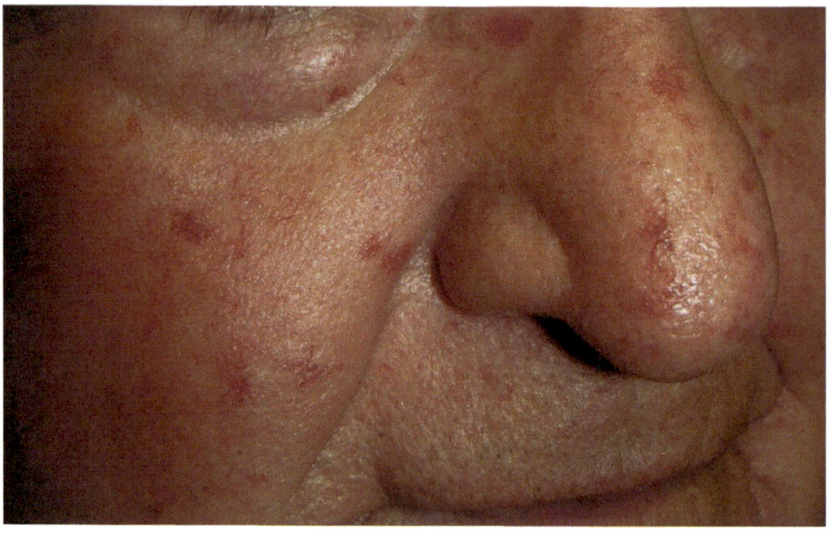

FIGURE 1.176 Telangiectatic mats: Scleroderma.

Evaluation and Management

A detailed history of the timing of lesions and associated systemic symptoms is indicated. The physical exam needs to focus on the distribution of the telangiectasias, with special attention to the oral mucosal and periungual skin. The skin exam should focus on other cutaneous signs of connective tissue disease or cutaneous lymphoma. Performing a skin biopsy is important to help differentiate whether lesions are aberrant blood vessels or have associated atypical lymphocytes, interface dermatitis, or increased mast cells. Evaluation parameters are summarized in **Table 1.21**. Treating the underlying disease may not resolve telangiectasia, so additional therapy such as pulse dye laser may be of benefit for those patients requesting removal.

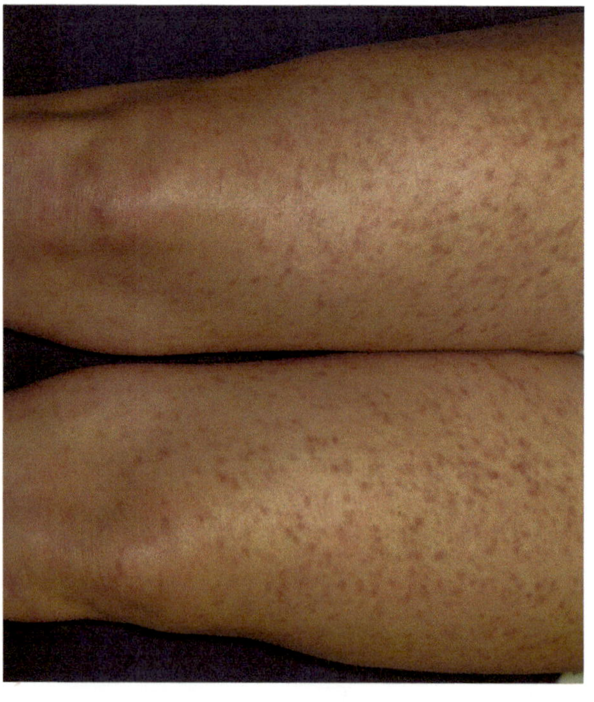

FIGURE 1.177 Cutaneous mastocytosis.

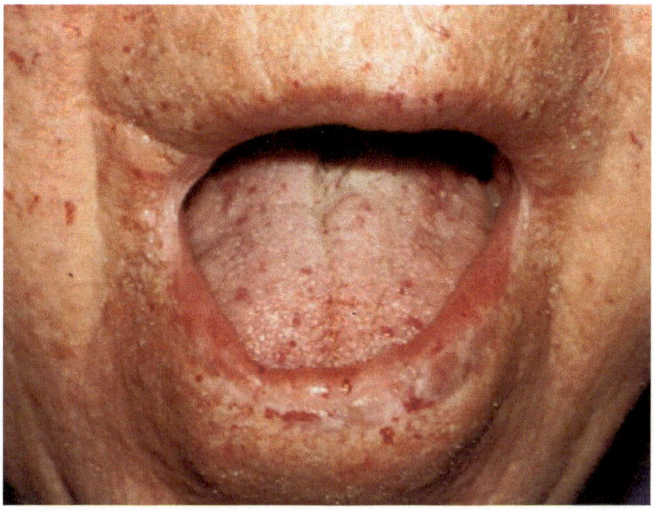

FIGURE 1.178 Hereditary hemorrhagic telangiectasia.

TABLE 1.21

Evaluation of Telangiectasia

Laboratory

- Complete blood count with platelets and differential
- Liver function tests
- Renal function tests
- Urinalysis
- Complement 3/4
- Antinuclear antibodies
- Anti-dsDNA antibodies
- Creatinine phosphokinase
- Aldolase
- Anti-centromere antibodies
- Anti-topoisomerase antibodies
- Serum tryptase
- Serum HCG and estrogen
- Hepatitis B/C
- HHT gene mutations (Endoglin and ACVRL1)

Radiographic

- CT and angiography will be contingent on the results of the above

BIBLIOGRAPHY

Hammill AM, Wusik K, Kasthuri RS. Hereditary hemorrhagic telangiectasia (HHT): A practical guide to management. Hematology Am Soc Hematol Educ Program 2021;2021(1):469–477.

Nofal A, Salah E. Acquired poikiloderma: Proposed classification and diagnostic approach. J AM Acad Dermatol 2013;69(3):e129-40.

Wiznia LE, Steuer AB, Penn LA, et al. Generalized essential telangiectasia. Dermatol Online J 2018;24(12):1030/qt2926z3f5.

Ulcers of Skin: Lower Extremities

Etiopathogenesis

Underlying arteriovenous disease or inflammatory conditions are often the cause of cutaneous ulceration of the lower leg in systemic disease. Venous insufficiency or arterial peripheral vascular disease with or without coexisting coagulopathies are the most common (85%). Atypical ulcerations (15%) are due to leukocytoclastic vasculitis, vasculopathy, hematologic disorders, infections, malignancy, trauma, or drug-induced or other inflammatory disorders. Several other ulcerating conditions, such as calciphylaxis, necrobiosis lipoidica, diabetic neurotrophic ulcers, and pyoderma gangrenosum, are discussed separately in Chapters 2, 5, 8, and 9.

Clinical Manifestations

Ulceration is defined as a full-thickness defect in the epidermis that can extend into or through the dermis. Peripheral edema and varicosities with ulceration suggest venous stasis (**Figure 1.179**), whereas ischemic ulcerations from arterial disease typically have jagged edges and a sharp cut-off appearance.

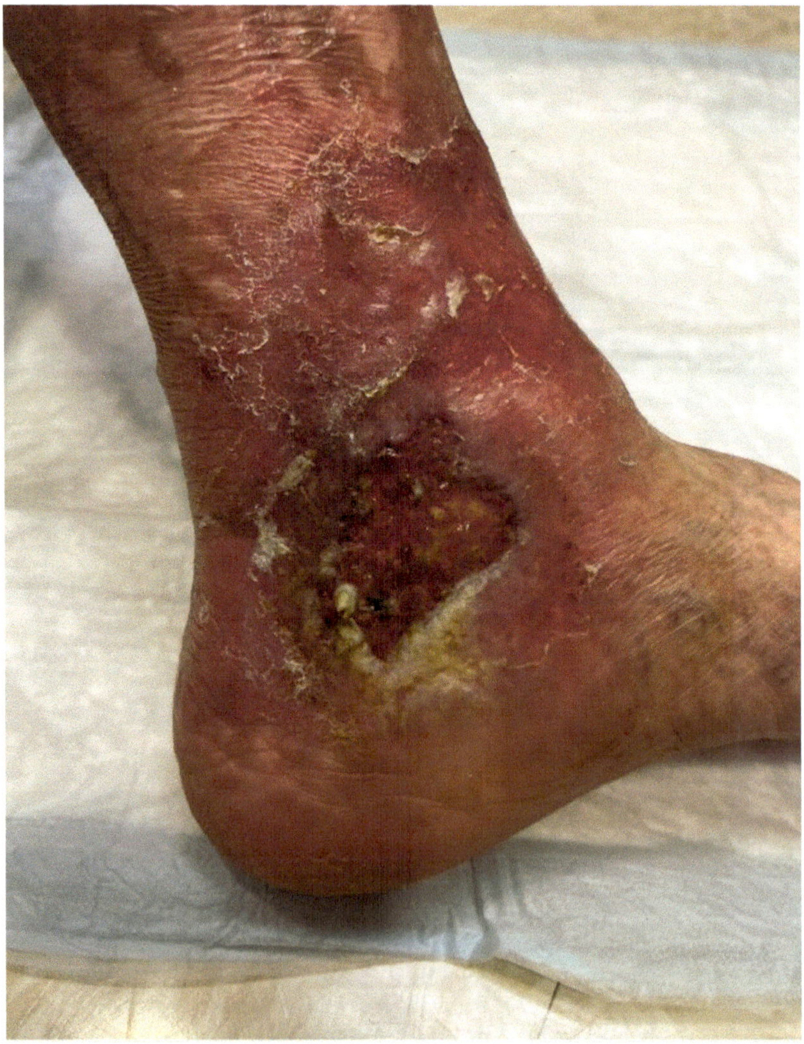

FIGURE 1.179 Venous stasis ulcer.

The white stellate scars of atrophie blanche (livedo vasculopathy) have been seen in ulcerations due to hypercoagulable states (**Figure 1.180**), whereas vasculitic ulcerations may present with purpura or be non-purpuric in nature (**Figures 1.181–1.183**). Associated findings may include pain, pallor, coolness, and purple papules with or without ulceration, which are known as pseudo-Kaposi sarcoma or acroangiodermatitis (**Figure 1.184**).

Systemic Manifestations

Venous insufficiency from deep venous varicosities may present with leg fatigue, swelling, and in some cases, recurrent thromboembolism. Arterial ulceration may be accompanied by symptoms or a history of claudication, exertional fatigue, or even angina. Autoimmune ulceration may include joint pain, fever, serositis, immunologic abnormality, neurologic abnormality, or photosensitivity. Hypercoagulable states such as the antiphospholipid antibody syndrome may present with chronic ulcerations of the extremities (**Figures 1.185**), stroke, venous and arterial thromboemboli, or recurrent fetal loss in women. Drugs used to treat systemic disease are also associated with ulceration (methotrexate, hydroxyurea).

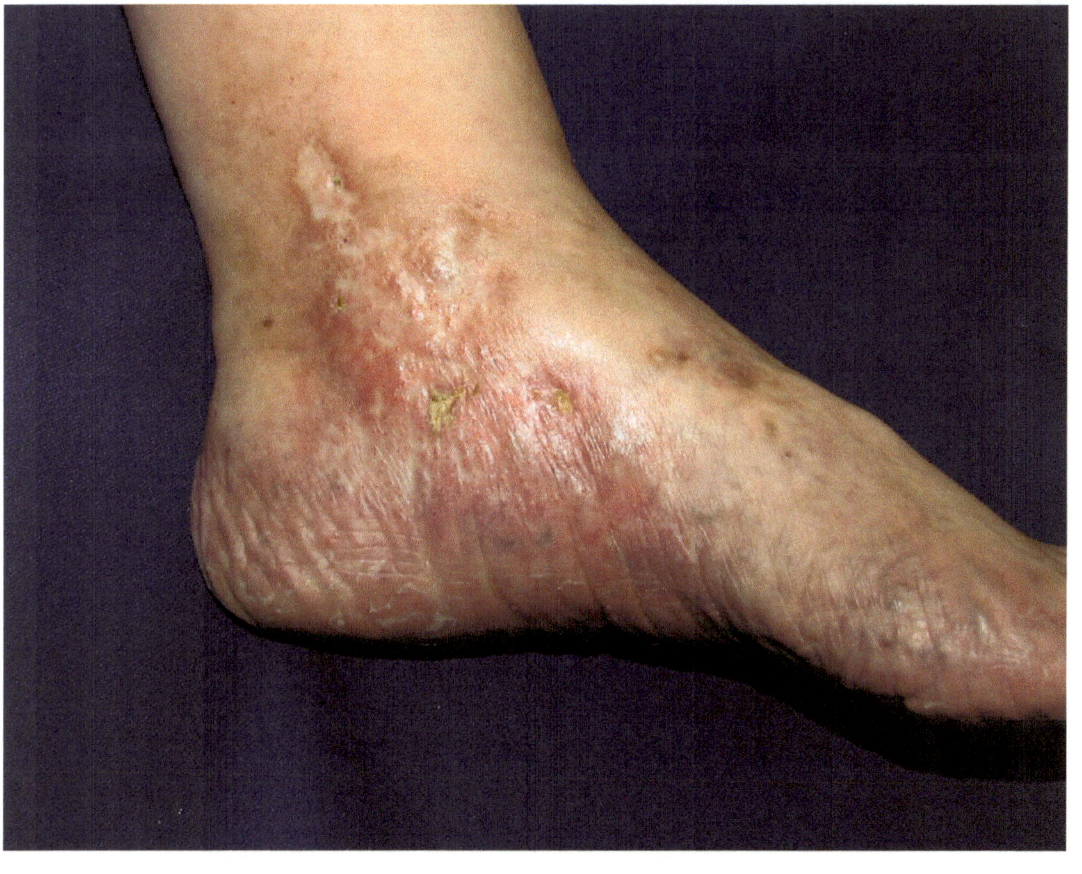

FIGURE 1.180 Atrophie blanche (livedo vasculopathy) with early venous ulceration.

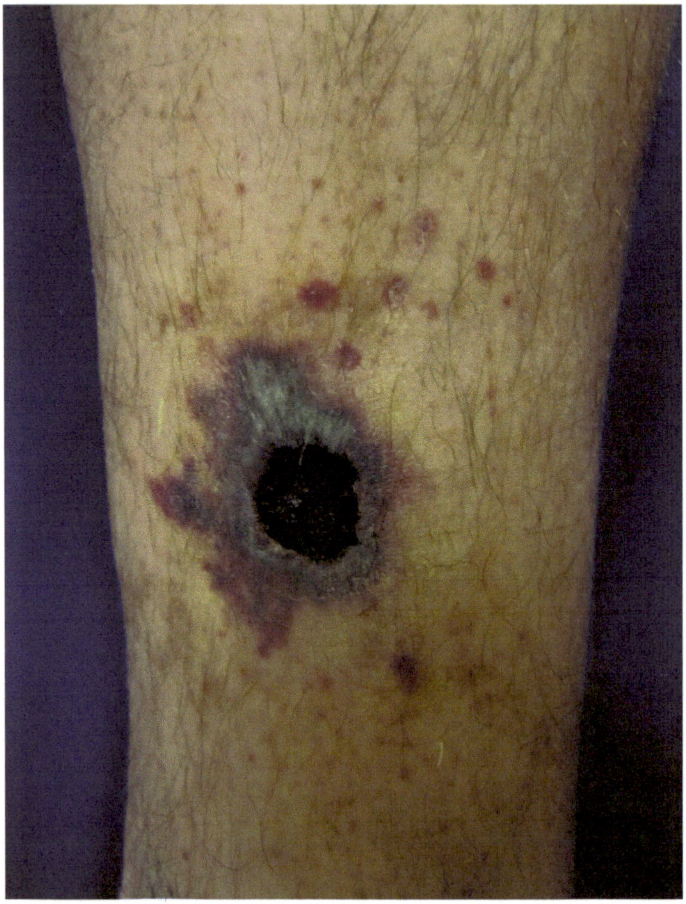

FIGURE 1.181 Vasculitic ulcer: Purpuric.

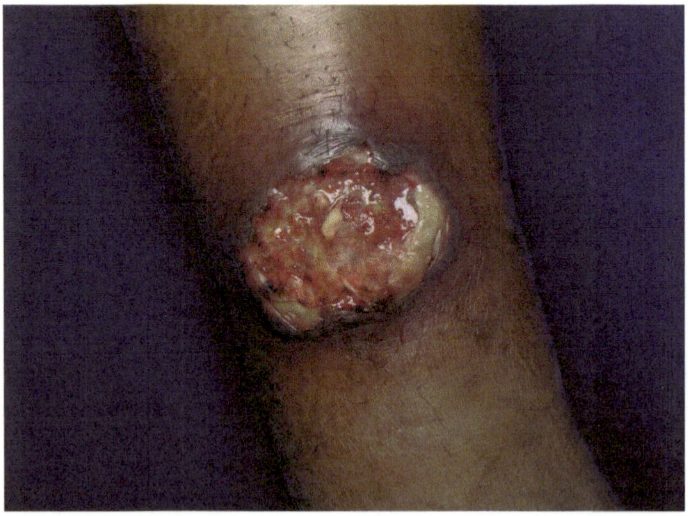

FIGURE 1.182 Vasculitic ulcer: Non-purpuric.

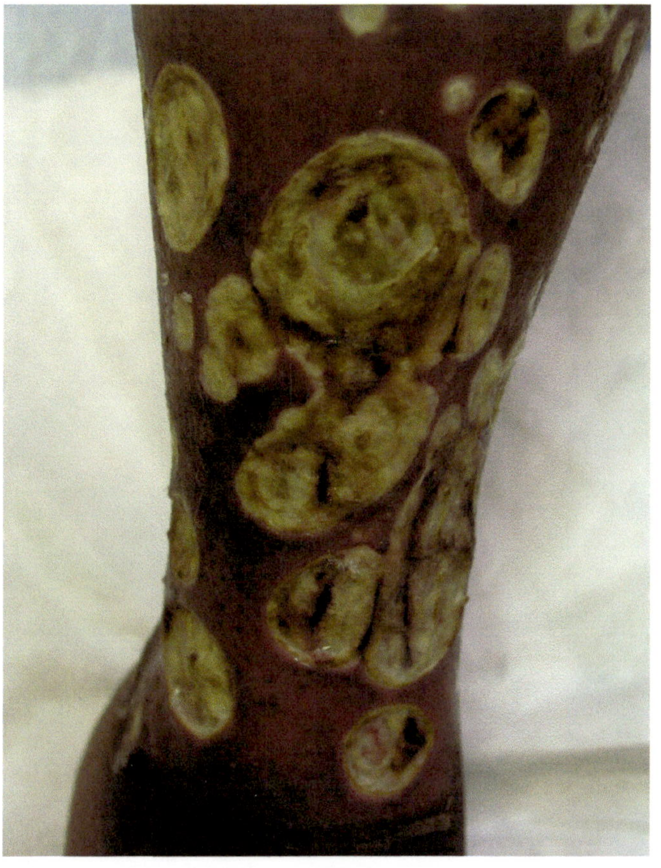

FIGURE 1.183 Vasculitic ulcer: Systemic lupus erythematosus.

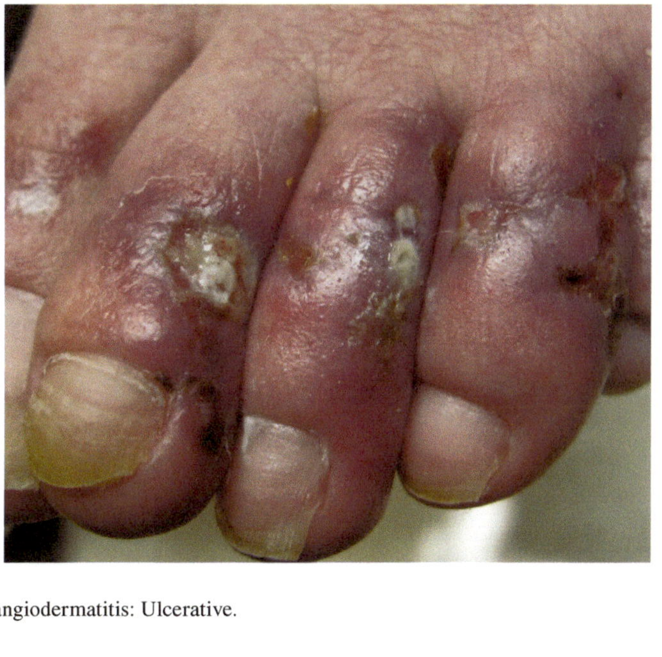

FIGURE 1.184 Acroangiodermatitis: Ulcerative.

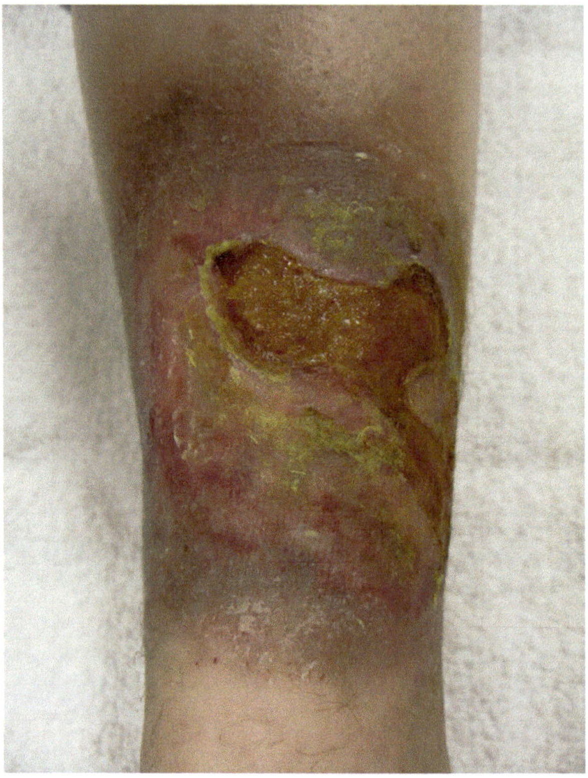

FIGURE 1.185 Chronic ulcer: Antiphospholipid antibody syndrome.

Evaluation and Management

A careful medical and drug history can help determine the cause of ulceration. The physical exam should include cardiac and vascular exams. A biopsy for histology and wound culture (to rule out an infectious cause) should be performed. Ancillary tests in the appropriate clinical settings, such as arterial or venous Doppler and Deep venous reflux studies, echocardiography, autoimmune serologic screening, and coagulopathy screening are also useful. Laboratory evaluation is summarized in **Table 1.22**. External compressive therapy or varicose vein ablation will be key for treatment of venous stasis ulceration. Arterial ulceration involves referral to vascular surgery for possible bypass or arterial grafting. Autoimmune disease treatment will typically involve chronic immunosuppression. If coagulopathy is present, chronic anticoagulation therapy may be needed.

TABLE 1.22

Leg Ulcer Evaluation

1. **Biopsy**
    - Histology of **active ulcer edge**
    - Bacterial, fungal and acid-fast bacillus (AFB)
2. **Autoimmunity**
    - Anti-nuclear antibody
    - Anti-dsDNA
    - Anti-smith antibody
    - Anti-centromere antibody
    - Anti-topoisomerase (Scl70)
    - Anti- ribonucleoprotein

(Continued)

TABLE 1.22 (*Continued*)

Leg Ulcer Evaluation

- Anti-SSA/B
- Rheumatoid factor
- Anti-cyclic citrullinated peptide
- Anti-neutrophilic cytoplasmic antibodies

3. **Prothrombotic states**
    - Factor V Leiden, prothrombin gene, and MTHFR mutations
    - Protein C/S
    - Anti-thrombin III
    - Lupus anticoagulant, anti-cardiolipin and beta2- glycoprotein antibodies
4. **Other**
    - Complete blood count with platelets and differential
    - Comprehensive metabolic panel
    - Urinalysis
    - HIV
    - Hepatitis B/C
    - Cryoglobulins
    - Chest X-ray

BIBLIOGRAPHY

Nickles MA, Tsoukas MM, Sweiss N, et al. Atypical ulcers: A stepwise approach for clinicians. Wounds 2022;34(10):236–244.

Schneider C, Stratman S, Kirsner R. Lower extremity ulcers. Med Clin North Am 2021;105:663–679.

Shanmugam VK, Angra D, Rahimi H, et al. Vasculitic and autoimmune wounds. J Vasc Surg Venous Lymphatic Disord 2017;5(2):280–292.

Thornsberry LA, LoSicco KI, English JC III. The skin and hypercoagulable states. J Am Acad Dermatol 2013;69(3):450–462.

Urticaria

Etiopathogenesis

Urticaria can be present in acute (<6 weeks) or chronic (>6 weeks) forms. The cellular mediator of all forms of urticaria is the mast cell. Upon degranulation, the mast cell releases mediators (histamine, leukotrienes, tryptase, chymase), which cause edema, inflammation, and itching. Acute urticaria can be caused by foods, infections, or medications. Chronic urticaria can be idiopathic, due to physical factors (**Table 1.23**; ultraviolet radiation [**Figure 1.186**]), or to an underlying autoimmune disorder (autoimmune thyroiditis, chronic autoimmune urticaria). Up to 30%–50% of patients with chronic autoimmune urticaria have antibodies to either a high-affinity immunoglobulin E (IgE) receptor on the mast cell or to IgE itself.

Clinical Manifestations

Urticaria (**Figure 1.187**) presents as pruritic, edematous, erythematous, nonscaling, minimally elevated plaques or wheals that vary in size from a few millimeters to several centimeters in diameter lasting less than 24 hours. Urticaria that burns instead of itches, lasts more than 24 hours, and resolves with petechia or purpura (**Figures 1.188** and **1.189**) may represent urticarial vasculitis (UV). Urticarial dermatitis (dermal hypersensitivity reaction) refers to an overlap of eczematoid dermatitis with a hive-like quality (**Figures 1.190** and **1.191**).

Systemic Manifestations

Acute urticaria can be associated with infections (*Streptococcus*, hepatitis, *Helicobacter pylori*). Photosensitivity produces solar urticaria, and cold urticaria can occur in patients with cryoglobulinemia. In patients with autoimmune urticaria, an association with thyroid autoimmunity, has been reported. Urticarial vasculitis may be normo- or hypocomplementemic in nature. Low complement with UV is often a forme fruste for developing SLE. Other associations are Sjögren syndrome and hepatitis C-induced cryoglobulinemia. Chronic urticaria, bone pain, hyperostosis, and immunoglobulin M (IgM) gammopathy is called Schnitzler syndrome. It has been reported to occur with a lymphoplasmacytic lymphoma in 10%–15% of cases. Dermal hypersensitivity reactions are associated with drug reactions, viral infections, and malignancy.

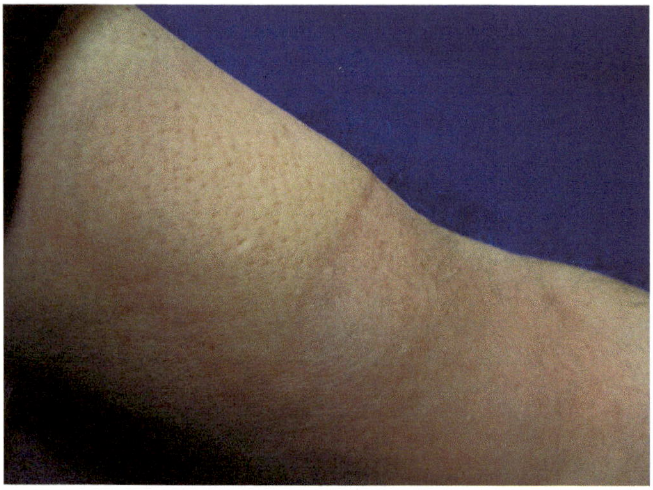

FIGURE 1.186 Solar urticaria.

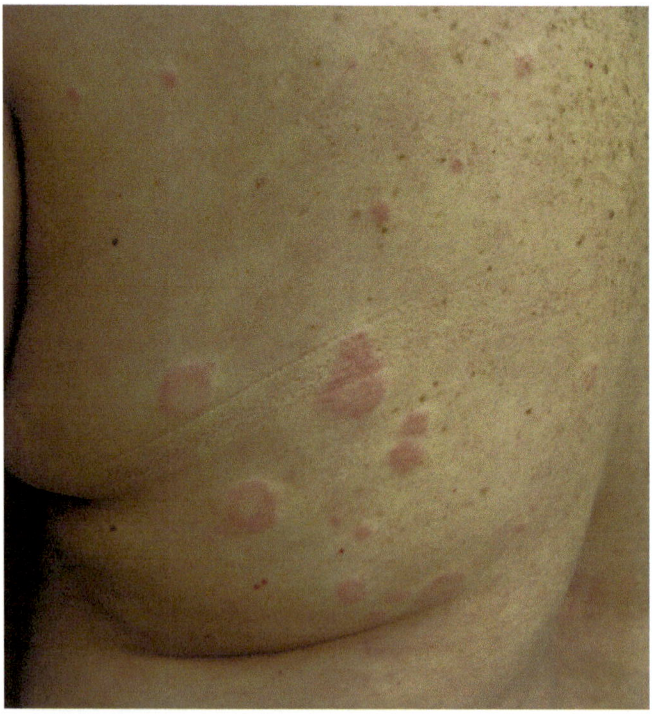

FIGURE 1.187 Chronic urticaria: Autoimmune thyroiditis.

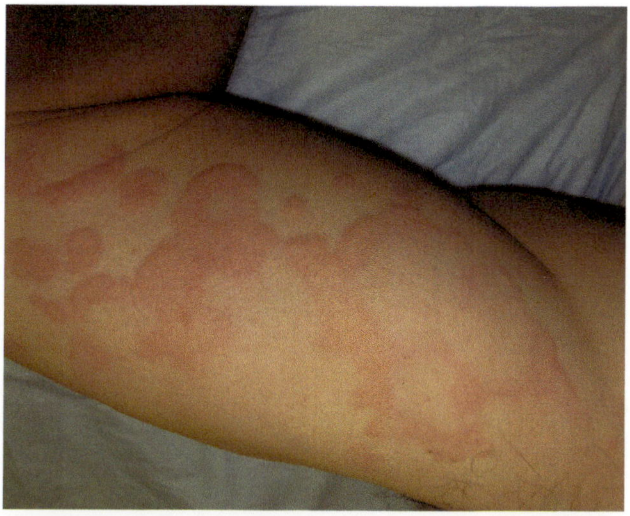

FIGURE 1.188 Urticarial vasculitis.

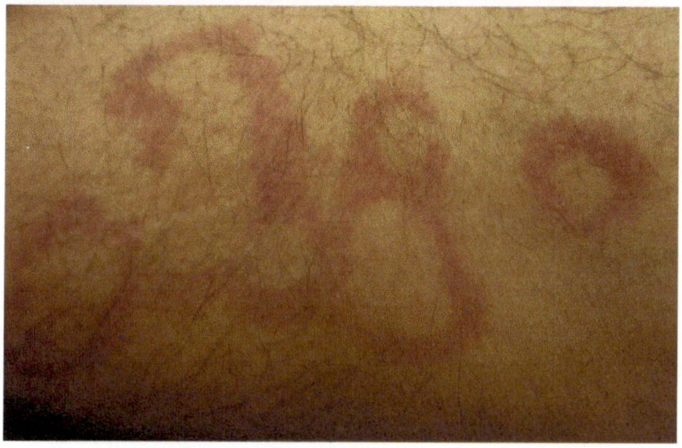

FIGURE 1.189 Urticarial vasculitis: Purpuric rings.

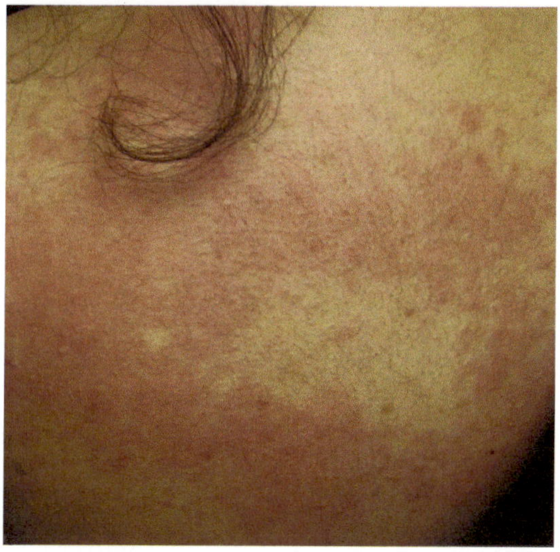

FIGURE 1.190 Dermal hypersensitivity reaction.

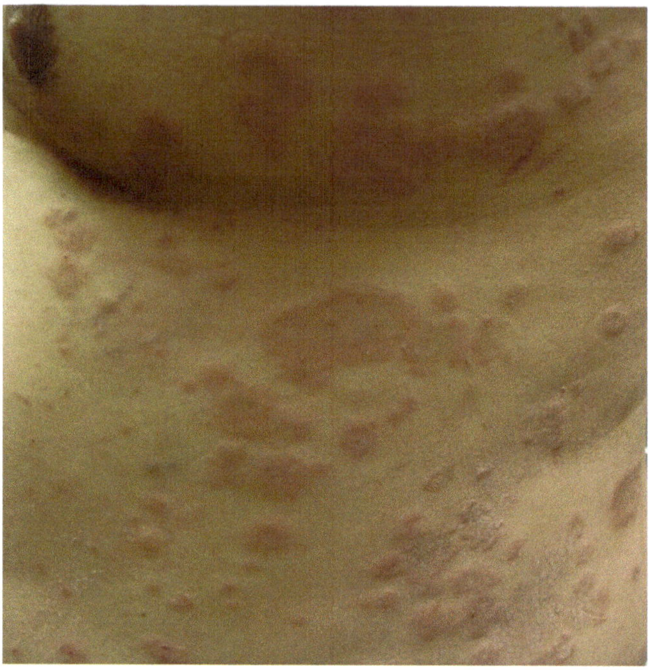

FIGURE 1.191 Dermal hypersensitivity reaction.

Evaluation and Management

In patients with acute urticaria, it is important to review recent illnesses, exposures to any recent foods, or medications. In chronic urticaria, provocative testing can be performed in the office, depending on the physical stimulus that is suspected. A chronic urticarial index (TPOs, TGs, and histamine-release assay) can be ordered to determine possible autoimmunity. If UV is suspected, a biopsy to look for evidence of leukocytoclastic vasculitis is needed. Laboratory evaluation consists of CBC, LFTs, RFTs, UA, C3/4, ANAs, Ro/La, Hep C, and CRYO, and a SPEP/SIFE and UPEP/UIFE should be obtained if Schnitzler syndrome is suspected. The first-line therapy for urticaria is treatment with antihistamines. First- or second-generation antihistamines are both effective. For UV and chronic urticaria that is unresponsive to these measures, immunosuppressive medications such as systemic corticosteroids, cyclosporine, mycophenolate mofetil, azathioprine, or omalizumab can be implemented.

TABLE 1.23

Physical Urticarias

Condition	History/Clinical Findings	Provocation Test
Symptomatic dermatographism	Itch often made worse with scratching, linear urticarial lesions	Wooden tip of cotton tipped applicator rubbed across skin
Delayed pressure urticaria	Appearance of wheals 4–6 hours following exposure	15lb weight applied to the skin or suspended by a strap on the skin for 15 minutes
Cold urticaria	Itching, wheals following exposure to cold	Apply ice cube in a bag to patient's forearm for 5–10 minutes
Heat urticaria	Itching, wheals following exposure to heat	Heat device or vial filled with warm water applied to the skin for 10 minutes
Solar urticaria	Wheals occurring within minutes of sun (or sometimes artificial light) exposure	UVA, UVB, visible light sources placed 10cm from patients back

(Continued)

TABLE 1.23 (*Continued*)

Physical Urticarias

Condition	History/Clinical Findings	Provocation Test
Aquagenic urticaria	Smaller 1–3mm wheals following exposure to water	Cloth soaked with room temperature water applied to the skin for 20–30 minutes
Vibratory urticaria	Localized angioedema, pruritus, wheals following exposure to vibratory stimuli	Vortex applied to forearm for 5 minutes, assess 10 minutes later
Cholinergic urticaria	Small 1–3mm wheals following exercise or with emotional stress	Exercise on treadmill or stationary bike for 15 minutes

BIBLIOGRAPHY

Bauer A, Dickel H, Jakob T, et al. Expert consensus on practical aspects in the treatment of chronic urticaria. Allergo J Int 2021;30(2):64–75.

He L, Yi W, Huang X, et al. Chronic urticaria: Advances in understanding of the disease and clinical management. Clin Rev Allergy Immunol 2021;61(3):424–448.

Zuberbier T, Bernstein JA, Maurer M. Chronic spontaneous urticaria guidelines: What is new? J Allergy Clin Immunol 2022;150(6):1249–1255. Erratum in: J Allergy Clin Immunol. 2023;151(2):580.

Xanthoderma

Etiopathogenesis

The term *xanthoderma* refers to the macular yellowish discoloration of skin. The most common causes of xanthoderma are jaundice, carotenemia, and lycopenemia. Jaundice can be differentiated clinically from carotenemia by the presence of yellowish discoloration of the conjunctiva and episclera (conjunctival icterus [**Figure 1.192**]), which will not occur in carotenemia. The pigmentation of the skin in jaundice is due to the presence of increased levels of bilirubin (either direct or indirect), while in carotenemia the pigmentation is due to increased levels of carotenoids in the lipid layer of the stratum corneum, which can be due to increased intake or impaired metabolism of carotenoids. Lycopene and carotene are chemical isomers. Lycopene is also lipophilic, which will cause carotenoderma with skin deposition.

Clinical Manifestations

Patients with xanthoderma have a diffuse discoloration of the skin. In patients with jaundice, yellowish discoloration will also be seen first on the oral mucous membranes (**Figures 1.193–1.195**) and the conjunctiva. Signs of associated liver disease such as spider angiomas may also be present (**Figure 1.196**). Significant pruritus may accompany jaundice in some patients. In carotenemia or lycopenemia, areas with thicker stratum corneum, such as the palms and soles (**Figures 1.197** and **1.198**), will have more prominent discoloration and are asymptomatic.

Systemic Manifestations

In patients with jaundice, patients may complain of fevers, weight loss, right upper quadrant pain, stool changes, or may be asymptomatic. The source of hyperbilirubinemia may be hepatocellular (viral hepatitis, autoimmune hepatitis, alcohol), cholestatic (viral hepatitis, primary biliary cirrhosis, malignancy), hemolytic (sickle-cell disease, hemolytic anemia), medication, or toxin-associated. Primary carotenemia and lycopenemia occur from increased intake of food with high levels of carotenoids/lycopenes (**Table 1.24**) and are generally asymptomatic. Secondary carotenemia is due to impaired metabolism that can be seen in certain disease states, such as diabetes, hypothyroidism (**Figure 1.199**), nephritic syndrome, anorexia, or liver disease, and may have systemic manifestations related to those underlying conditions. Exposure to occupational compounds, medications (dihydroxyacetone, dipyridamole), and a rare multiple myeloma producing anti-flavin antibodies are also among the differential diagnoses.

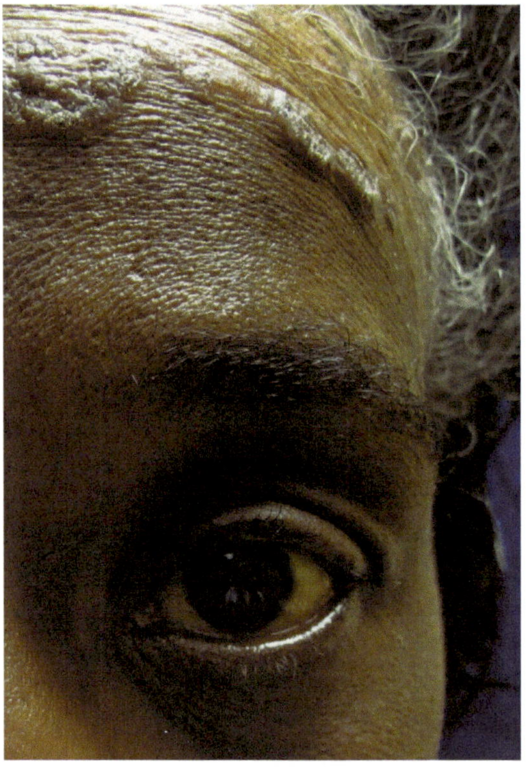

FIGURE 1.192 Conjunctival icterus: Sarcoidosis and primary biliary cirrhosis.

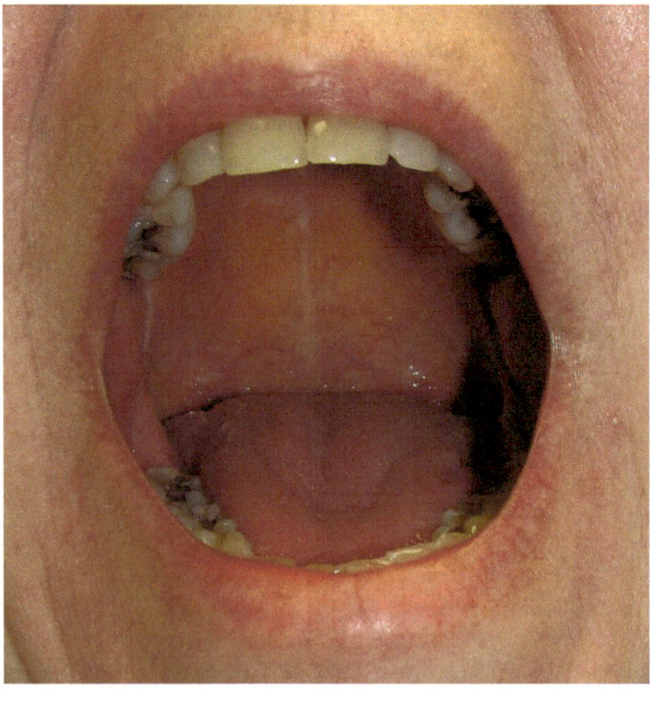

FIGURE 1.193 Jaundice: Upper palate.

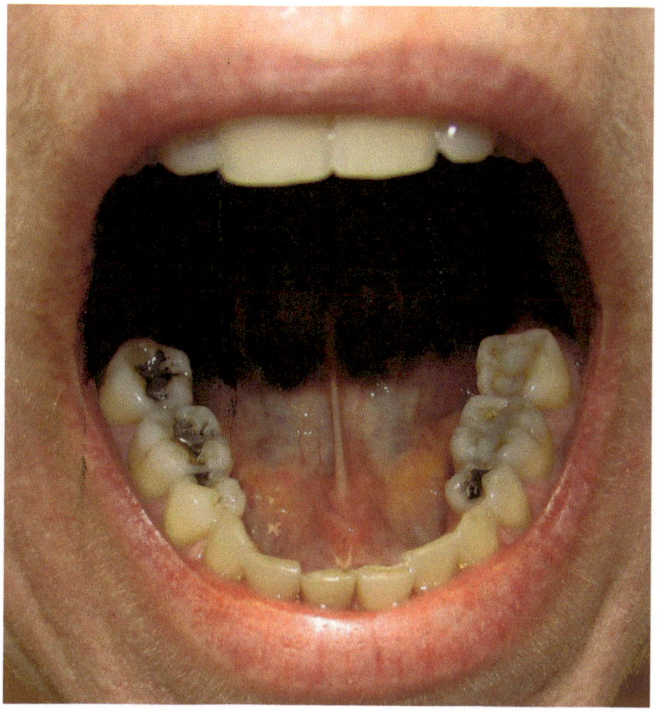

FIGURE 1.194 Jaundice: Floor of mouth.

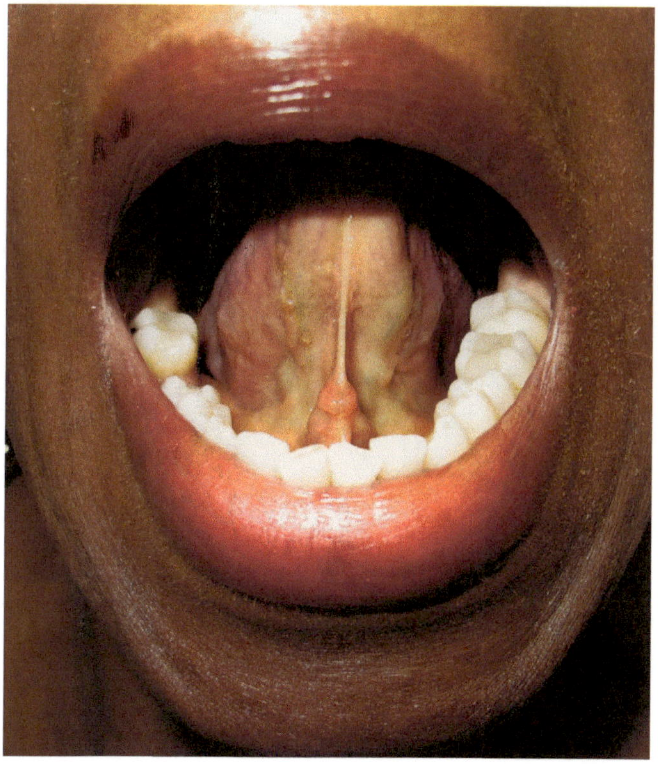

FIGURE 1.195 Jaundice: Base of tongue.

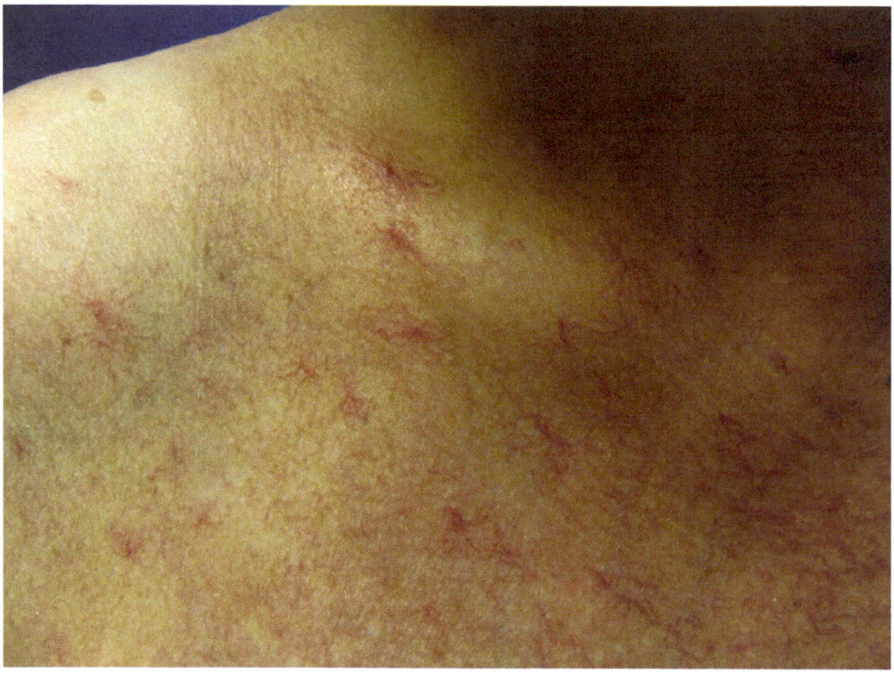

FIGURE 1.196 Jaundice with spider angiomas.

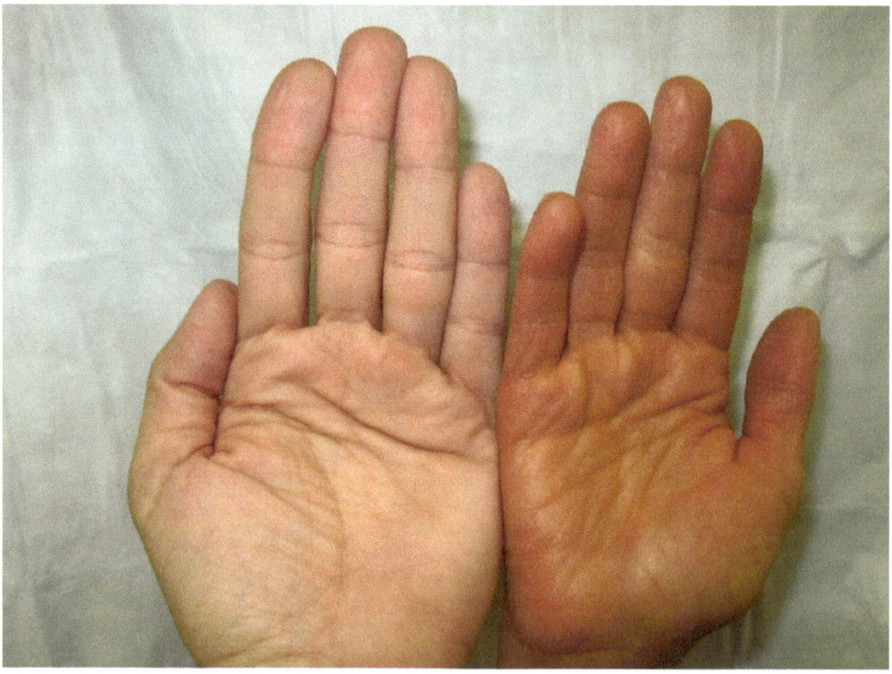

FIGURE 1.197 Primary hypercarotenoderma: Normal on left.

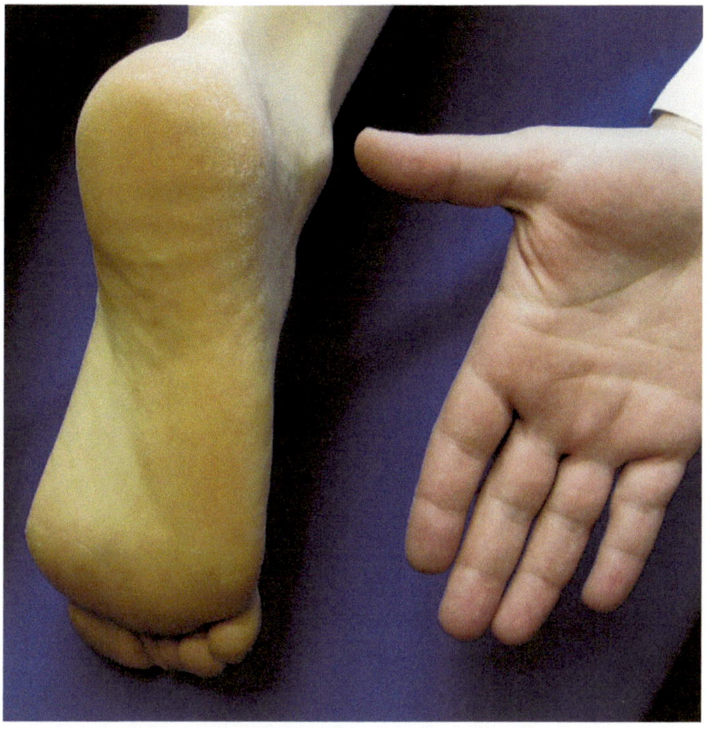

FIGURE 1.198 Primary hypercarotenoderma: Normal on right.

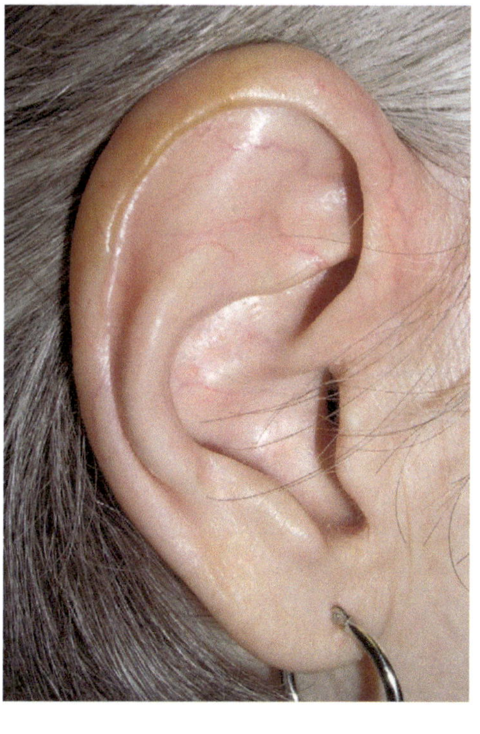

FIGURE 1.199 Secondary hypercarotenoderma: Hypothyroidism.

Evaluation and Management

Patients with xanthoderma need a careful history, medication review, review of symptoms, and examination of the eyes and mucous membranes. If conjunctival/mucous membrane icterus is present, laboratory investigation should include LFTs, haptoglobin, Hep B, Hep C, PT/PTT, albumin, and CBC. In patients with clinical findings more consistent with carotenemia, history should be focused on the patient's diet. Laboratory evaluation with serum beta carotene, TFTs, FBG, HA1c, Flip (fasting lipid), prealbumin, UA, LFTs, and SPEP will allow differentiation between primary and secondary carotenoderma. Treatment of xanthoderma is directed at the underlying cause.

TABLE 1.24

Xanthoderma Due to Dietary Consumption

1. **Carotenemia**
Alfalfa, apricots, asparagus, beans, beets, broccoli, butter, cantaloupe, carrots, chard, collard greens, cucumber, eggs, endive, escarole, kale, Romaine lettuce, mango, milk, mustard, oranges papaya, palm oil, parsley, peaches, podded peas prunes, pumpkin, red bell peppers, rutabaga, spinach, butternut squash, sweet potatoes, turnips, watercress, yellow corn.
2. **Lycopenemia**
Apricots, asparagus, grapefruit, guavas, mangos, papaya, persimmon, red cabbage, sweet red peppers, tomatoes, watermelon.

BIBLIOGRAPHY

Haught JM, Patel S, English JC III. Xanthoderma: A clinical review. J Am Acad Dermatol 2007;57: 1051–1058.

Soundararajan V, Charny JW, Bain MA et al. The color of skin: Orange diseases of the skin, nails, and mucosa. Clin Dermatol 2019;37(5):520–527.

Tanaka A, Miyauchi T, Kitamura S et al. Carotenoderma due to lycopenemia: A case report and evaluation of lycopene deposition in the skin. J Dermatol 2022;49(12):1320–1324.

Xanthomas

Etiopathogenesis

Xanthomas occur from the deposition of lipids into the skin. These include eruptive, tuberous, tendinous, palmar, planar, xanthelasma, and verruciform xanthomas. They frequently occur in the setting of hyper- or dyslipidemia. Although the exact mechanisms are unknown, circulating lipoproteins or lipoprotein–immunoglobulin complexes become deposited in the skin, where they are phagocytosed by macrophages and present histologically as "foam cells."

Clinical Manifestations

The characteristic finding seen in xanthomas, regardless of type, is a yellow to orange discoloration. Eruptive xanthomas appear as multiple red to yellow papules (**Figures 1.200** and **1.201**), often with pruritus. Tuberous and tendinous xanthomas are red to pink papulonodules that occur on extensor surfaces, such as the elbows, knees, and hands. Yellowish discoloration of palmar creases is called xanthoma striata palmaris. Planar xanthomas are noninflammatory yellow macules to plaques that can occur diffusely on the skin (**Figure 1.202**). Xanthomas commonly seen on the eyelids are called xanthelasmata (**Figure 1.203**). If the xanthoma encompasses the entire eyelids, it must be distinguished from a planar xanthoma. Verruciform xanthomas are plaques commonly seen in the mouth.

Systemic Manifestations

Eruptive xanthomas are associated with hypertriglyceridemia. Triglyceride levels in these patients can exceed 4000 mg/mL. Tuberous xanthomas can be seen in dysbetalipoproteinemia (broad beta disease) and familial hypercholesterolemia. Tendinous xanthomas are most often seen in the setting of familial hypercholesterolemia. Other disorders associated with tendinous xanthomas include cerebrotendinous xanthomatosis and β-sitosterolemia. Palmar xanthoma is pathognomonic for Type III hyperlipoproteinemia. Planar xanthomas are associated with hematologic disorders (monoclonal gammopathy and multiple myeloma). Xanthelasmata are common; their presence warrants lipid evaluation (although approximately 50% of patients are normolipemic). Of note, it has been recently associated as an independent risk factor, such as diagonal earlobe creases (**Figure 1.204**) and severe male androgenetic alopecia, for coronary artery disease.

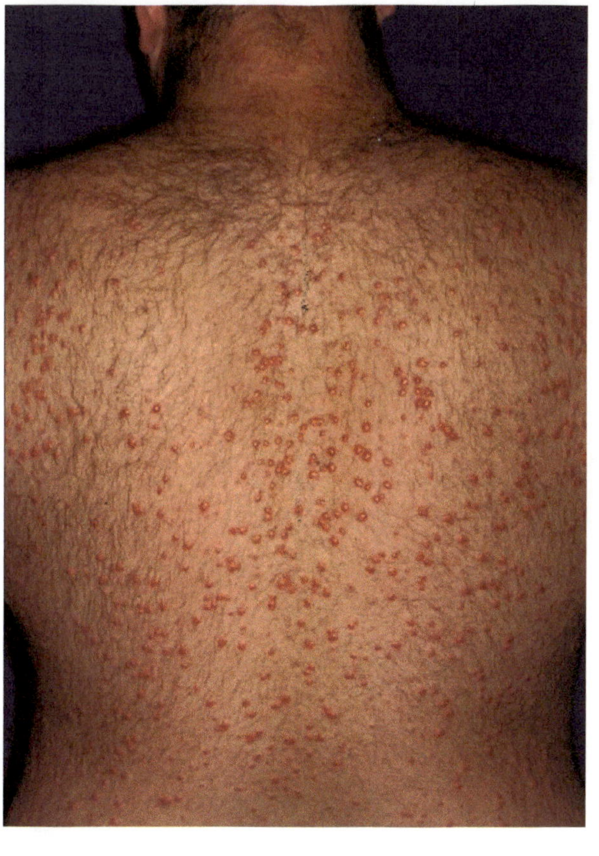

FIGURE 1.200 Eruptive xanthoma.

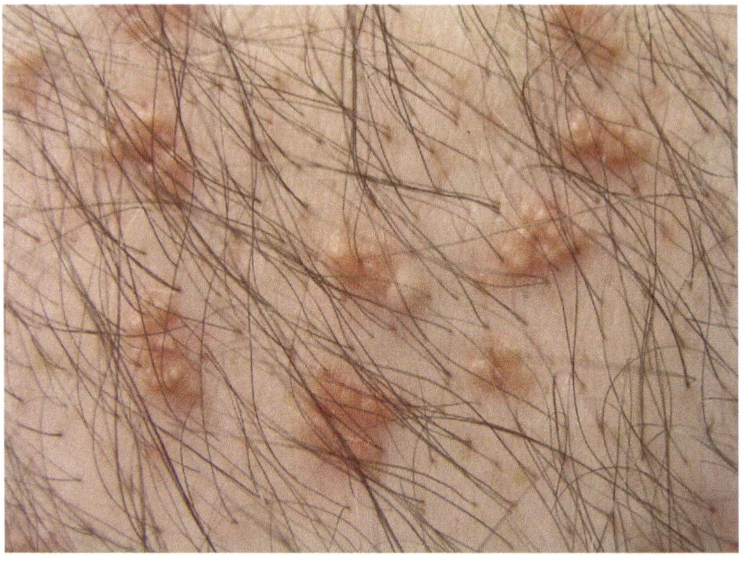

FIGURE 1.201 Eruptive xanthoma.

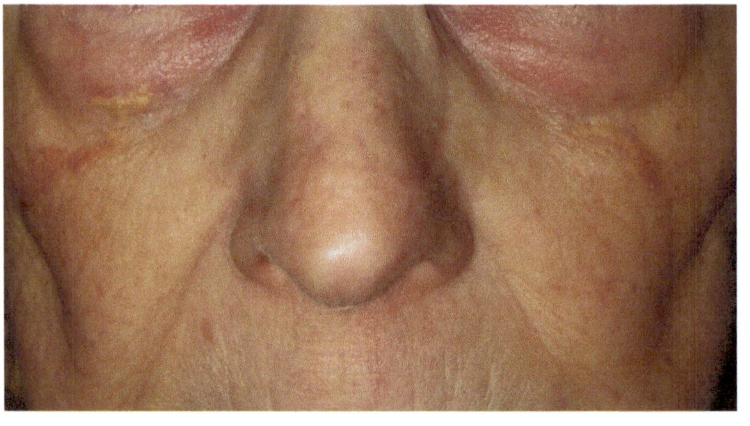

FIGURE 1.202 Planar xanthoma.

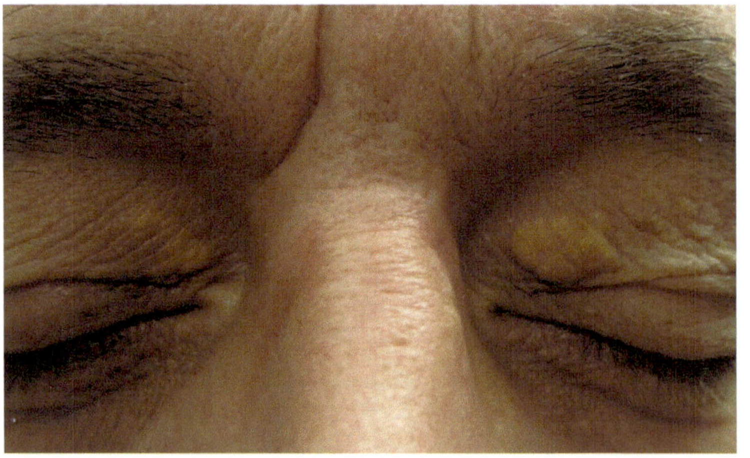

FIGURE 1.203 Xanthelasmata.

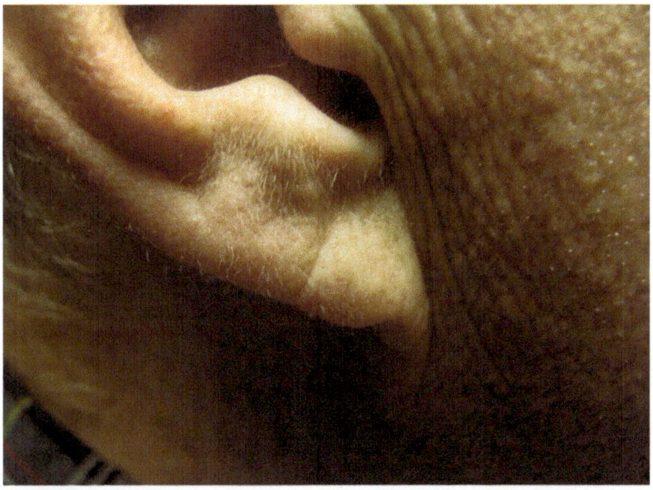

FIGURE 1.204 Diagonal earlobe crease.

Evaluation and Management

Evaluation usually requires a multidisciplinary approach and is aimed at identifying and treating the underlying cause of the xanthomas. Laboratory evaluation of FBG, HA1c, and FLip is indicated. Dietary measures, along with antihyperlipidemic medications (3-hydroxy-3-methylglutaryl coenzyme A [HMG-CoA] reductase inhibitors, bile acid-binding resins, niacin, probucol, fibric acid derivatives) and cardiac evaluation are suggested. However, in the setting of planar xanthomas, a CBC, SPEP/SIFE, and UPEP/UIFE should be obtained. A detected monoclonal gammopathy requires evaluation by hematology. Surgical excision, ablative laser techniques, trichloroacetic acid, and cryosurgery have all been reported for improving the clinical appearance of xanthomas.

BIBLIOGRAPHY

Alnouri F, Al-Allaf FA, Athar M, et al. Xanthomas can be misdiagnosed and mistreated in homozygous familial hypercholesterolemia patients: A call for increased awareness among dermatologists and healthcare practitioners. Glob Heart 2020;15(1):19.

Booken N, Goerdt S, Goebeler M. Diffuse plane normolipemic xanthomatosis associated with monoclonal gammopathy. Dermatol 2009;219(1):91–92.

Edston E. The earlobe crease, coronary artery disease, and sudden cardiac death: An autopsy study of 520 individuals. Am J Forensic Med Pathol 2006;27:129–133.

Marogi EP, Ohiomoba RO, Stone RJ. Eruptive xanthomas: Importance of recognition to reduce delay of effective triglyceride reduction. Am J Med 2022;135(4):444–447.

Tang K, Wu M, Li J. Eruptive xanthomas. JAMA Dermatol 2023;159(4):449.

Theodosiou G, Zafeiriadou V, Baimpa E. Diffuse plane xanthoma in patient with monoclonal gammopathy. Br J Haematol 2024;205(6):2109–2110.

2

Calcifying, Perforating, and Atrophic Disorders

Anetoderma

Etiopathogenesis

Anetoderma describes well-demarcated regions of flaccid skin caused by loss of dermal elastic fibers. The etiology is unknown, but mechanisms may include defective elastic synthesis, uncontrolled elastolytic enzymes, elastophagocytosis, ischemia, or shared autoimmune antigenicity.

Clinical Manifestations

Typical lesions are 1- to 2-cm oval-shaped, well-demarcated regions of skin characterized by flaccid skin, which may appear atrophic or protuberant compared to normal surrounding skin (**Figures 2.1–2.5**). Lesions may appear anywhere but most commonly on the torso and extremities. The appearance of these lesions may or may not be preceded by an erythematous dermatitis. Primary anetoderma occurs with no previous skin pathology, whereas secondary anetoderma occurs with previous skin inflammation.

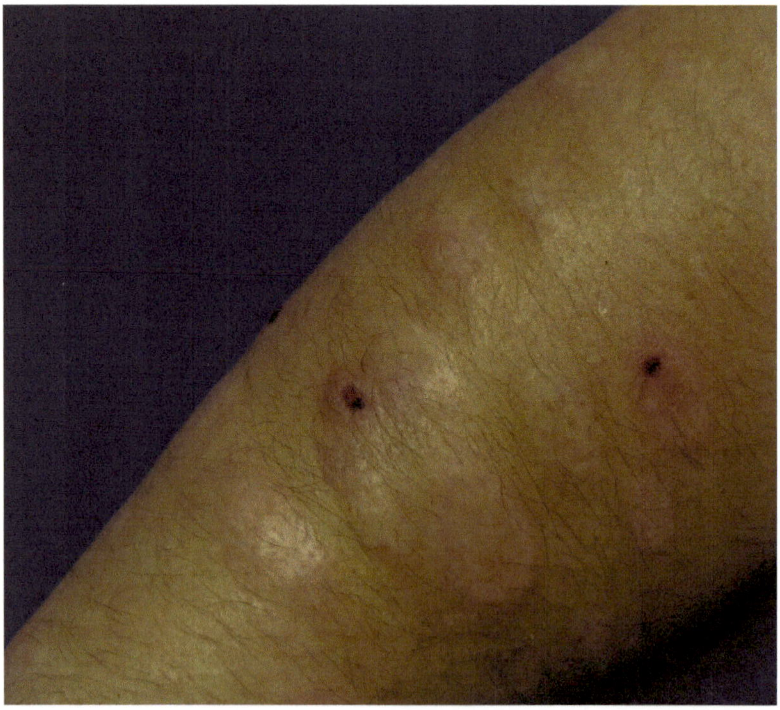

FIGURE 2.1 Primary anetoderma: Antiphospholipid antibody syndrome.

DOI: 10.1201/9781003492665-2

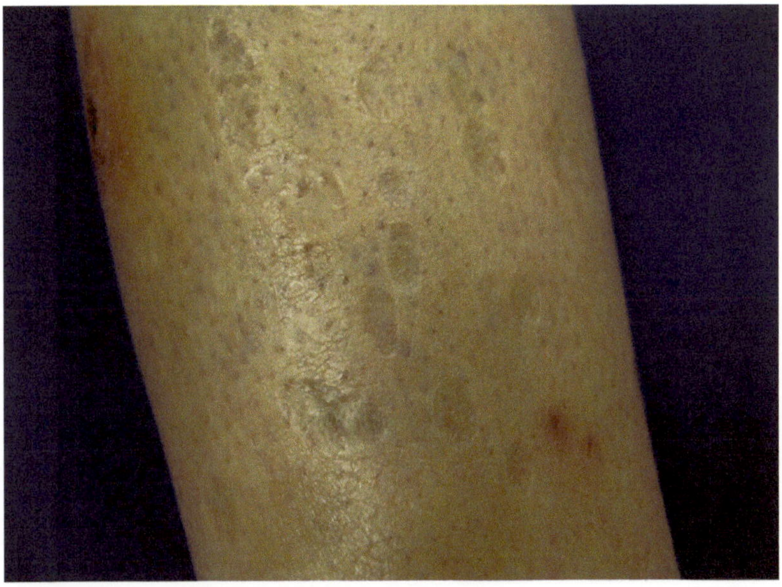

FIGURE 2.2 Primary anetoderma: Antiphospholipid antibody syndrome.

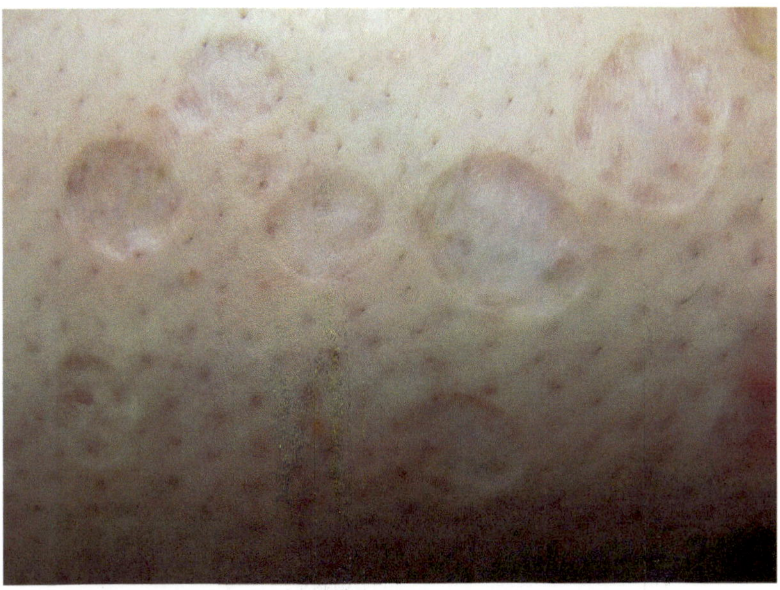

FIGURE 2.3 Primary anetoderma: Antiphospholipid antibody syndrome.

Systemic Manifestations

Primary anetoderma has been associated with systemic lupus erythematosus (SLE), Sjögren syndrome, autoimmune thyroiditis, autoimmune hemolytic anemia, adrenal insufficiency, human immunodeficiency virus (HIV), and penicillamine exposure. A growing body of evidence suggests that a hypercoagulable state such as antiphospholipid antibody (APLA) production $\pm$ APLA syndrome may underlie primary anetoderma. Causes of secondary anetoderma include inflammatory disorders caused by infections (varicella, syphilis, Lyme disease, leprosy), neoplastic disorders (pilomatricoma, cutaneous B-cell lymphoma, juvenile xanthogranuloma), or inflammatory disorders (lupus profundus, granuloma annulare, acne). Familial/congenital anetoderma has rarely been described.

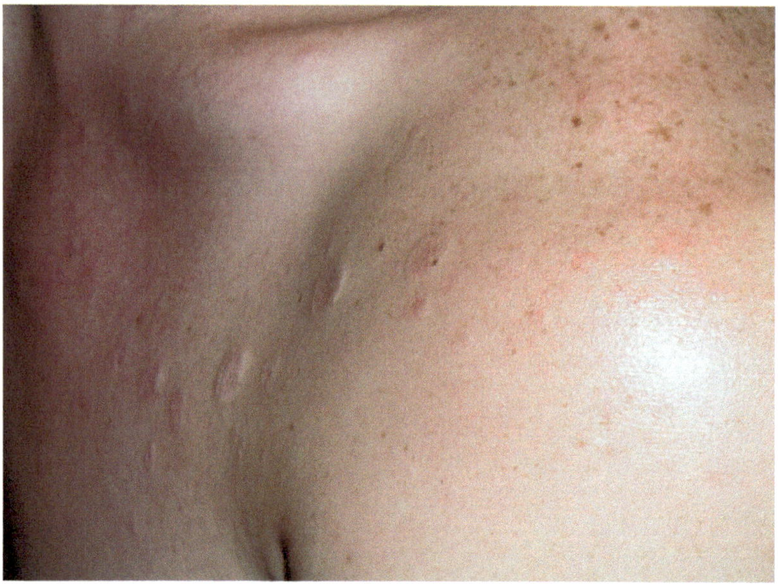

FIGURE 2.4 Primary anetoderma: Systemic lupus erythematosus.

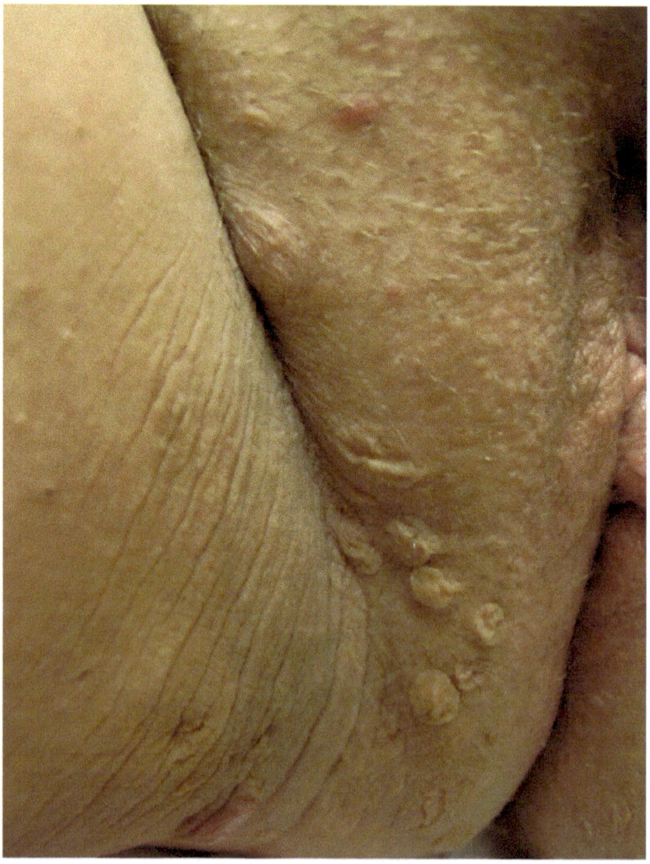

FIGURE 2.5 Secondary anetoderma: Groin folliculitis.

Evaluation and Management

Clinical suspicion of anetoderma should prompt a diagnostic skin biopsy with elastic tissue stains demonstrating loss or fragmentation of elastic fibers in the dermis. The workup is reviewed in **Table 2.1** and should include evaluation for coagulopathy and rheumatic and endocrine disorders. A thorough medication, sexual, and travel history may help uncover an infectious etiology. There is no treatment for this skin lesion, but identifying the underlying cause and providing appropriate treatment may prevent the development of additional lesions.

TABLE 2.1

Evaluation of Anetoderma

Laboratory
• Lupus anticoagulant
• APLAs
• Proteins C and S
• Gene mutations (Factor V Leiden, prothrombin, methyl tetrahydrofolate reductase)
• Antithrombin III activity
• Homocysteine
• Antinuclear antibodies
• Anti-double-stranded DNA antibodies
• Anti-Smith antibodies
• Anti-Ro/SSA and anti-La/SSB antibodies
• Complement 3 and 4
• Thyroid function tests
• Antithyroglobulin antibodies
• Antithyroid peroxidase antibodies
• AM cortisol level
• HIV
• Rapid plasma reagin (RPR)

BIBLIOGRAPHY

Cook JC, Puckett Y. Anetoderma. In: StatPearls [internet]. Treasure Island (FL): StatPearls Publishing 2023.

Esquivel-Valerio JA, Cardenas-de la Garza JA, Arvizu-Rivera RI, et al. Disseminated anetoderma associated with antiphospholipid antibodies. Clin Rheumatol 2020;39(12):3887–3888.

Iglesias-Puizas A, Batalla A, Peon G, et al. Anetoderma and systemic lupus erythematosus: Case report and literature review. Acta Derm Venereol 2019;99(3):335–336.

Thornsberry LA, LoSicco KI, English JC III. The skin and hypercoagulable states. J Am Acad Dermatol 2013;69(3):450–462.

Atrophie Blanche (Livedo Vasculopathy)

Etiopathogenesis

Atrophie blanche (AB), also known as livedo vasculopathy (LV), is a condition that may be present as a result of chronic venous stasis, abnormalities causing endothelial damage, or hypercoagulable states. AB may represent an abnormal scarring reaction due to vascular damage in combination with hypercoagulable states.

Clinical Manifestations

AB presents with livedoid discoloration, erythema to purpura, with subsequent development of the characteristic stellate, "porcelain-white," atrophic scars (**Figure 2.6**). Chronic lesions may develop ulcerations (**Figures 2.7** and **2.8**). Although the classic presentation involves the appearance of lesions of bilateral malleoli, involvement of dorsal feet and toes (**Figure 2.9**) can also occur. Pain may be severe and is often due to ulceration or to ongoing microthrombotic events.

Systemic Manifestations

Venous stasis from varicosities with venous reflux, cardiac failure, or low intravascular protein oncotic pressure may lead to AB. Connective tissue disease (SLE, rheumatoid arthritis, paraproteinemia, cryofibrinogenemia) and infections (hepatitis B and hepatitis C) have been reported with AB. Associated thromboembolic events such as superficial thrombophlebitis (**Figure 2.10**), deep vein thrombosis, pulmonary emboli, and transient ischemic/stroke have occurred in patients with AB in the setting of a Factor V Leiden mutation, prothrombin gene mutation, antithrombin III deficiency, homocysteinemia, protein C and S deficiency, and the APLA syndrome. Neurologic involvement can also manifest as pain and paresthesia if there is ischemic damage to peripheral nerves.

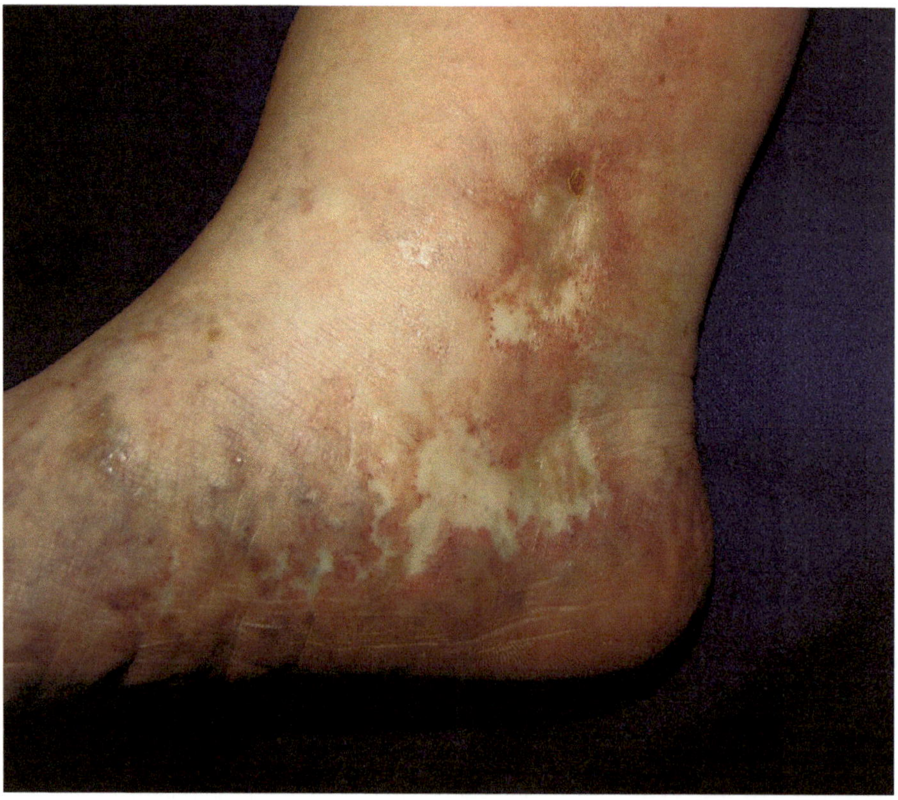

FIGURE 2.6 Atrophie blanche: Medial malleolus.

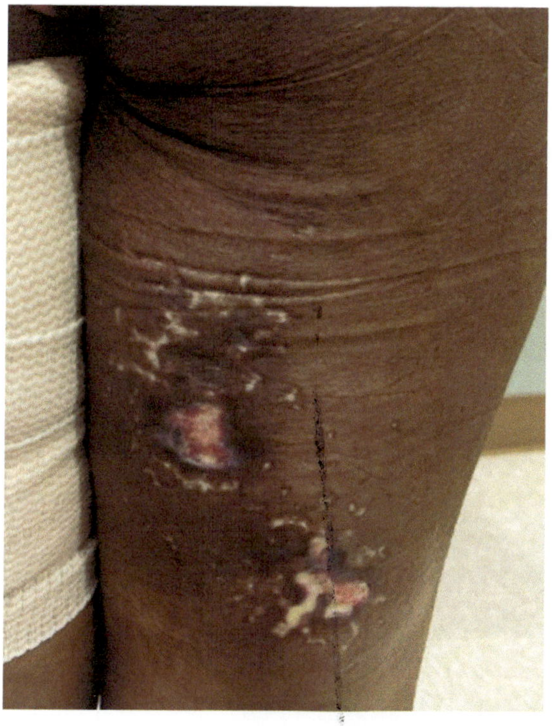

FIGURE 2.7 Livedo vasculopathy associated with systemic lupus erythematosus.

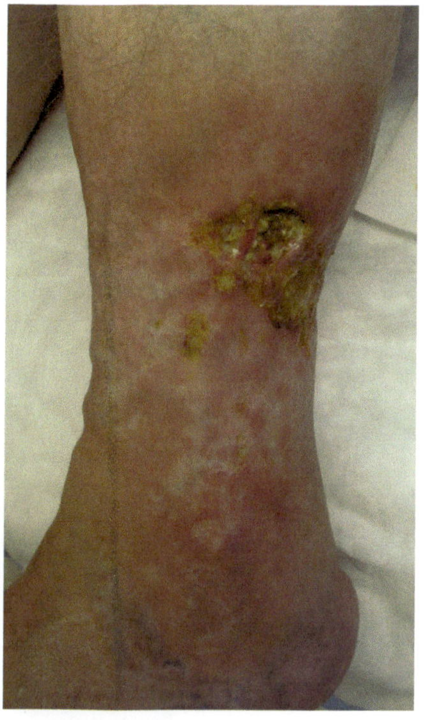

FIGURE 2.8 Atrophie blanche: Chronic venous insufficiency ulcer.

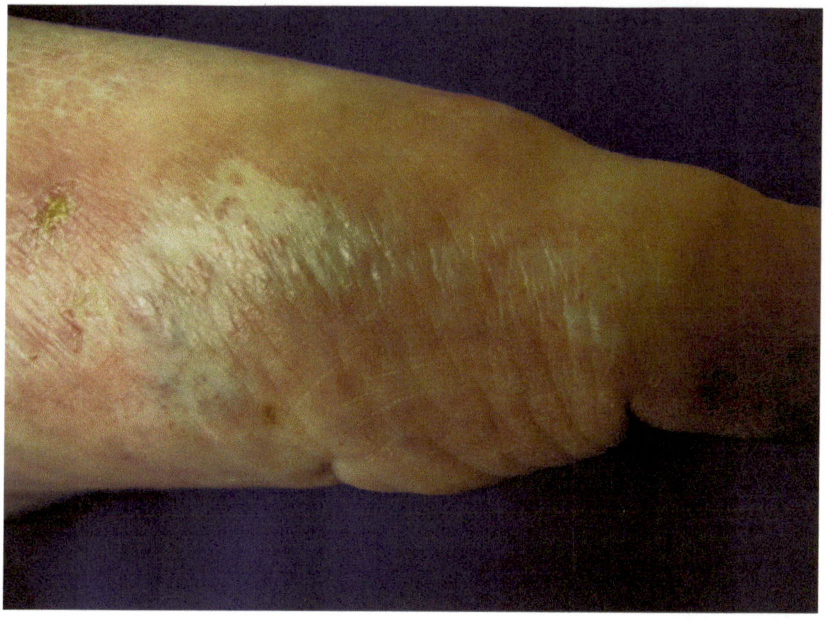

FIGURE 2.9 Atrophie blanche: Foot and toe.

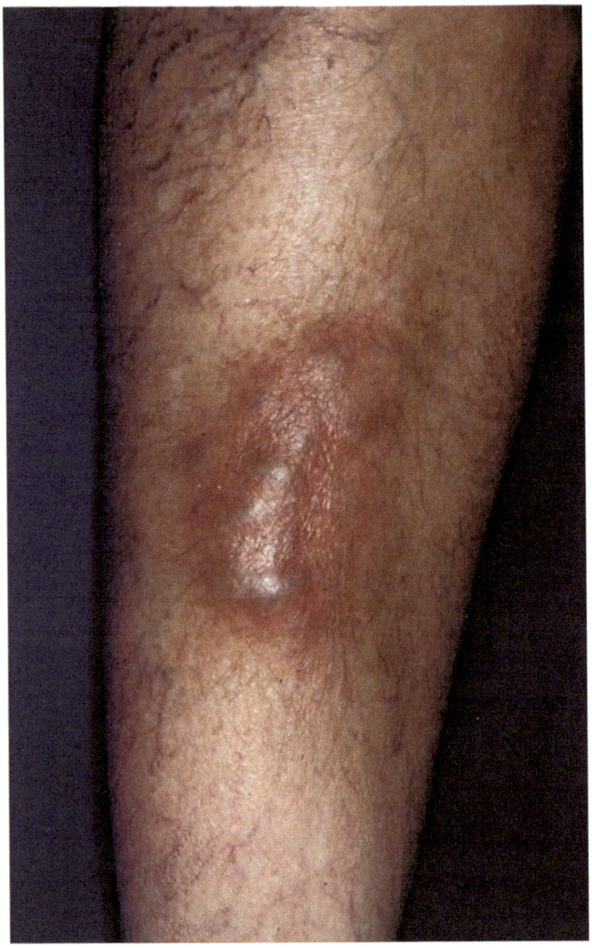

FIGURE 2.10 Superficial thrombophlebitis.

Evaluation and Management

Recommended screening is summarized in **Table 2.2**. Treatment of AB is often dissatisfying; however, anticoagulation with warfarin, pentoxifylline, aspirin, or low-molecular-weight heparin; direct oral anticoagulants (apixaban/rivaroxaban); and iloprost have been reported to provide relatively good results. Immunosuppression with cyclosporine, tumor necrosis factor alpha (TNFα) and Janus kinase (JAK) inhibitors, and intravenous immunoglobulin (IVIG) therapy has also been reported. Vasodilatory medications such as nifedipine or nicotinic acid can be attempted. Compression therapy for underlying venous abnormalities such as varicose veins or venous stasis can decrease the risk of ulceration.

TABLE 2.2

Evaluation of Atrophie Blanche (Livedo Vasculopathy)

Laboratory

- Lupus anticoagulant
- Antiphospholipid antibodies
- Proteins C and S
- Gene mutations (Factor V Leiden, prothrombin, methyl tetrahydrofolate reductase)
- Antithrombin III activity

(Continued)

TABLE 2.2 (*Continued*)

Evaluation of Atrophie Blanche (Livedo Vasculopathy)

Laboratory
• Homocysteine
• Anti-nuclear antibody
• Rheumatoid factor
• Anticyclic citrullinated protein antibodies
• Hepatitis B and hepatitis C antibodies
• Serum protein electrophoresis/Serum immunofixation electrophoresis/serum free light chains
• 24-h urine protein electrophoresis/Urine immunofixation electrophoresis
• Cryoglobulin

BIBLIOGRAPHY

Burg MR, Mitschang C, Goerge T, et al. Livedo vasculopathy – A diagnostic and therapeutic challenge. Front Med (Lausanne) 2022;9:10012178.

Eswaran H, Googe P, Vedak P, et al. Livedoid vasculopathy: A review with focus on terminology and pathogenesis. Vasc Med 2022;27(6):593–603.

Micieli R, Alavi A. Treatment for livedoid vasculopathy: A systematic review. JAMA Dermatol 2018;154(2):193–202.

Thornsberry LA, LoSicco KI, English JC III. The skin and hypercoagulable states. J Am Acad Dermatol 2013;69(3):450–462.

Calcinosis Cutis

Etiopathogenesis

When serum calcium and phosphate equilibrium are disturbed, calcinosis cutis, the abnormal formation of calcium phosphate crystals in the skin, can occur. Calcinosis cutis is categorized as dystrophic, metastatic, iatrogenic/traumatic, idiopathic, or calciphylactic. Calciphylaxis is discussed in this chapter in the next section.

Clinical Manifestations

Presentation typically includes firm, painless, or exquisitely tender dermal nodules that may perforate or ulcerate. Dystrophic calcification is calcium salt deposition in the presence of inflammation (calcium and phosphate levels are normal), as seen in SLE, scleroderma, mixed connective tissue disease (**Figures 2.11** and **2.12**), dermatomyositis, (**Figures 2.13** and **2.14**), panniculitis, and skin neoplasms. Metastatic calcification is due to abnormal calcium and phosphate balance from derangement of hormonal control (hyperparathyroidism), abnormal absorption (milk alkali syndrome), hypervitaminosis D, familial hyperphosphatemia (tumoral calcinosis), or renal failure (**Figure 2.15**). Iatrogenic calcinosis results from therapeutically elevated serum or locally induced tissue calcium. Idiopathic calcinosis describes skin calcification with neither trauma nor abnormality in calcium/phosphate homeostasis.

Systemic Manifestations

Idiopathic, iatrogenic, and dystrophic calcification due to skin neoplasms are typically incidental and generally do not feature systemic manifestations. On the other hand, calcinosis cutis, in general, should prompt an examination searching for signs of rheumatologic disease (heliotrope rash, malar rash, shawl sign, Gottron papules, Raynaud phenomenon, joint pain, skin thickening/tightening), endocrinopathies, nephrogenic disease, or dietary abnormalities. Metastatic calcifications may feature symptoms of fatigue, psychosis, nausea/vomiting, symptoms of renal insufficiency, bone pain, nephrolithiasis, or gout, the so-called "bones, stones, abdominal groans, and psychic overtones."

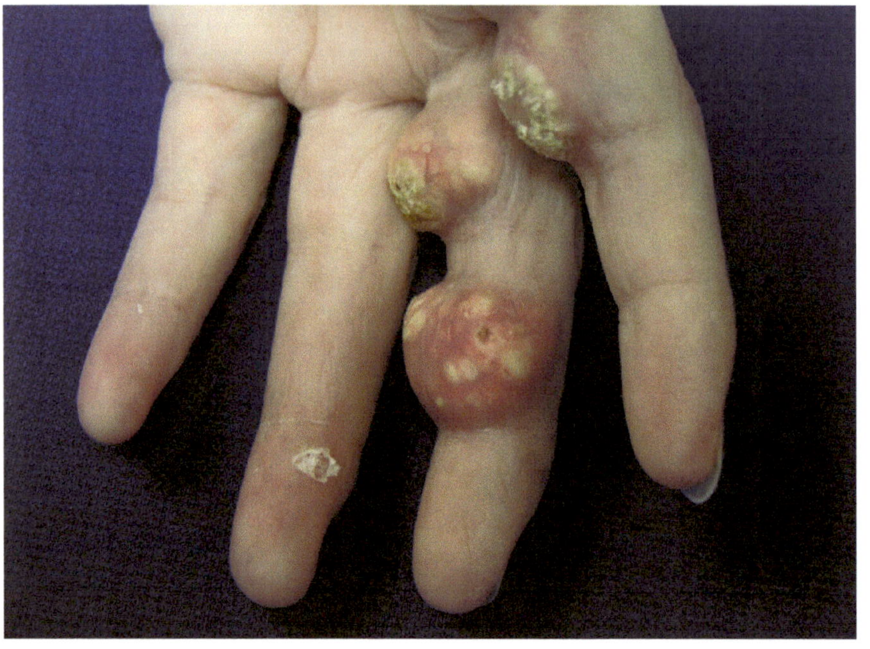

FIGURE 2.11 Dystrophic calcifications: Mixed connective tissue disease.

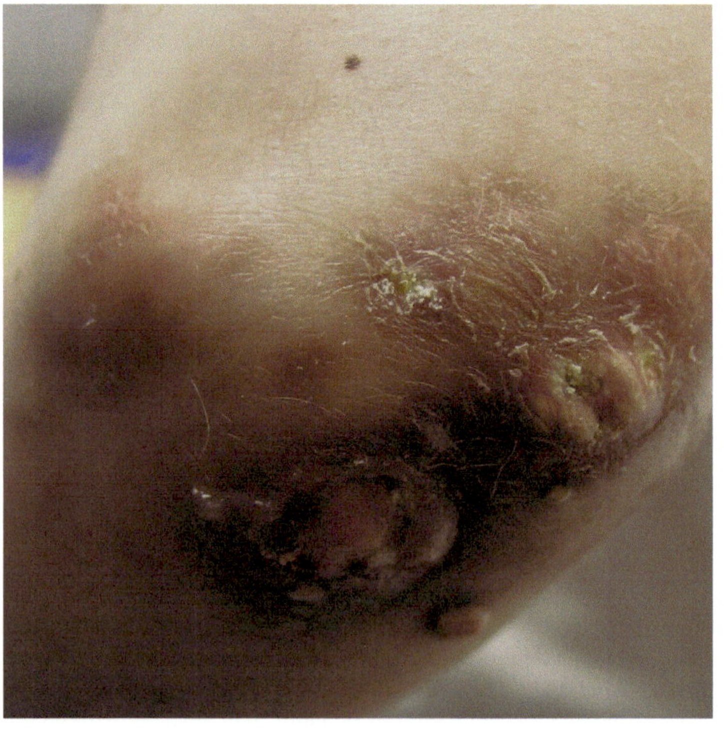

FIGURE 2.12 Dystrophic calcifications (ulcerated): Mixed connective tissue disease.

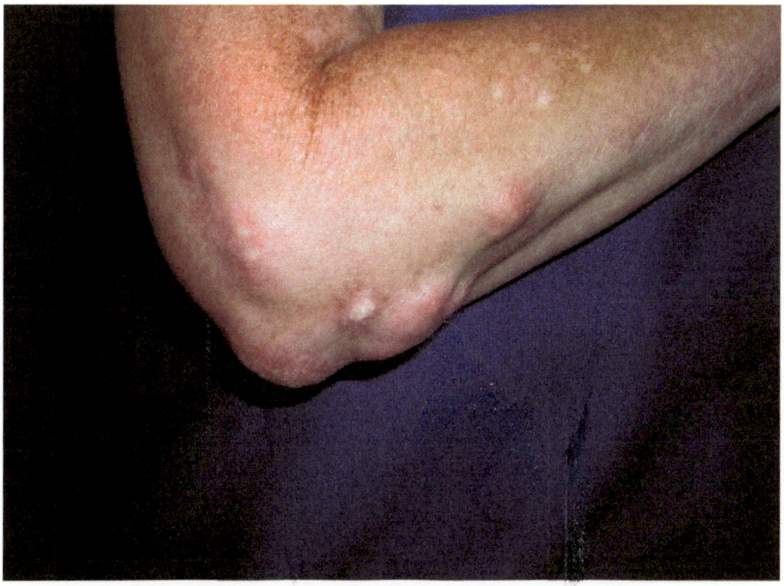

FIGURE 2.13 Dystrophic calcifications: Dermatomyositis.

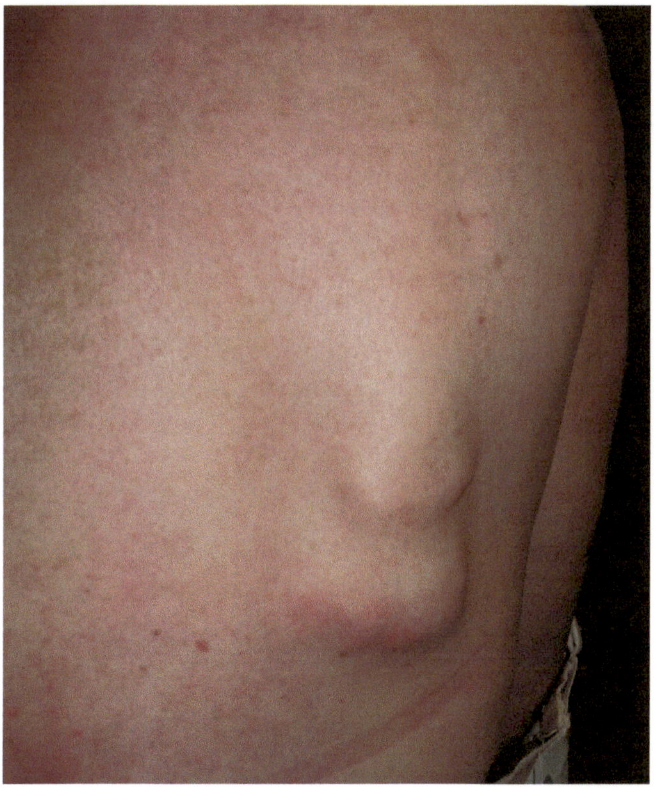

FIGURE 2.14 Dystrophic calcifications: Dermatomyositis.

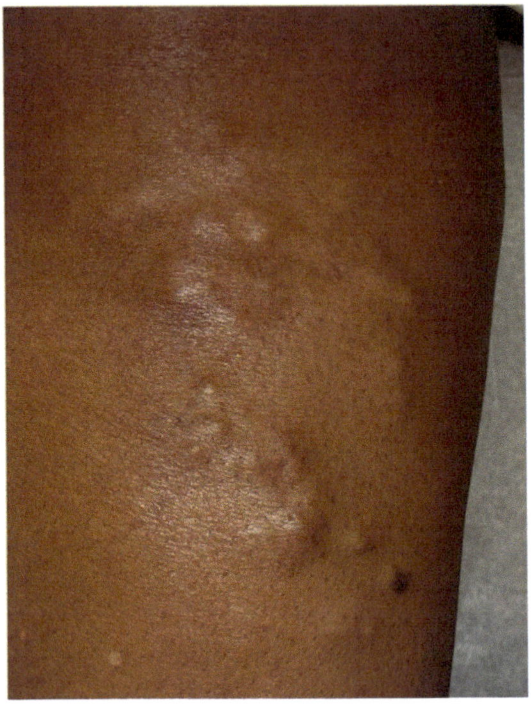

FIGURE 2.15 Metastatic calcifications: Chronic renal disease.

Evaluation and Management

Skin biopsy can confirm the diagnosis with an incisional or wedge biopsy in cases of panniculitis. An interview and review of systems can reveal clues suggesting rheumatologic, endocrinologic, or nephrogenic disease risk. The distribution and location of lesions suggest iatrogenic/traumatic causes. Calcinosis cutis should prompt the laboratory testing summarized in **Table 2.3**. Treatment is aimed at treating the underlying disease state and by calcium-lowering agents (diltiazem, bisphosphonates) and surgical, laser, or extracorporeal lithotripsy procedures. In patients with calcinosis associated with rheumatologic diseases, improvements have been reported with biologic agents such as infliximab or rituximab.

TABLE 2.3

Evaluation of Calcinosis Cutis

Laboratory
• Serum calcium (Ca^{2}+)
• Serum phosphate (PO_4)
• Ca^{2}+/PO_4 product
• Parathyroid hormone (PTH)
• Vitamin D 25-hydroxy
• Renal function tests
• Urinalysis
• Creatinine phosphokinase
• Aldolase
• Anti-nuclear antibody
• Anti-double stranded antibody DNA,
• Anti-Smith antibody Sm,
• Anti-Ro/SSA and anti-La/SSB antibodies
• Anti-toposimerase antibodies
• Anticentromere antibody

BIBLIOGRAPHY

Lau CB, Smith GP. Treatment of calcinosis cutis associated with autoimmune connective tissue diseases. Arch Dermatol Res 2024;316(7):390.

Le C, Bedocs PM. Calcinosis Cutis. In: StatPearls [Internet]. Treasure Island (FL): StatPearls Publishing; 2023.

Reiter N, El-Shabrawi L, Leinweber B, et al. Calcinosis cutis: Part I. Diagnostic pathway. J Am Acad Dermatol 2011;65(1):1–12.

Reiter N, El-Shabrawi L, Leinweber B, et al. Calcinosis cutis: Part II. Treatment options. J Am Acad Dermatol 2011;65(1):15–22.

Calciphylaxis

Etiopathogenesis

Calciphylaxis, or calcific uremic arteriolopathy, results from catastrophic deposition of calcium within the intima of arteries and arterioles. This leads to vascular occlusion with subsequent tissue destruction.

Clinical Manifestations

Calcification within arterioles results in vascular damage, leading to purpura, skin necrosis, and ulceration with severe pain (**Figures 2.16–2.20**). Purpura often presents as a retiform purpura; however, indurated plaques or even bullous lesions have been described. Skin necrosis and ulceration typically form due to disrupted arteriolar flow, resulting in severe pain, increased risk of infection or sepsis, and multisystem organ failure. Lesions typically develop on the lower extremities, torso, and genitals.

Systemic Manifestations

End-stage renal disease requiring hemodialysis is the most common disorder associated with the development of calciphylaxis but may be seen in the setting of renal transplantation and drug-induced nephropathy or acute kidney injury. Nonuremic cases have also been reported and are summarized in **Table 2.4**.

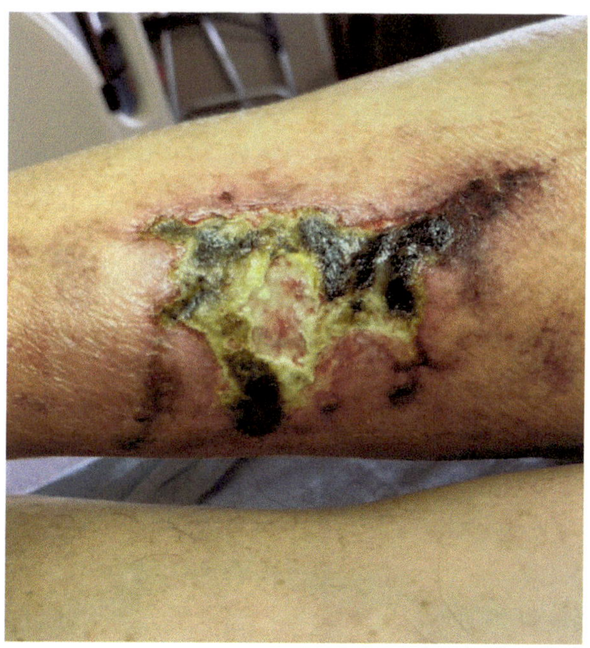

FIGURE 2.16 Calciphylaxis: Leg.

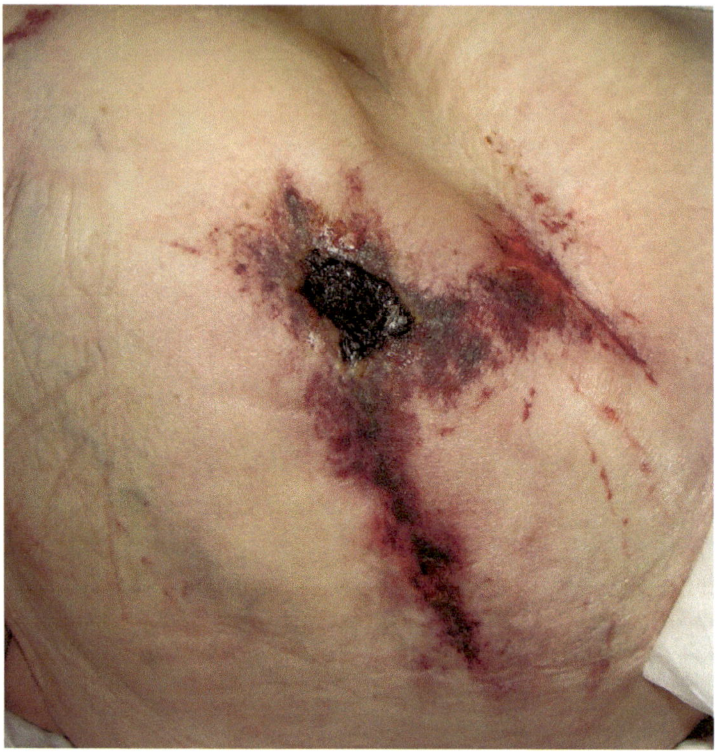

FIGURE 2.17 Calciphylaxis: Thigh/hip.

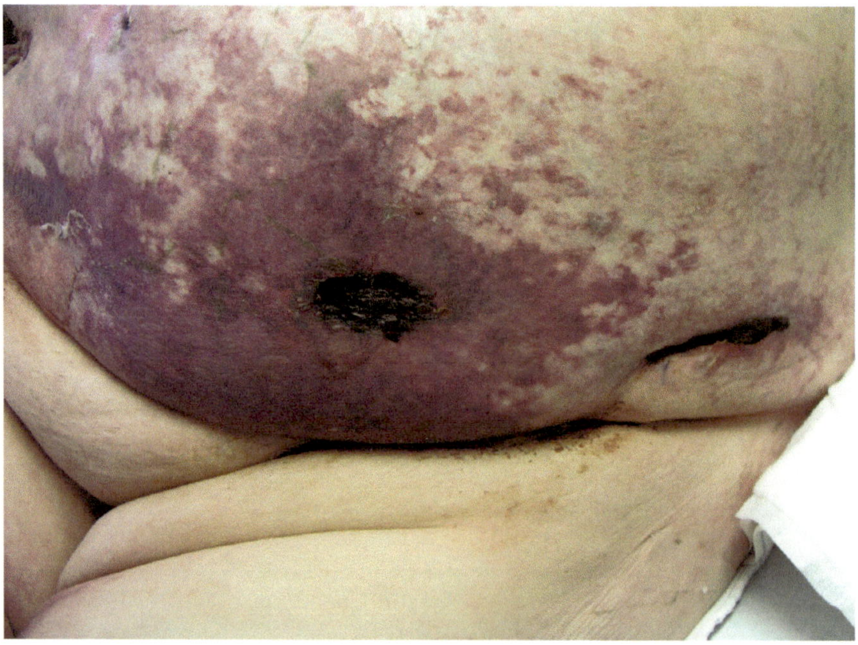

FIGURE 2.18 Calciphylaxis: Abdomen; ulcerative with bullae.

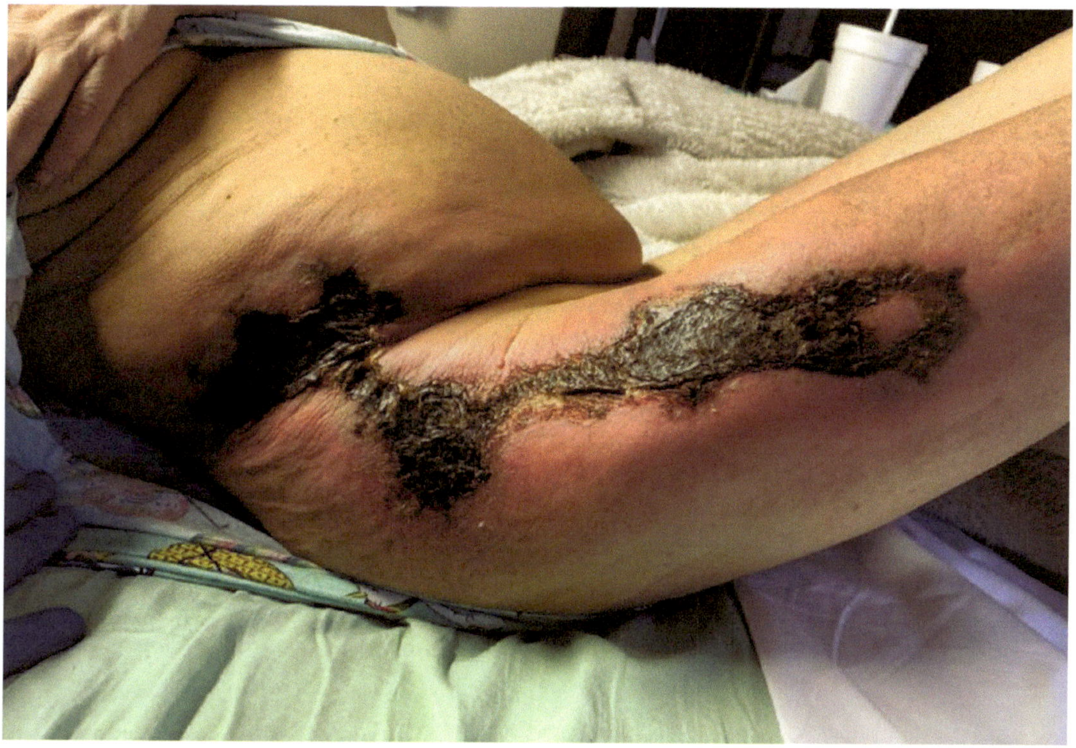

FIGURE 2.19 Calciphylaxis: Abdomen/thigh.

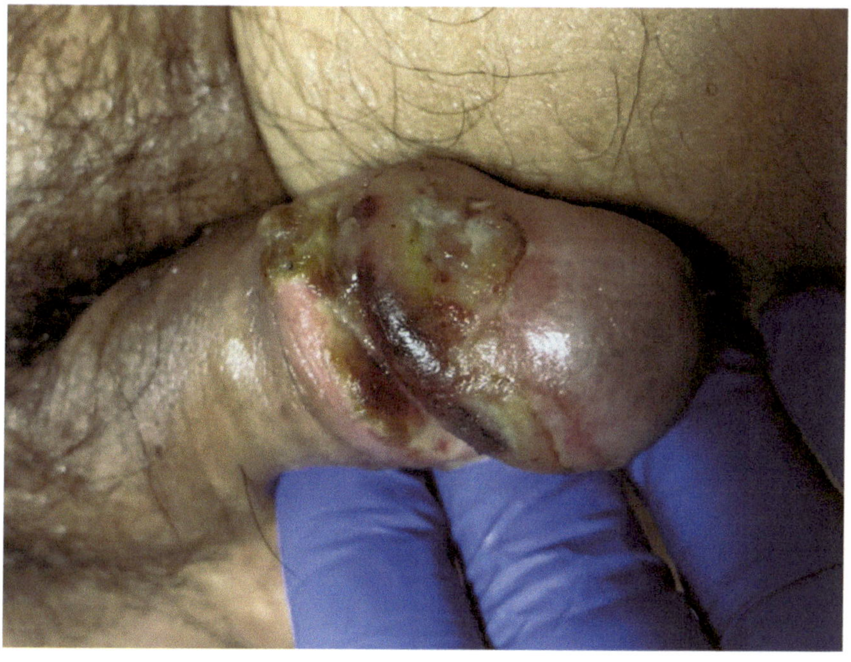

FIGURE 2.20 Calciphylaxis: Penile.

Evaluation and Management

A skin biopsy showing calcification of the media of arterioles, often with accompanying panniculitis, is diagnostic for calciphylaxis. However, because uncontrolled bleeding may be a complication, biopsy in a controlled surgical environment should be considered. Although an elevated $Ca^{2}+/PO_4$ product greater than 70 mg^2/dL^2 is a specific finding, it is, nonetheless, not sensitive for the diagnosis of calciphylaxis. PTH-level abnormalities may be high or low. Treatments include low-calcium dialysis, intravenous sodium thiosulfate, bisphosphonates, and cinacalcet. With the possible role of a hypercoagulable state in calciphylaxis, therapy with tissue plasminogen activator or low-molecular-weight heparin has also been reported. Surgical intervention by parathyroidectomy has been studied; however, the lack of large study populations makes the overall benefit of parathyroidectomy questionable.

Overall outcomes of treatment remain disappointing. Acral calciphylaxis has a better prognosis than truncal calciphylaxis; however, median survival was typically less than 1 year, with median survival among dialysis patients being 2–3 months, whereas median survival for patients not requiring dialysis was 8–9 months.

TABLE 2.4

Causes of Nonuremic Calciphylaxis

Causes
- Hyperparathyroidism
- Secondary hyperparathyroidism due to vitamin D deficiency
- Diabetes mellitus
- Alcoholic liver disease
- Vitamin D and K deficiency
- Autoimmunity
- Thrombophilia (APLA)
- Malignancy

Medications
- Warfarin
- Calcium
- Prednisone
- Iron
- Recombinant PTH

BIBLIOGRAPHY

Kodumudi V, Jeha GM, Mydlo N, et al. Management of cutaneous calciphylaxis. Adv Ther 2020;37(12):4797–4807.

Marin BG, Aghagoli G, Hu SL, et al. Calciphylaxis and kidney disease: A review. Am J Kidney Dis 2023;81(2):232–239.

Yousuf S, Busch D, Renner R, et al. Clinical characteristics and treatment modalities in uremic and non-uremic calciphylaxis – A dermatological single-center experience. Ren Fail 2024;46(1):2297566.

Nigwekar SU, Thadhani R, Brandenburg VM. Calciphylaxis. N Engl J Med 2018;378(18):1704–1714.

Cutis Laxa

Etiopathogenesis

Cutis laxa results from the loss of or destruction of elastin fibers of the skin, causing loss of elasticity of the epidermis. Several genetic disorders from mutations in fibulin 5, fibulin 4, ATP7A, and lysyl oxidase cause inherited cutis laxa. Acquired destruction of elastin fibers has been associated with medications, malignancies, infections, connective tissue disease, nephropathy, enzyme deficiency, and inflammatory disorders.

Clinical Manifestations

Acquired cutis laxa presents with the cutaneous finding of loose, pliable skin, resulting in the appearance of redundant or pendulous skin (**Figure 2.21**). Wrinkles of skin develop prematurely and are often exaggerated, giving patients a characteristic "bloodhound" appearance. Exaggerated wrinkling of the facial skin and laxity of the earlobes are commonly initially encountered. Localized disease has been reported, limited to the fingertips (**Figure 2.22**) or face. The skin in acquired cutis laxa does not easily bruise or develop scars, as seen in Ehlers–Danlos syndrome (**Figure 2.23**).

Systemic Manifestations

In inherited cutis laxa, the loss of elastic tissue can result in several systemic manifestations. Herniation (inguinal and hiatal hernias) and diverticulosis of the gastrointestinal and urinary systems can occur. More catastrophically, vascular aneurysms such as aortic aneurysm or rupture can develop. Lung involvement typically presents as emphysema, whereas some patients may develop joint laxity, skeletal malformations, and osteopenia. Acquired cutis laxa has several causes, which are summarized in **Table 2.5**. Type I acquired cutis laxa is localized or generalized skin involvement with visceral organ involvement (pulmonary, cardiovascular, gastrointestinal, and urogenital). Type II acquired cutis laxa is without visceral organ involvement.

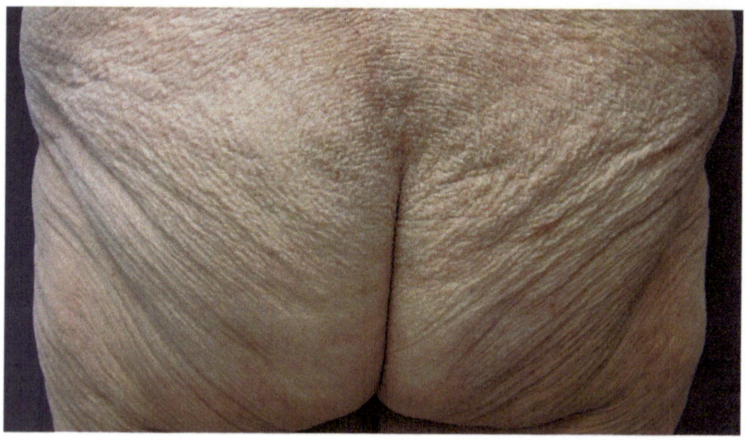

FIGURE 2.21 Acquired cutis laxa.

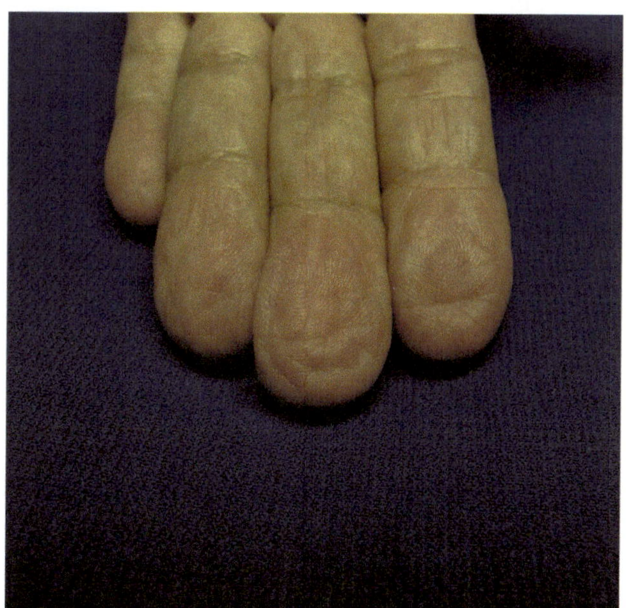

FIGURE 2.22 Acral localized acquired cutis laxa: Rheumatoid arthritis.

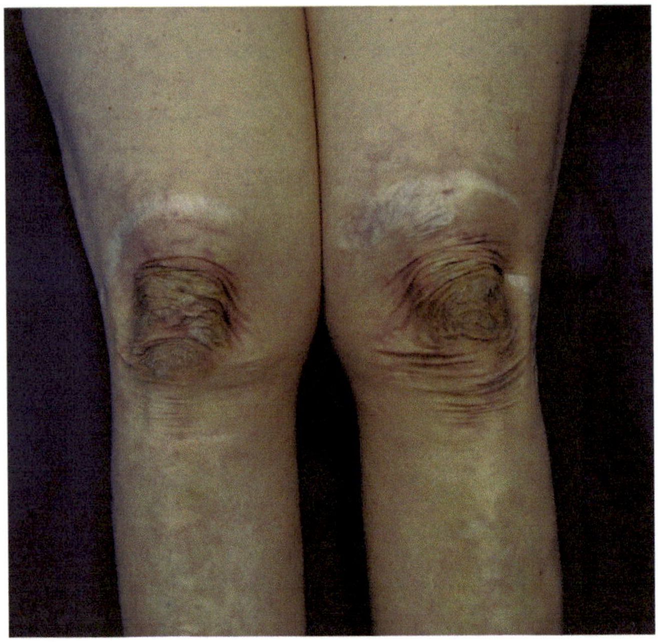

FIGURE 2.23 Ehlers–Danlos syndrome: Fish-mouth scarring.

Evaluation and Management

A skin biopsy with histologic loss of staining of elastin fibers can confirm the diagnosis. Workup of cutis laxa should include screening for possible connective tissue disease, including antinuclear antibodies (ANAs), complement 3 and 4 (C3/4), and rheumatoid factor (RF) if there is clinical suspicion. Complete blood count (CBC) with platelets and differential, chest X-ray (CXR), computed tomography (CT), serum protein electrophoresis/serum immunofixation electrophoresis (SPEP/SIFE), and urine protein electrophoresis/urine immunofixation electrophoresis (UPEP/UIFE) can be helpful in identifying lymphoma or multiple myeloma. A serum tryptase assessment is recommended if systemic mastocytosis is suspected. For possible infectious etiologies, it is important to obtain a sexual/travel/exposure history with laboratory testing with an RPR, Lyme titer, and stool/ova examination. Unfortunately, there is no medical treatment for acquired cutis laxa aside from identifying and treating the underlying disease or discontinuing medications. Surgical excision of pendulous or redundant skin can offer cosmetic improvement.

TABLE 2.5

Causes of Acquired Cutis Laxa
Inflammatory disorders
• Neutrophilic dermatoses
• Mastocytosis
• Urticaria
• Leukocytoclastic vasculitis
• Wells syndrome
• Sarcoidosis
• Rheumatoid arthritis
• Amyloidosis
• Systemic lupus erythematosus
• Marshall–Stickler syndrome
• Alpha 1- antitrypsin deficiency

(Continued)

TABLE 2.5 (*Continued*)

Causes of Acquired Cutis Laxa

Causes of Acquired Cutis Laxa
Neoplasia
• Multiple myeloma
• Lymphoma
Medications
• Penicillamine
• Penicillin
• Amoxicillin
• Escitalopram
• Sertraline
• Isoniazid
• Levonorgestrel intrauterine device
Infections
• Treponema
• Borrelia
• Onchocerca
• Toxocara

BIBLIOGRAPHY

Khodeir J, Ohanian P, Feghali J. Acquired cutis laxa: A clinical review. Int J Dermatol 2024;63(10): 1334–1356.

Mohamed M, Voet M, Gardeitchik T, et al. Cutis laxa. Adv Exp Med Biol 2014;802:161-184.

Peralta-Amaro AL, Quintal-Ramirez MJ, Esteban-Prado A, et al. Type I acquired cutis laxa: Report of a unique progressive case and short review. Am J Med Sci 2024;367(4):268–273.

Perforating Disorders

Etiopathogenesis

Acquired perforating disorders (APDs) comprise the perforating disorders that occur in adulthood and may present as elastosis perforans serpiginosa (EPS), reactive perforating collagenosis (RPC), perforating folliculitis (PF), or Kyrle disease. In all of these cases, an abnormal dermal component is extruded through the epidermis: elastic fibers, collagen, hair or follicular infundibulum, or keratin, respectively. Other inflammatory skin diseases can feature a secondary perforating phenomenon. The precise biochemical mechanism of action is unknown.

It is thought that local mechanical or chemical trauma resulting in a reactive but abnormal deposition of elastin, collagen, or keratin may trigger the perforating disorder. Microangiopathy is considered an etiology for APDs associated with diabetes. Medication-induced APDs have been reported with the use of biologic agents such as natalizumab, risankizumab, and necitumumab.

Clinical Manifestations

APDs clinically present as pruritic, keratotic papulonodular lesions. EPS features small flesh-colored to red papules that can be isolated or become confluent arcuate plaques. EPS lesions favor the face, upper trunk, and extremities. RPC starts as small firm papules that can quickly grow to a larger size and often feature a necrotic core. Lesions favor sites predisposed to trauma: the dorsum of hands, face, and extensor surfaces of extremities. Lesions of perforating folliculitis and Kyrle disease tend to appear on hair-bearing skin. These develop as folliculocentric firm papules with a keratotic central core and may have an entrapped hair.

Systemic Manifestations

APDs (**Figures 2.24** and **2.25**) are strongly associated with diabetes mellitus and chronic renal failure (diabetic nephropathy), especially for those undergoing hemodialysis or with a history of renal transplantation. Other associations include metabolic syndrome, atherosclerotic disease, hepatitis C, hypothyroidism, tuberculous lymphadenitis, and psoriasis. APDs may also occur in otherwise healthy patients. EPS has been associated with penicillamine therapy (**Figures 2.26** and **2.27**) and genodermatoses (Rothmund–Thomson syndrome, osteogenesis imperfecta, Marfan syndrome, Ehlers–Danlos syndrome, and Down syndrome). See **Table 2.6** for details.

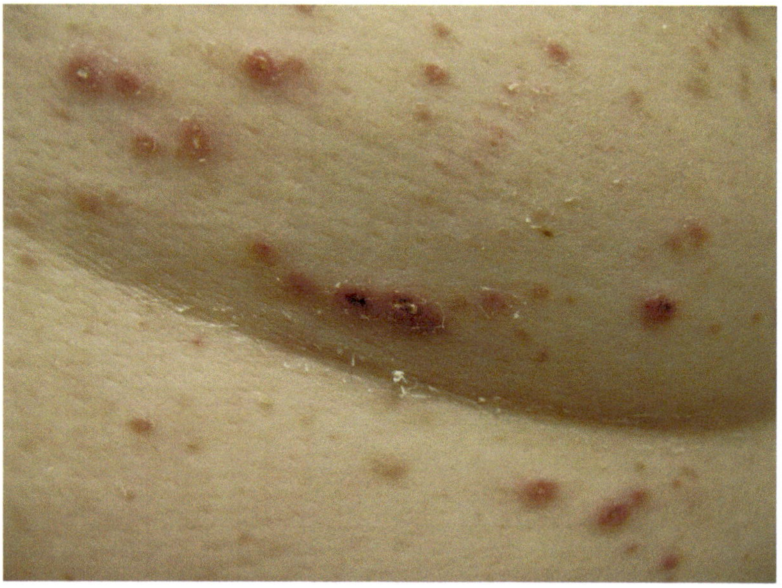

FIGURE 2.24 Acquired perforating disorder: Diabetes.

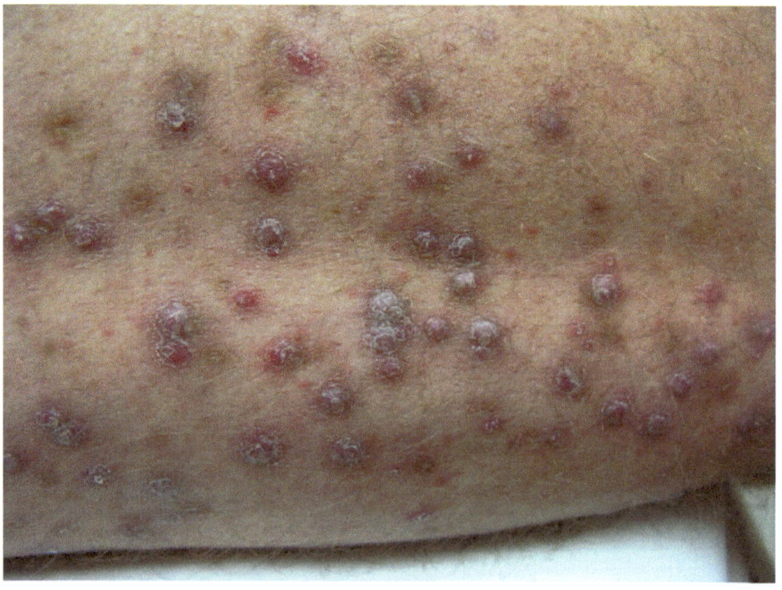

FIGURE 2.25 Acquired perforating disorder: Diabetic nephropathy.

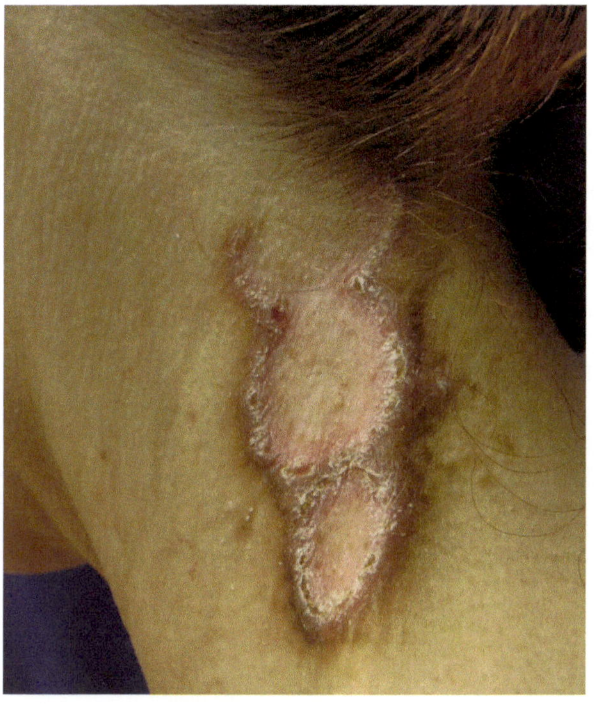

FIGURE 2.26 Acquired perforating disorder: Penicillamine-induced elastosis perforans serpiginosa.

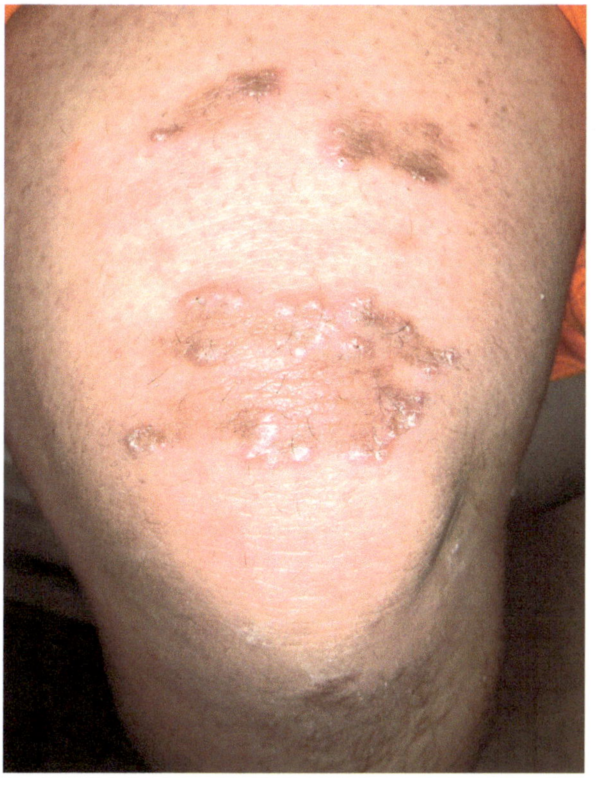

FIGURE 2.27 Acquired perforating disorder: Down syndrome-associated elastosis perforans serpiginosa.

Evaluation and Management

A skin biopsy can determine if perforation is occurring. Screening fasting blood glucose (FBG), hemoglobin A1c (HA1c), and renal function tests (RFTs) is prudent if there is no preceding history of glucose intolerance or chronic renal failure. Alternative testing may include thyroid function tests (TFTs), liver function tests (LFTs), Hep C, purified protein derivative (PPD), or QuantiFERON Gold. Treatment options tend to be limited for these disorders; however, a trial of topical or oral retinoids with keratolytics may aid in symptomatic relief. Systemic immunosuppression with mycophenolate mofetil and dupilumab has been reported as an effective treatment in some cases.

TABLE 2.6

Summary of Calcifying, Perforating, and Atrophic Disorders

Disorder	Clinical Features	Histologic Features	Associated Conditions
Anetoderma	Oval-shaped, flaccid plaques Can be atrophic or protuberant	Loss or fragmentation of elastic fibers	Anti-phospholipid antibody syndrome, SLE, hypercoagulable states
Atrophie blanche	Stellate, "porcelain white" scarring ulceration in chronic lesions	Microthrombi present in superficial vessels	Venous stasis, hypercoagulable states
Calcinosis cutis	Firm, dermal nodules Can be painless or tender	Fibrosis and calcification	Connective tissue disease
Calciphylaxis	Stellate, purpuric exquisitely tender indurated plaques In older lesions, ulceration may be present	Epidermal and dermal necrosis, calcification in the media of arterioles	End-stage renal disease
Cutis laxa	Loose, pliable skin	Loss of elastic tissue	Sarcoidosis, amyloidosis, RA, SLE, multiple myeloma, lymphoma
Perforating disorders	Pruritic, hyperkeratotic papules and nodules	Transepidermal elimination of collagen, elastin	Diabetes, metabolic syndrome, hepatitis, chronic renal failure

BIBLIOGRAPHY

Guo L, Zeng YP, Jin HZ. Reactive perforating collagenosis treated with dupilumab: A case report and literature review. Dermatol Ther 2022;35(12):e15916.

Harabaoui S, Litaiem N. Acquired perforating dermatosis. In StatPearls [internet]. Treasure Island (Fl): StatPearls Publishing; 2023.

Nieto-Benito LM, Pulido-Pérez A, Bergón-Sendín M. Acquired perforating dermatosis: A sign of systemic disease. Actas Dermosifiliogr 2021;112(Suppl 1):4.

3

Connective Tissue Disorders

Behcet's Syndrome

Etiopathogenesis

Behcet's syndrome (BS) is an autoimmune disorder of unknown etiology that causes systemic vasculitis. The disease is unique for causing a combination of arterial and venous inflammation affecting all vessel types (aorta to superficial veins), leading to impairment of activities of daily living and mortality. Although seen primarily through the Mediterranean to the Middle East, it has occurred worldwide. Men and women are equally affected; however, males may have more severe disease. The strongest genetic associations are with human leukocyte antigen (HLA)-B51 and the endoplasmic reticulum aminopeptidase 1 (ERAP1). NK cells and M1 polarized macrophages may be associated with inflammation. Neutrophilic activation and formation of neutrophil extracellular traps cause vascular thrombosis. Lymphatic vessel endothelial hyaluronan receptor 1 and podoplanin causing lymphangiogenesis may be the cause of uveitis.

Clinical Manifestations

The diagnostic criteria for BS include recurrent oral ulcerations (minor, major, or herpetiform aphthous ulceration recurring every 3 months over a 12-month period [**Figure 3.1**]) and at least two of the following: recurrent genital ulceration (**Figure 3.2**), eye inflammation, positive pathergy test (**Figure 3.3**), or other skin lesions (erythema nodosum, pseudofolliculitis, papulopustular, or acneiform lesions).

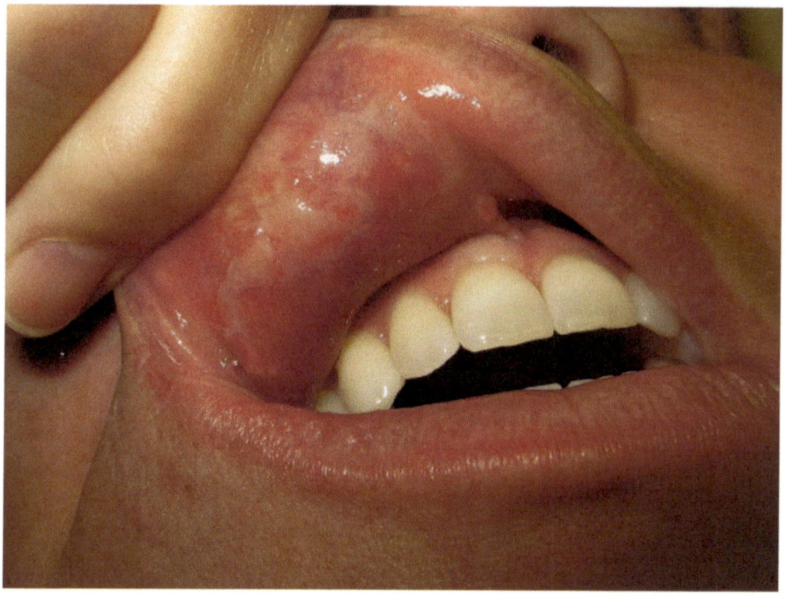

FIGURE 3.1 Behcet's syndrome: Oral aphthous.

DOI: 10.1201/9781003492665-3

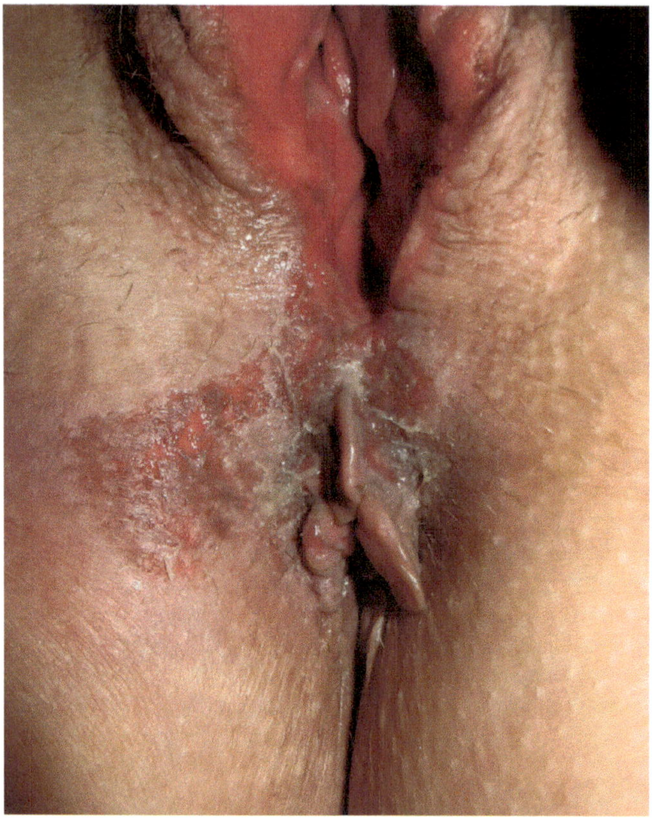

FIGURE 3.2 Behcet's syndrome: Anogenital ulcerations.

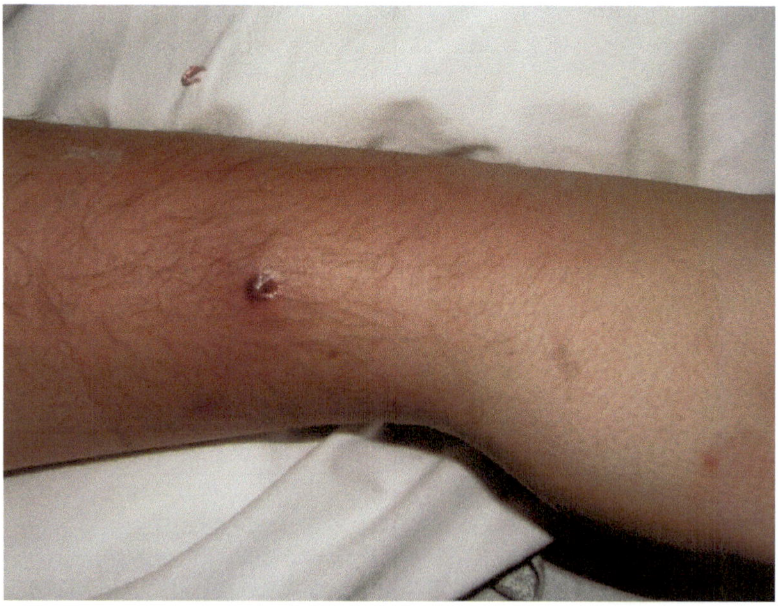

FIGURE 3.3 Behcet's syndrome: Pathergy.

Systemic Manifestations

Ocular inflammation from panuveitis may lead to rapid visual decline. Eventual ocular hypertension, cataracts, and retinal vasculitis may lead to blindness. Patients may develop arthritis/arthralgias. Involvement of the central nervous system (parenchymal inflammation and cerebral venous sinus thrombosis) may cause severe headaches, pyramidal signs, hemiparesis, mood changes, sphincter incompetence, and sensorineural hearing loss. BS is a procoagulant state with increased risk for deep venous thrombosis and arterial aneurysm (aorta and pulmonary artery). Diarrhea, abdominal pain, and rectal bleeding suggest gastrointestinal (GI) disease.

Evaluation and Management

Recurring episodes of oral/genital ulcerations with systemic symptoms should raise concern for BS. Complex aphthous may appear with similar ulcerations, but patients do not manifest ocular or systemic symptoms. A multispecialty approach with rheumatology and ophthalmology is often required to confirm the diagnosis. There is no standard serologic biomarker for the disease, but HLA-B51 can be ordered (only positive 20% of the time). Pathergy positivity may be increased using patient salvia or the pneumococcal vaccine. Treatment consists of immunosuppressive agents that include corticosteroids, colchicine, azathioprine, cyclosporine, interferon-alpha, cyclophosphamide, apremilast, anti-tumor necrosis factor (TNF) agents, and anti-interleukin-1 (IL-1), 6, 17, 23 inhibitors. Cyclosporine should be avoided in patients with neurologic involvement.

BIBLIOGRAPHY

Emmi G, Bettiol A, Hatemi G, et al. Behcet's syndrome. Lancet 2024;403(10431):1093–1108.

Hatemi G, Seyahi E, Fresko I, et al. Behcet's syndrome: One year in review 2023. Clin Exp Rheumatol 2023;41(10):1945–1954.

Hatemi G, Ucar D, Uygunoglu U, et al. Behcet syndrome. Rheum Dis Clin North Am 2023;49(3):585–602.

Dermatomyositis

Etiopathogenesis

Dermatomyositis (DMM) is an idiopathic inflammatory myopathy (IIM) of unknown etiology that involves a cytokine-mediated (upregulation of type I interferon pathways) lymphocytic process that damages muscle and skin. In addition, myositis autoantigens drive a B-cell antigen-specific immune response in muscles. The subsequent development of myositis-specific autoantibodies is specific to diseases within the spectrum of IIM.

Clinical Manifestations

Patients present with pruritic rash, fatigue, and muscle weakness. Proximal muscle strength is easily overcome on resistance testing. Pathognomonic skin findings include Gottron's papules (violaceous papules over interphalangeal joints [**Figure 3.4**]) and Gottron's signs (violaceous erythema along the hands, elbows, knees [**Figure 3.5**], and lateral thighs). Other characteristic findings include scalp rash with a nonscarring alopecia (**Figure 3.6**), heliotrope rash (violaceous erythema with edema of eyelids [**Figures 3.7** and **3.8**]), shawl sign (violaceous macular erythema around neck and back that may develop a sandpaper-like texture [**Figures 3.9–3.11**]), Samitz's sign (ragged cuticles with globular telangiectasia in proximal nail fold [**Figure 3.12**]), and mechanics' hands, which refers to scales and roughness of the lateral digits (**Figure 3.13**). Secondary changes often include poikiloderma, bullae, erosions, and calcinosis cutis. Wong's DMM (**Figure 3.14**) refers to an overlap between pityriasis rubra pilaris and DMM.

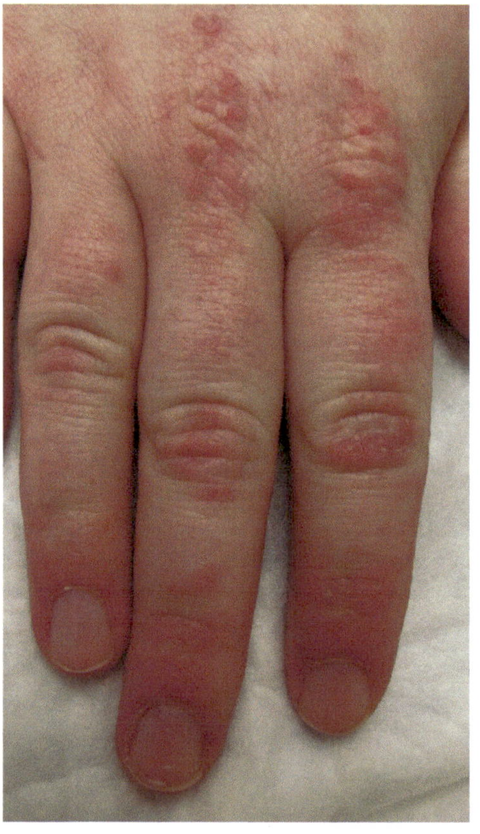

FIGURE 3.4 Dermatomyositis: Gottron's papules.

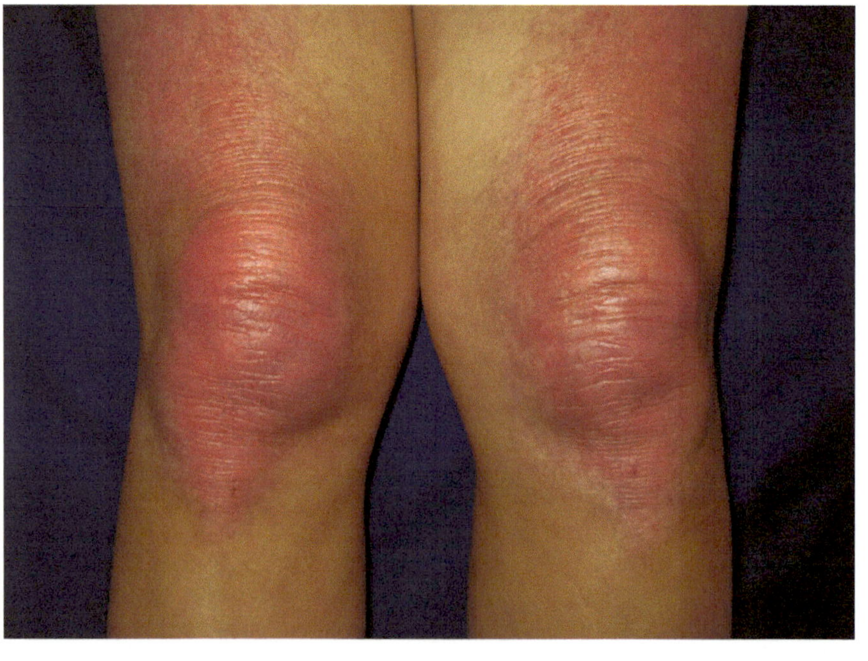

FIGURE 3.5 Dermatomyositis: Gottron's sign.

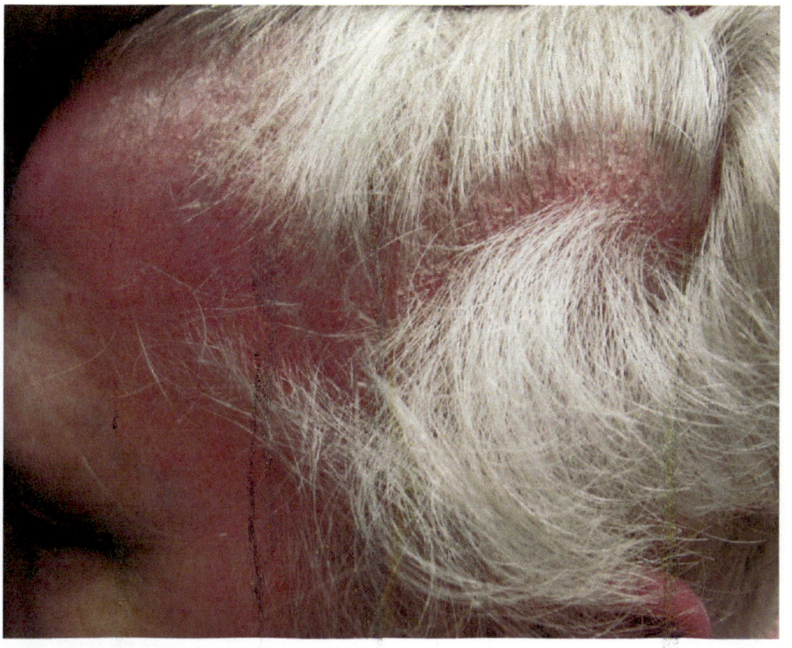

FIGURE 3.6 Dermatomyositis: Scalp.

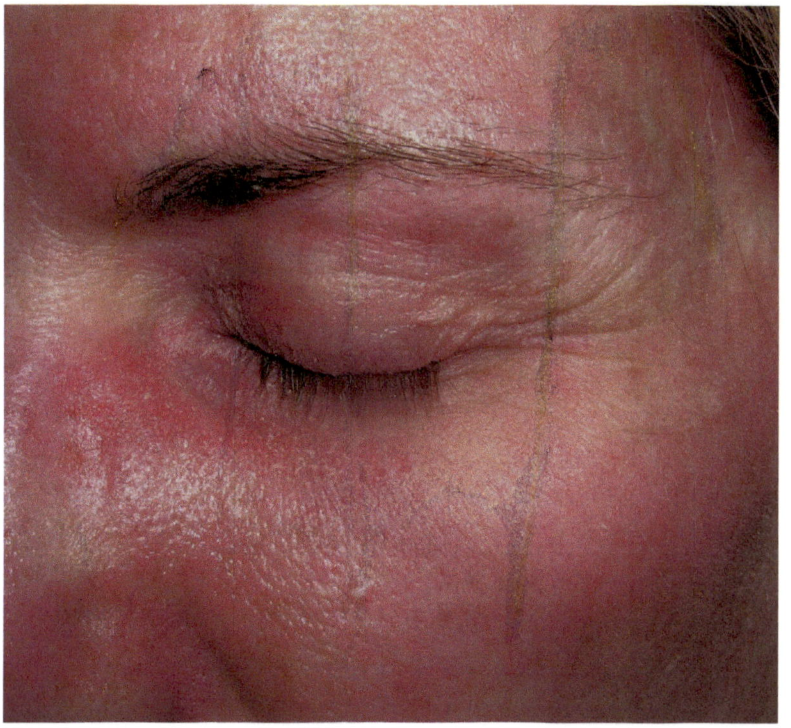

FIGURE 3.7 Dermatomyositis: Heliotrope rash.

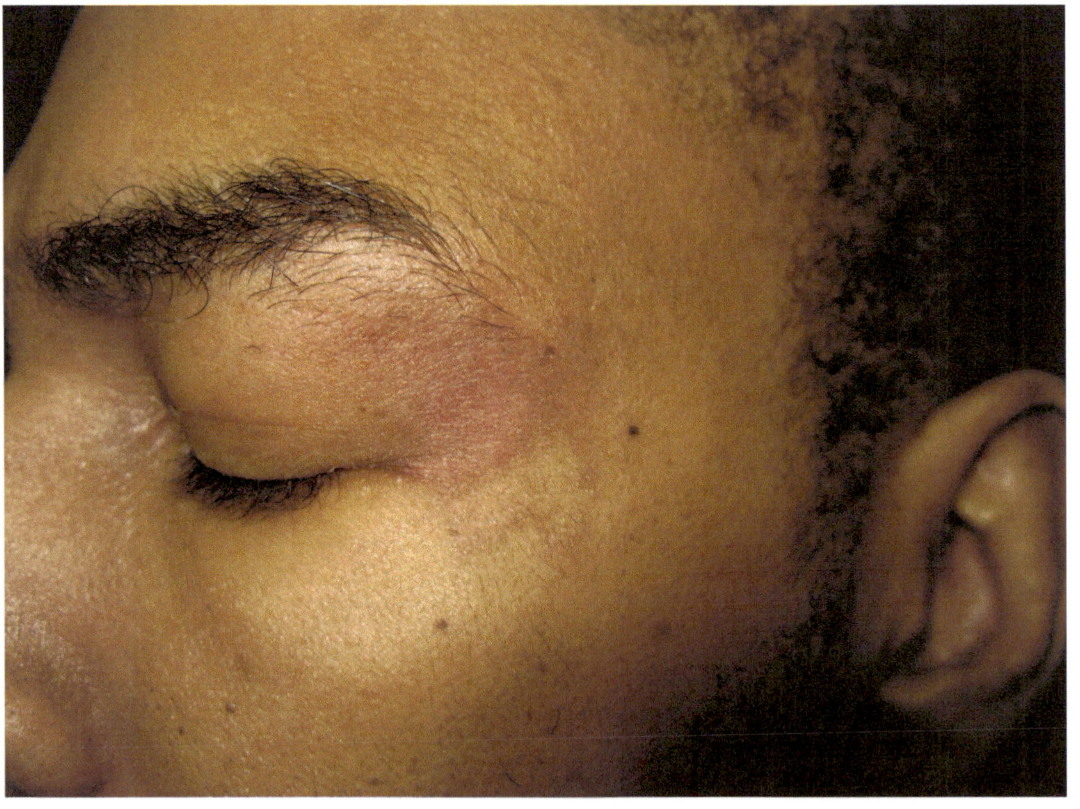

FIGURE 3.8 Dermatomyositis: Heliotrope rash.

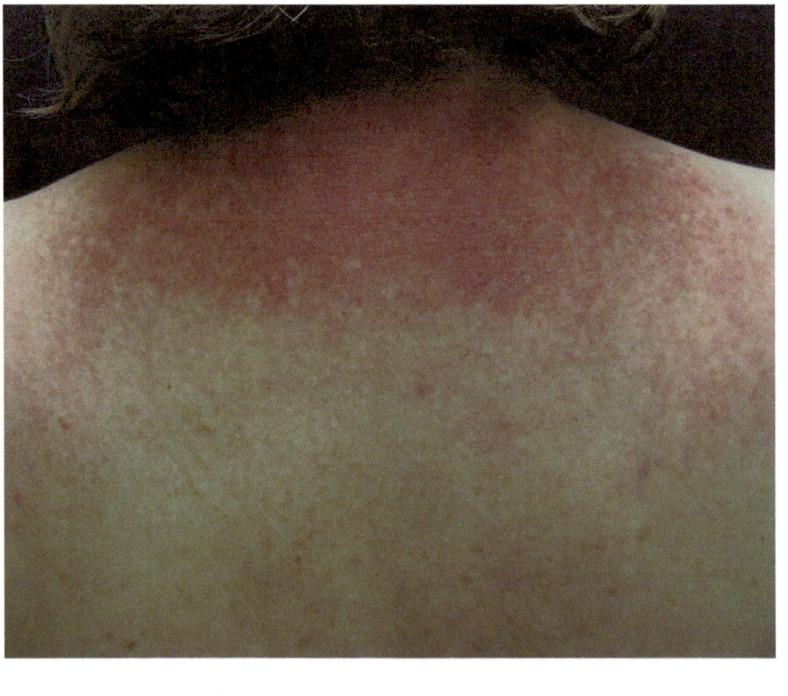

FIGURE 3.9 Dermatomyositis: Shawl sign.

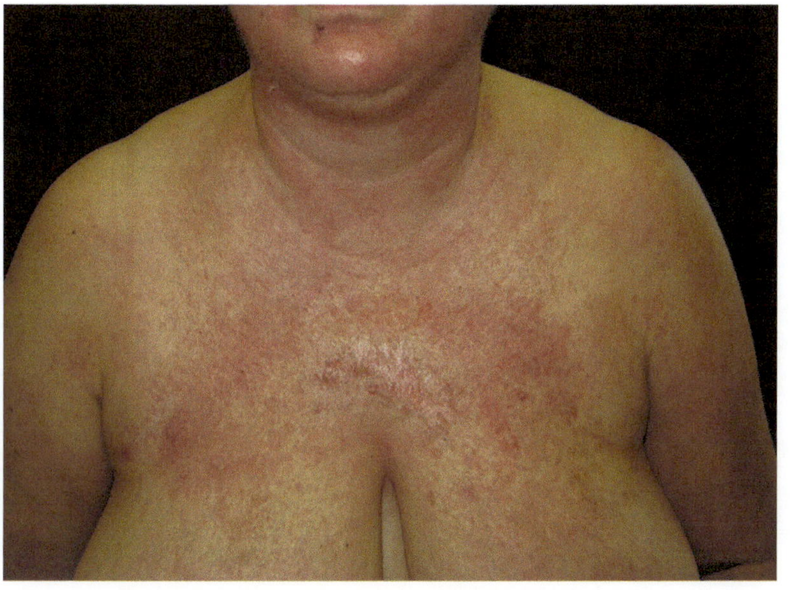

FIGURE 3.10 Dermatomyositis: Poikilodermatous shawl sign.

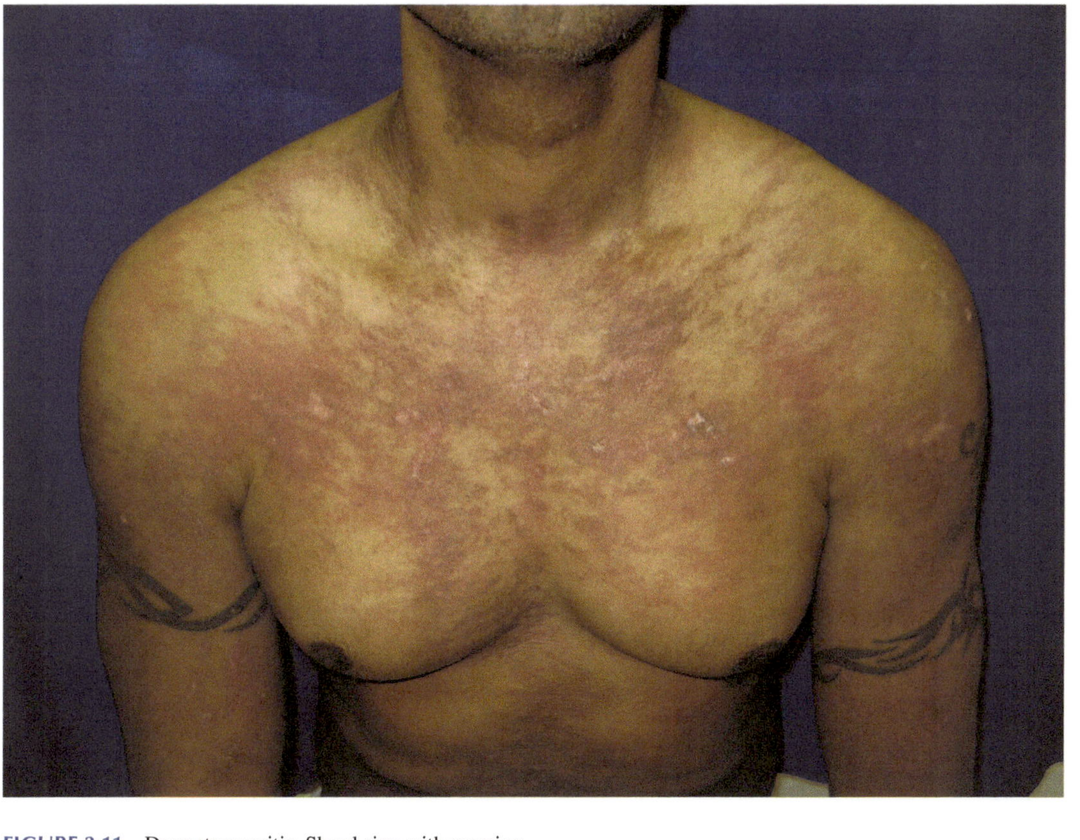

FIGURE 3.11 Dermatomyositis: Shawl sign with scarring.

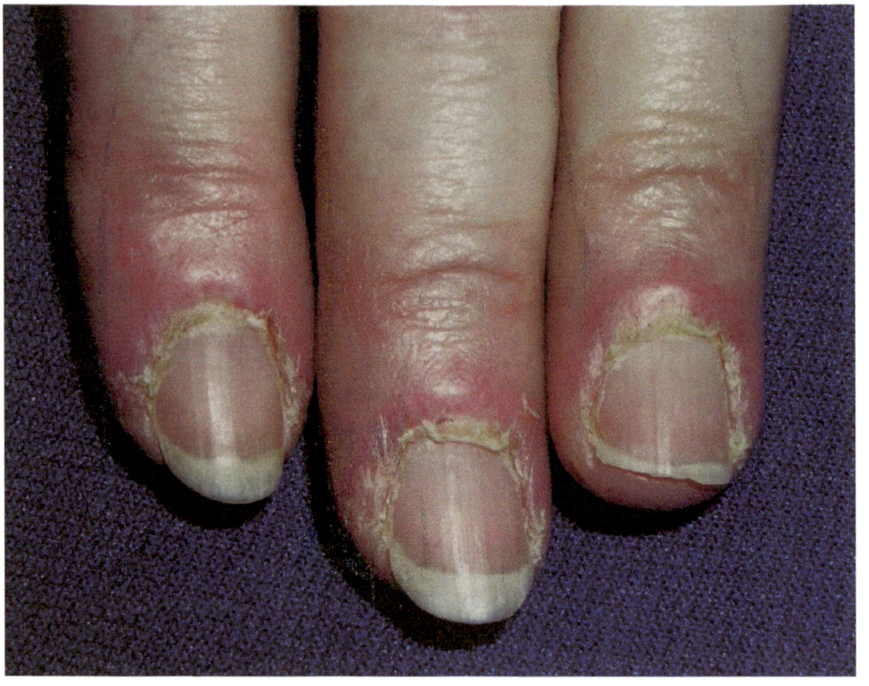

FIGURE 3.12 Dermatomyositis: Samitz's sign.

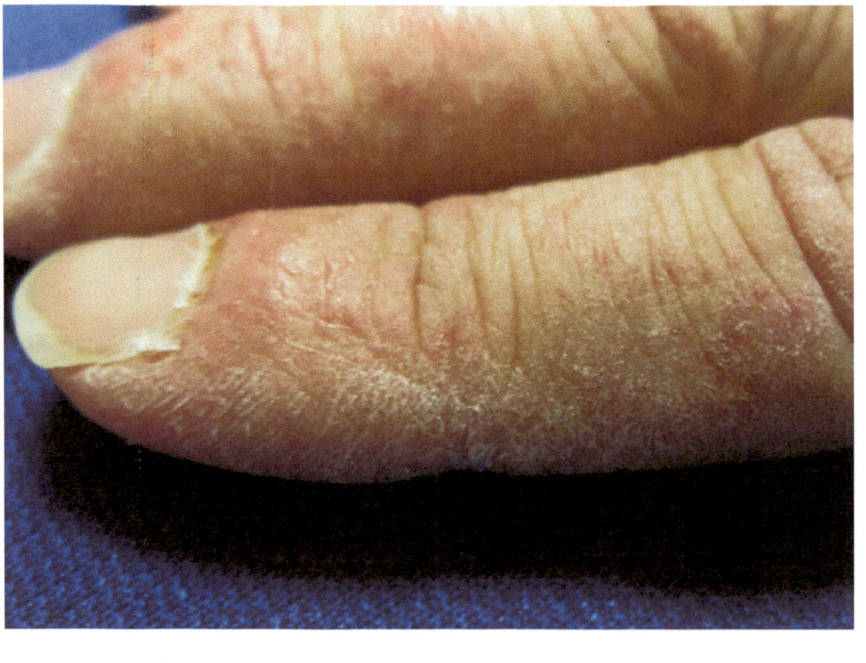

FIGURE 3.13 Dermatomyositis: Mechanics' hands.

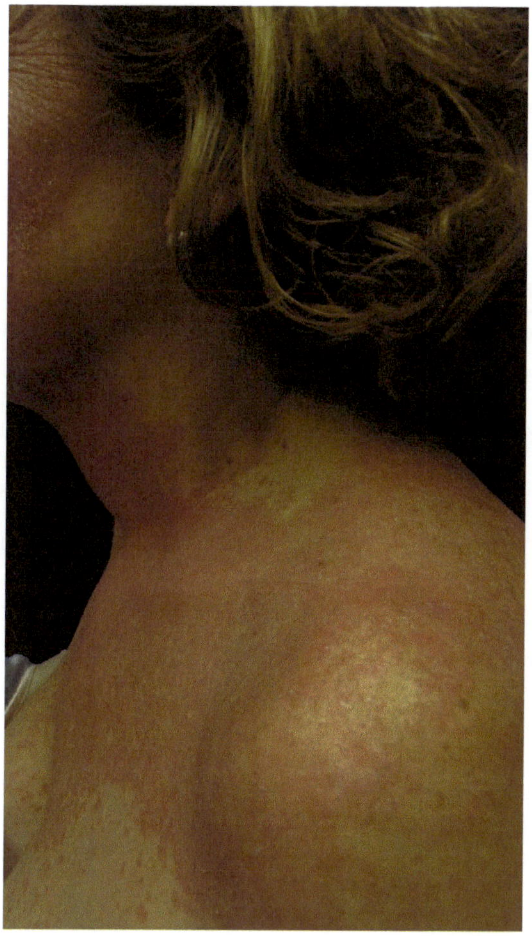

FIGURE 3.14 Dermatomyositis: Wong's type.

Systemic Manifestations

The extent of muscle inflammation varies from classic DMM to clinically amyopathic DMM. However, both are considered paraneoplastic syndromes, with 25% having or developing an adenocarcinoma (ovarian cancer—most common in women; lung cancer—most in men; and nasopharyngeal cancer—southeastern Asian patients). Anti-transcription intermediary factor 1 (anti-TIF1-γ; anti-p155) antibodies are associated with increased risk of cancer, whereas anti-Mi-2 antibodies are associated with a better prognosis. Patients may develop significant pulmonary morbidity from interstitial lung disease (ILD) if positive for anti-Jo1, anti-melanoma differentiation-associated protein 5 (anti-MDA5), or anti-clinically amyopathic dermatomyositis (anti-CADM-140) antibodies. Post-myopathic DMM (skin predominate disease despite control of muscle disease) occurs in 40% of classic DMM.

Evaluation and Management

A thorough history and physical review of age-appropriate malignancy screening is indicated. Skin biopsy with immunohistochemical staining for PMAC can help differentiate DMM from cutaneous lupus. A pan-computed tomography (CT) of chest/abdomen/pelvis and transvaginal pelvic ultrasound in females may look for occult disease not identified from initial screening. Some institutions monitor blood counts, myositis-specific antibodies (**Table 3.1**), and tumor markers (CA-125, CA19-9). A consultation to otolaryngology is recommended in DMM patients with southeastern Asian ethnicity. Malignancy screening should be done annually for 3–5 years. Screening for ILD is done with a pulmonary function test (PFT) with diffuse lung capacity carbon monoxide (DLCO). If there is a decrease in DLCO, a consultation with a pulmonologist for management is prudent. Treatment consists of topical corticosteroids and calcineurin inhibitors with strict photoprotection. Stepwise progression for systemic therapy includes methotrexate, mycophenolate mofetil, intravenous immunoglobulin (IVIG), anti-TNF agents, rituximab, plasmapheresis, and Janus kinase/signal transducer of activation (JAK/STAT) inhibitors.

TABLE 3.1

Myositis-Specific Autoantibodies

Antibody	Characteristics
Anti-Mi2	Classic skin presentation Responds to treatment
Anti-MDA5 (Anti-CADMI40)	Cutaneous ulcerations Interstitial lung disease
Anti-NXP-2	Classic skin presentations Calcinosis cutis
Anti-TIFI1-γ	Severe cutaneous disease Malignancy
Anti-SAE1/2	Severe cutaneous disease Skin ulcers, dysphagia
Anti Jo-1, PL-7, PL-12	Mechanics hands Interstitial lung disease

BIBLIOGRAPHY

Cassard L, Seraly N, Riegert M, et al. Dermatomyositis: Practical guidance and unmet needs. Immunotargets Ther 2024;13:151–172.

Lu X, Peng Q, Wang G. Anti-MDA5 antibody-positive dermatomyositis: Pathogenesis and clinic progress. Nat Rev Rheumatol 2024;20(1):48–62.

Pandya R, Fleitsch J, Lim D, et al. Clinical characteristic and symptom progression of dermatomyositis subtypes: A retrospective analysis of a prospective database. J Am Acad Dermatol 2024;91(1):31–36.

Sevim E, Kobrin D, Casal-Dominquez M, et al. A comprehensive review of dermatomyositis treatments – From rediscovered classics to promising horizons. Expert Rev Clin Immunol 2024;20(2):197–209.

Lupus Erythematosus

Etiopathogenesis

Lupus erythematosus (LE) is an autoimmune condition with a spectrum of skin lesions, systemic disease, or a combination of both. In genetically susceptible patients (HLA-DRB1*0301/1501), ultraviolet light induces an accumulation of apoptotic cells that activate proinflammatory cytokines (interferon-α, TNF-α), causing activation of B and T lymphocytes with plasmacytoid and myeloid dendritic cell production of B-cell-dependent antibody production that produced the skin lesions of acute lupus erythematosus (ACLE), subacute lupus erythematosus (SCLE), and chronic cutaneous lupus erythematosus (CCLE).

Clinical Manifestations

CCLE may present in several forms. Discoid LE (DLE) presents with localized (**Figures 3.15** and **3.16**), generalized, and hypertrophic erythematous plaques (**Figures 3.17–3.19**) with follicular plugging, dyschromia, hyperkeratosis, atrophy, and scarring on the scalp, ears, head, neck, and upper torso. Lupus panniculitis induces indurated plaques on the upper extremities and face. If there is an overlying DLE, it is referred to as lupus profundus. LE tumidus (**Figures 3.20–3.22**) presents as indurated to boggy erythematous plaques due to extensive mucin deposition in the dermis. Acral LE may present with violaceous papules of perniosis (chilblains LE [**Figure 3.23**]), atrophic macules of Degos-like (livedo vasculopathy) CCLE (**Figure 3.24**), periungual telangiectasia, livedo reticularis, and Raynaud's phenomenon. SCLE is a photodistributed eruption presenting with psoriasiform annular to polycyclic plaques (**Figure 3.25**). Drug-induced SCLE (i.e., thiazides, terbinafine [**Figure 3.26**]) most often appears like SCLE. ACLE is a malar rash (**Figure 3.27**) in patients presenting with an active flare of systemic lupus erythematosus (SLE).

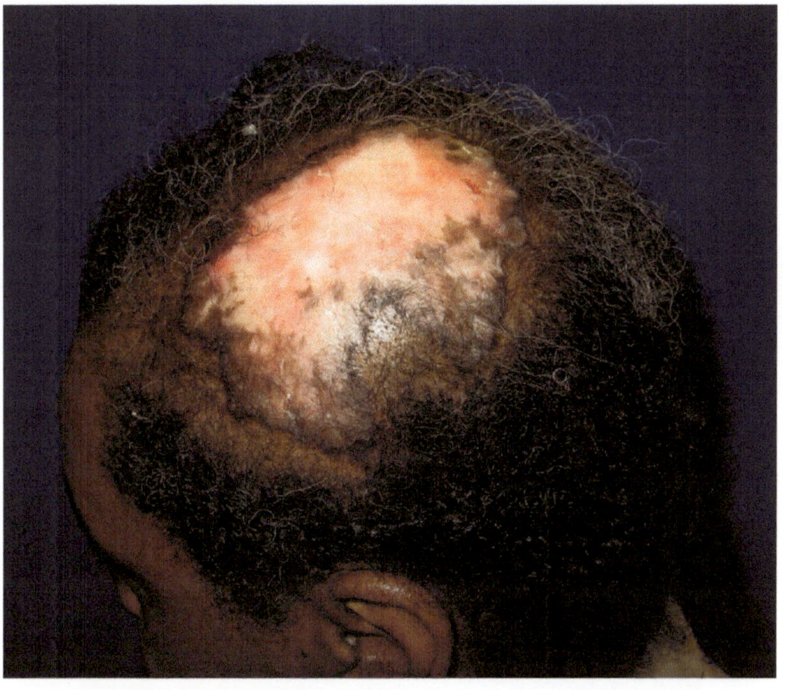

FIGURE 3.15 Localized discoid lupus erythematosus.

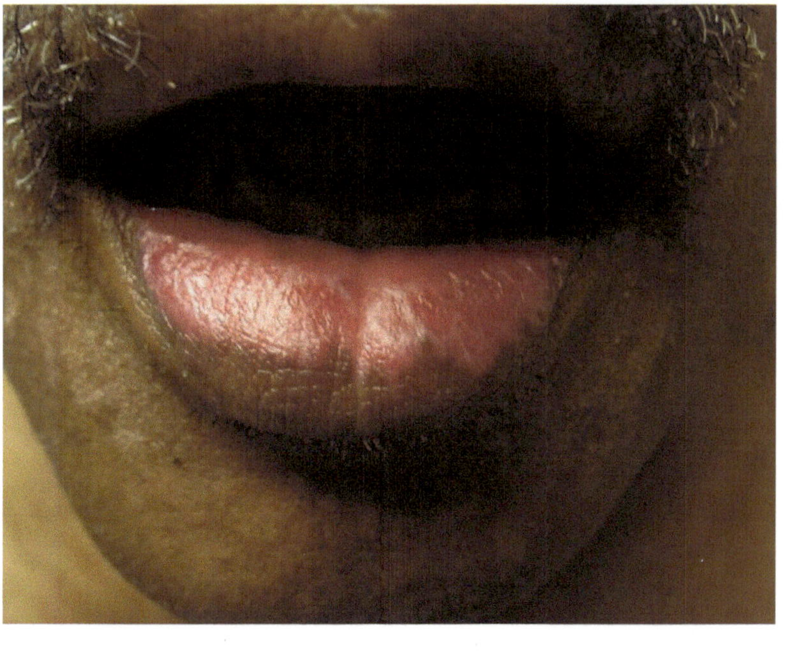

FIGURE 3.16 Localized discoid lupus erythematosus.

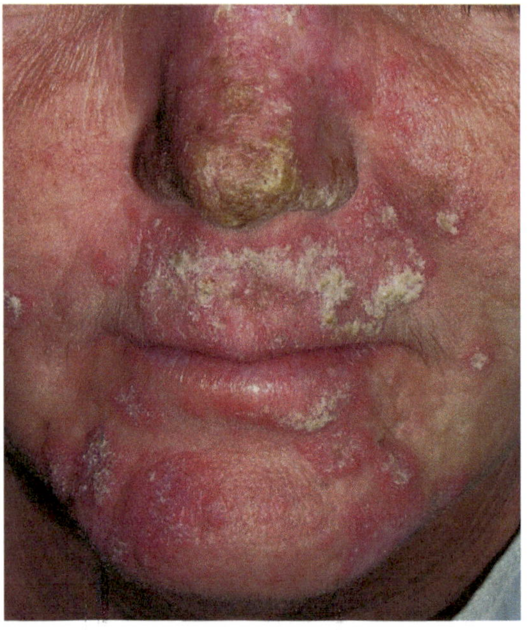

FIGURE 3.17 Hypertrophic discoid lupus erythematosus.

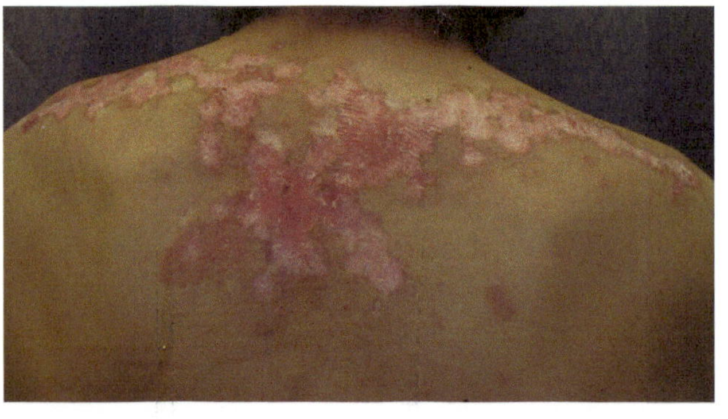

FIGURE 3.18 Generalized discoid lupus erythematosus.

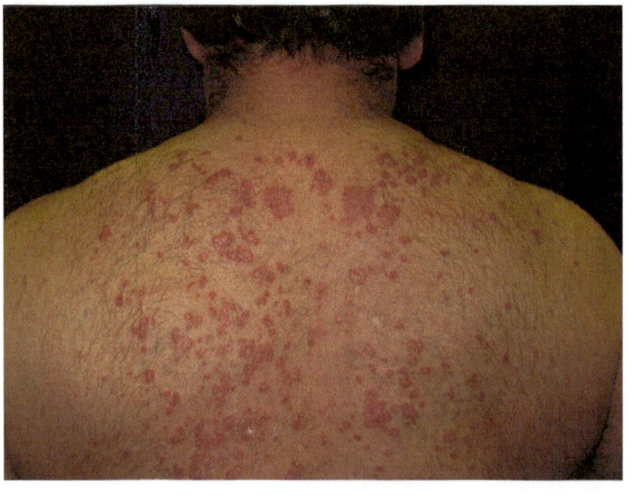

FIGURE 3.19 Generalized hypertrophic discoid lupus erythematosus.

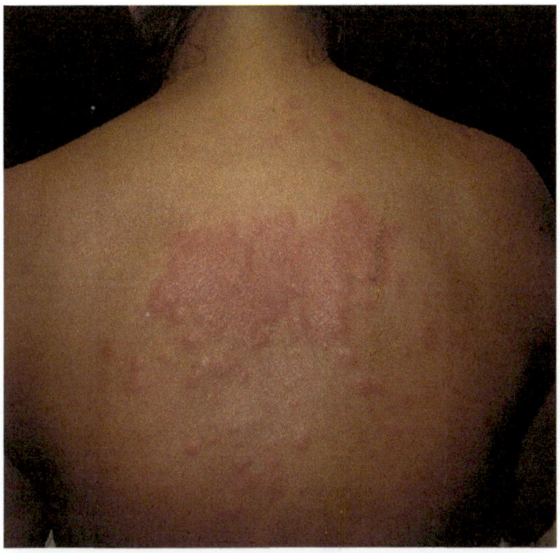

FIGURE 3.20 Lupus erythematosus tumidus.

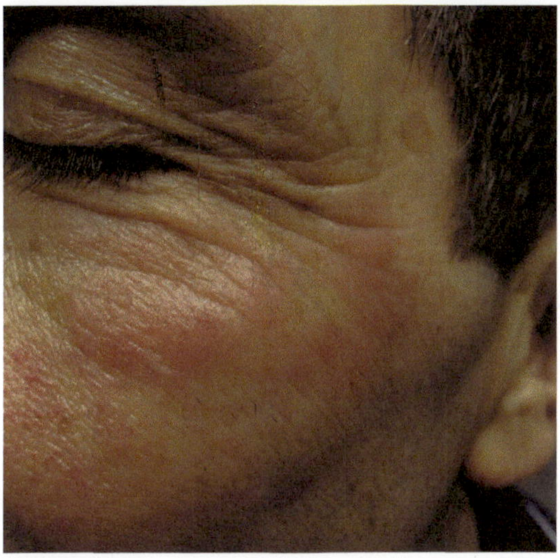

FIGURE 3.21 Lupus erythematosus tumidus.

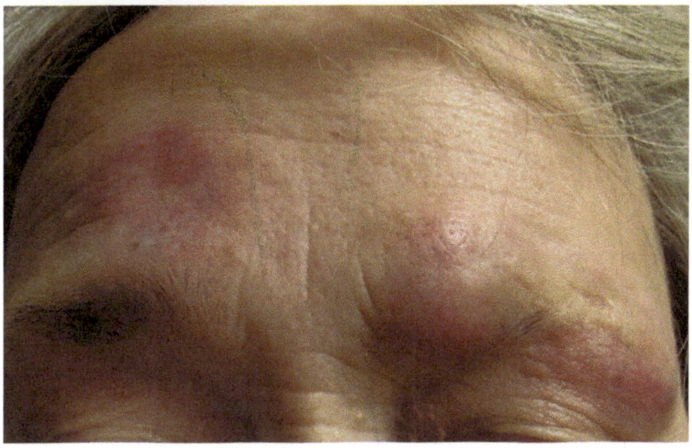

FIGURE 3.22 Lupus erythematosus tumidus with lupus panniculitis.

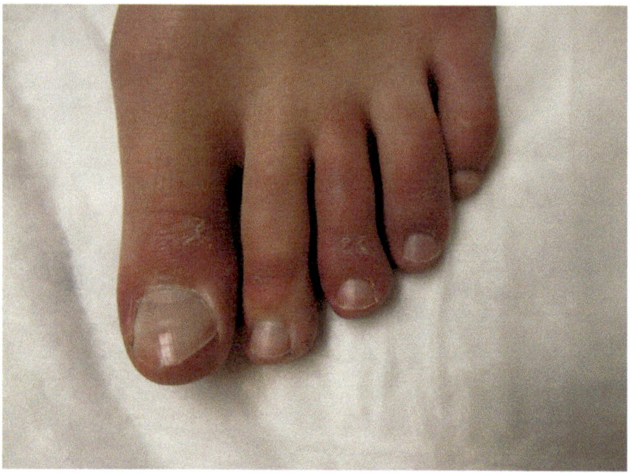

FIGURE 3.23 Chilblains lupus erythematosus.

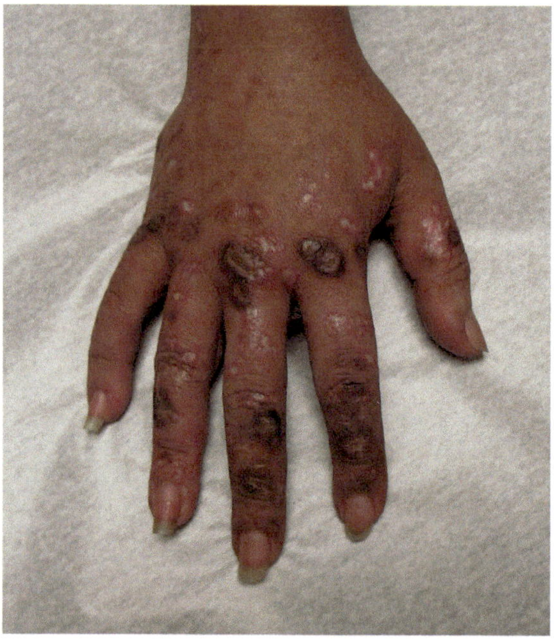

FIGURE 3.24 Acral chronic cutaneous lupus erythematosus with livedo vasculopathy (Degos-like).

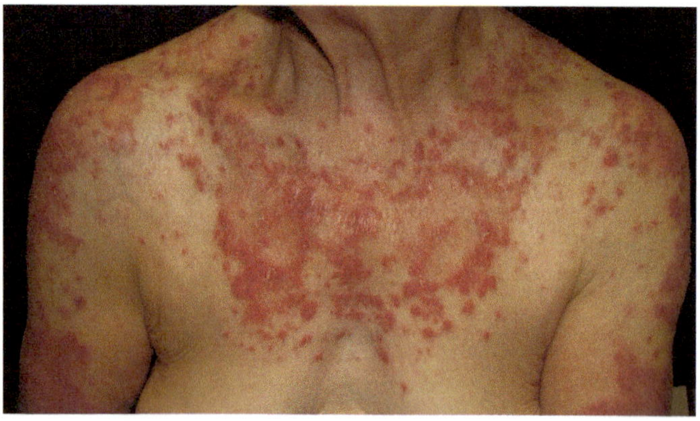

FIGURE 3.25 Subacute cutaneous lupus erythematosus.

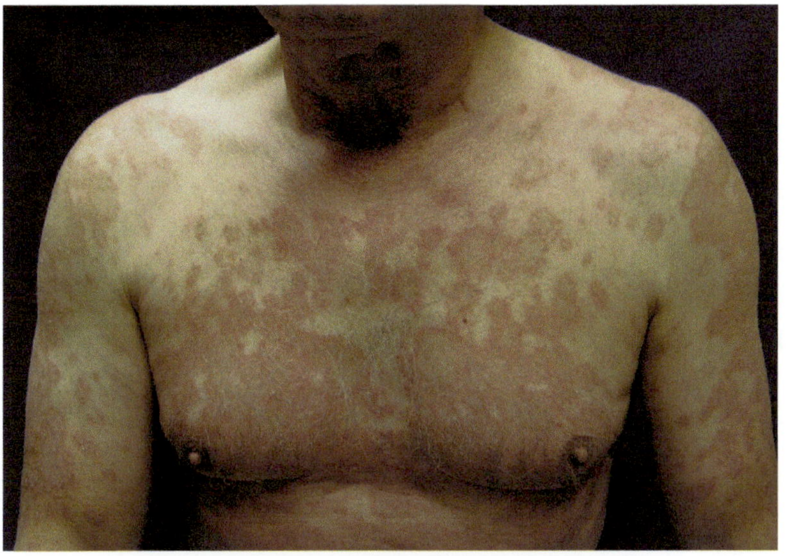

FIGURE 3.26 Drug-induced subacute cutaneous lupus erythematosus: Terbinafine.

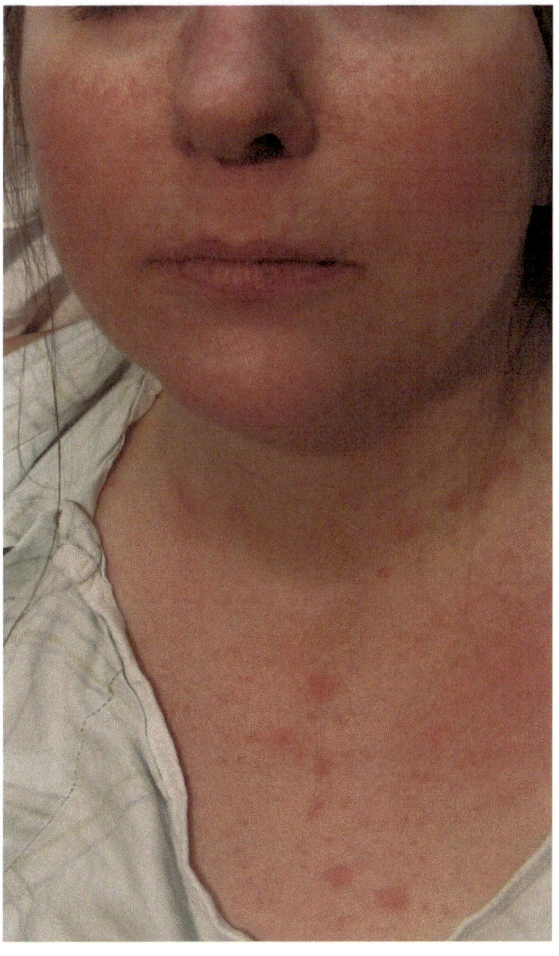

FIGURE 3.27 Acute cutaneous lupus erythematosus.

Systemic Manifestations

One hundred percent of patients with ACLE have SLE with concurrent oral ulcers, arthritis, serositis, glomerulonephritis, cerebritis, or bone marrow suppression. Up to 25% of patients with generalized DLE develop SLE, and indicators include periungual telangiectasia, anemia, leukopenia, arthralgias/arthritis, elevated erythrocyte sedimentation rate, and antinuclear antibodies. Localized DLE patients have a 5% chance of developing SLE. Seventy percent of DLE patients that develop SLE will do so within 5 years of diagnosis. Ten percent of SCLE patients are at risk for developing SLE. Patients with livedo reticularis, nonhealing leg ulcers, anetoderma, and pseudovasculitis lesions may have associated antiphospholipid antibodies and risk for thromboembolic disease. TNF-α has demonstrated the potential as a biomarker for ACLE.

Evaluation and Management

Cutaneous LE patients need a history and physical review of signs and symptoms of SLE. A skin biopsy will demonstrate vacuolar interface dermatitis, with thickened basement membrane and intense periadnexal/vascular lymphocytic infiltrate. Initial and annual lab testing for complete blood count (CBC), liver function test (LFT), renal function test (RFT), urinalysis (UA), complement 3 and 4 (C3/4), antinuclear antibodies (ANA), anti-double-stranded DNA (dsDNA), anti-Smith antibodies (Sm), and anti-Ro/SSA and anti-La/SSB antibodies (Ro/La) is recommended. Refer to rheumatology as needed. Management includes sun protection and sunscreens, including topical steroids or calcineurin inhibitors, in addition to oral steroids, antimalarials, nonsteroidal immunosuppressants/modulators (methotrexate, azathioprine, mycophenolate mofetil, dapsone, thalidomide), or biologic agents (IVIG, rituximab, belimumab, anifrolumab, litifilimab), based on severity.

BIBLIOGRAPHY

Gunther C, Wenzel J. Lupus erythematosus. J Dtsch Dermatol Ges 2023;21(4):426–430.

Jinshan Z, Yong Q, Fangpi C, et al. The role of TNF-α as a potential marker for acute lupus erythematosus in patients with systemic lupus erythematosus. J Dermatol 2024;51(11):1481–1491.

Nieble D, de Vos L, Fetter T, et al. Cutaneous lupus erythematosus: An update on pathogenesis and future therapeutic directions. Am J Clin Dermatol 2023;24(4):521–540.

Zhou W, Wu H, Zhao M, et al. New insights into the progression from cutaneous lupus to systemic lupus erythematosus. Expert Rev Clin Immunol 2020;16(8):829–837.

Psoriasis and Psoriatic Arthritis

Etiopathogenesis

Psoriasis is a chronic inflammatory disorder of the skin and joints. The etiology is unknown, but is thought to occur when some trigger (physical trauma, bacterial product, cellular stress) causes DNA release from keratinocytes. This leads to activation of myeloid dendritic cells, which speeds keratinocyte proliferation and initiates a systemic inflammatory reaction.

Clinical Manifestations

Localized, guttate, generalized (**Figures 3.28** and **3.29**), and inverse psoriasis presents with pink-to-red plaques of various size and scale with a relatively symmetric distribution. Psoriasis can also affect the nails, causing nail pitting, oil spotting, and onycholysis. Erythrodermic psoriasis presents as generalized erythema associated with desquamation, hair loss, and nail dystrophy. Pustular psoriasis, localized to hands/feet/nails (**Figures 3.30** and **3.31**) or generalized (**Figure 3.32**), presents large collections of sterile confluent pustules with erythema and/or scaling. Psoriatic arthritis can affect any joint with mild to severe erosive arthropathy (**Figures 3.33** and **3.34**). Psoriatic nailing pitting and crumbling is associated with development of psoriatic arthritis.

Systemic Manifestations

Psoriasis (early onset, extensive) is associated with a metabolic syndrome (hypertension, hyperlipidemia, obesity, and glucose intolerance) from chronically elevated levels of Th1 and Th17 cytokines with subsequent risk for cardiac and peripheral vascular disease. Other diseases that are seen more frequently with psoriasis include diabetes, fatty liver disease, Crohn's disease, ulcerative colitis, lymphoma, fibromyalgia, and depression. Pustular and erythrodermic psoriasis may present with signs of electrolyte imbalance, protein wasting, and high cardiac output failure. Pustular psoriasis may occur initially in pregnancy or chronic psoriasis patients who have been tapered off steroids too rapidly. Hypocalcemia classically occurs with pustular psoriasis. Localized pustular psoriasis has been associated with autoimmune thyroiditis, gluten enteropathy, biologic agents, smoking, and SAPHO syndrome (synovitis, acne [**Figure 3.35**], pustulosis, hyperostosis, osteitis).

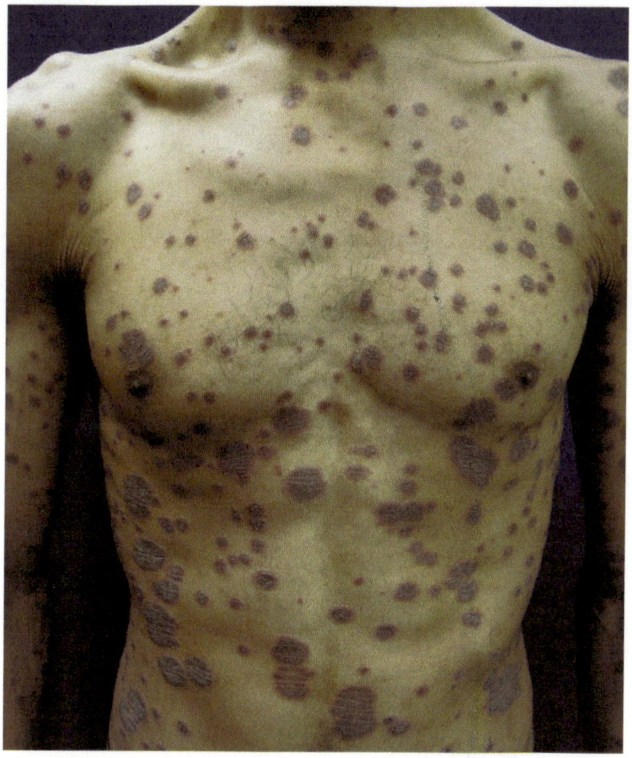

FIGURE 3.28 Psoriasis: Early/extensive.

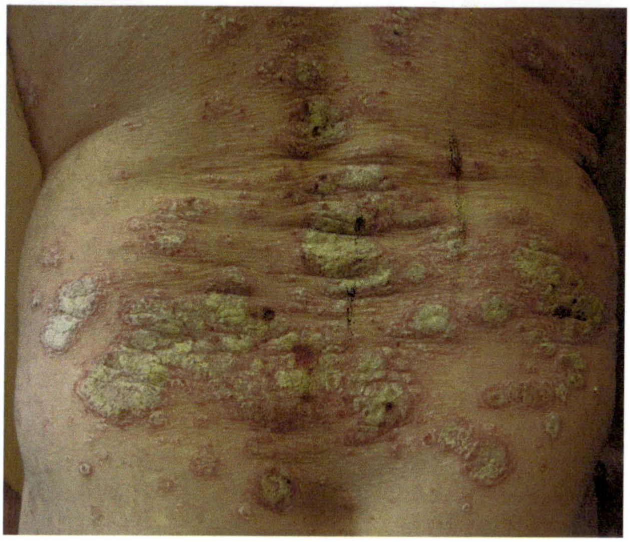

FIGURE 3.29 Psoriasis: Metabolic syndrome.

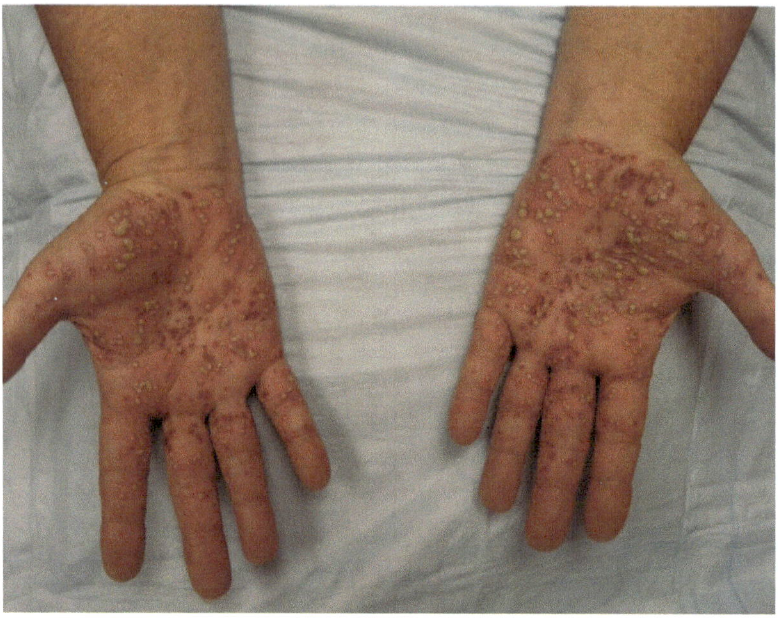

FIGURE 3.30 Psoriasis: Localized palmar pustular.

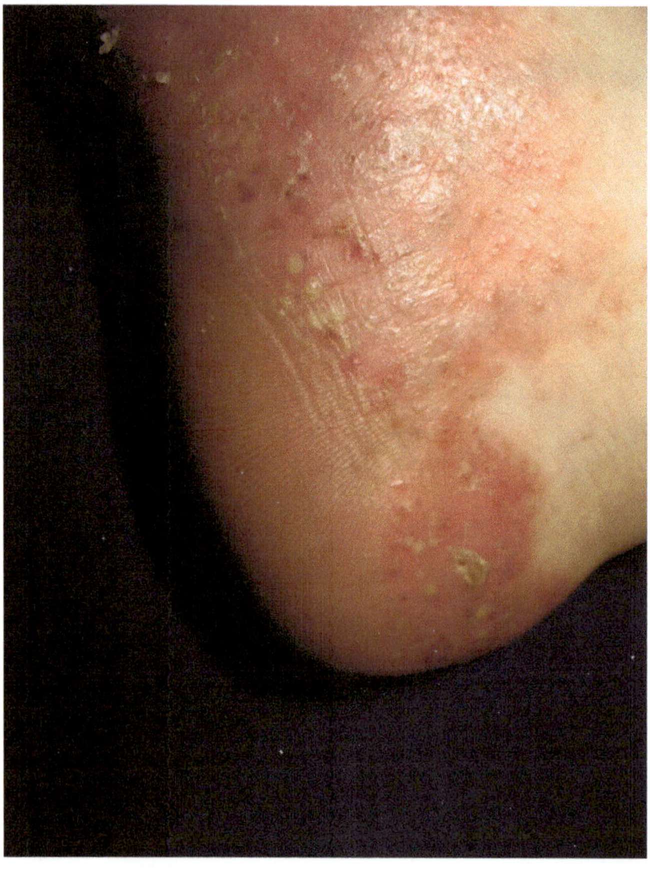

FIGURE 3.31 Psoriasis: Localized plantar pustular.

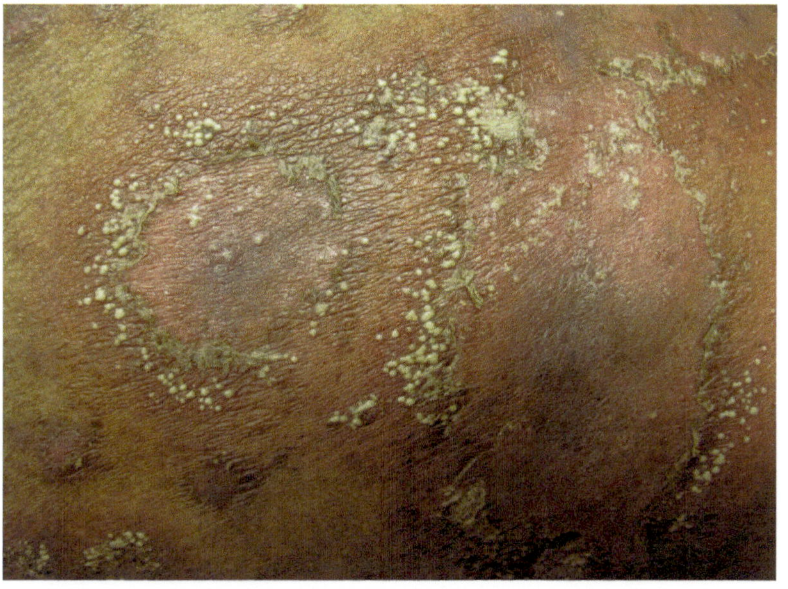

FIGURE 3.32 Psoriasis: Generalized pustular.

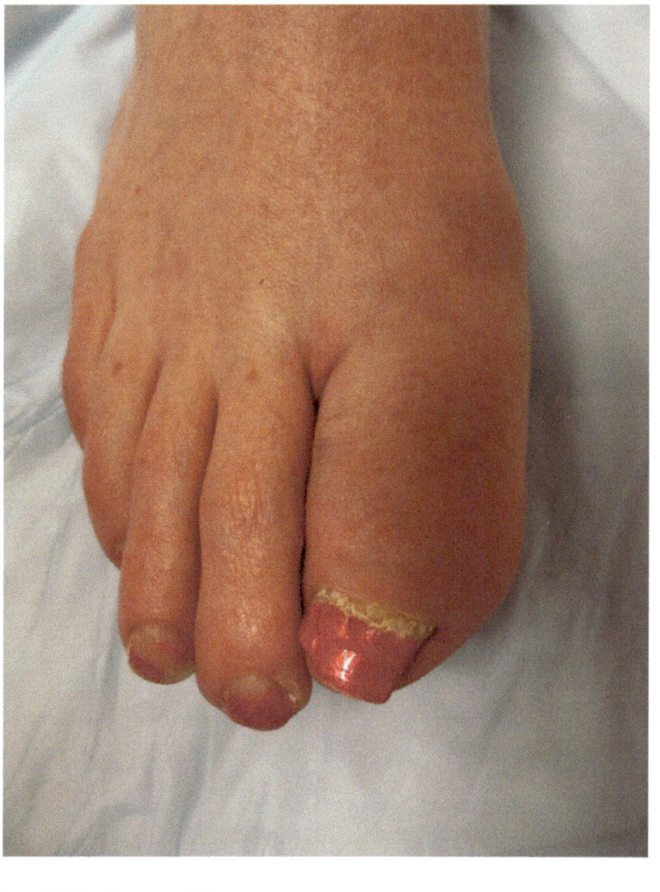

FIGURE 3.33 Psoriatic arthritis: Sausage digit.

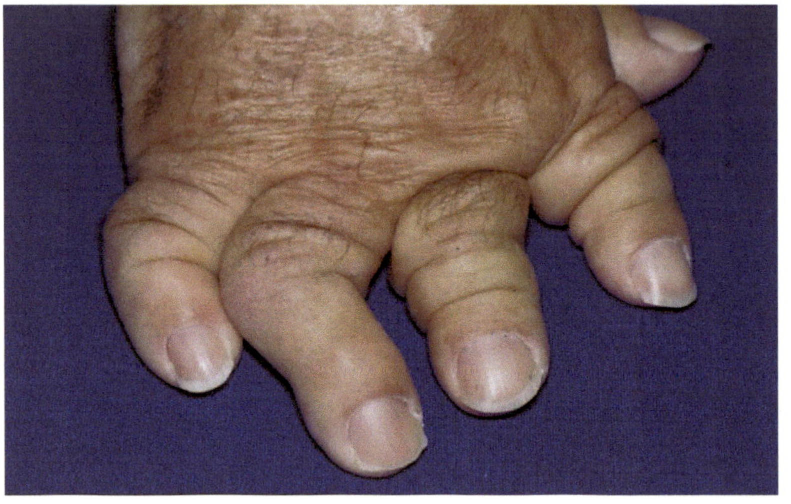

FIGURE 3.34 Psoriatic arthritis: End-stage arthritis mutilans.

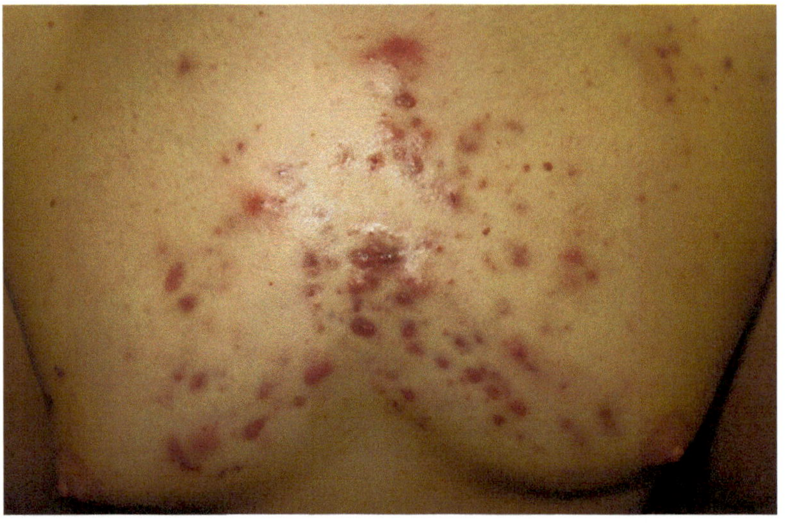

FIGURE 3.35 SAPHO syndrome: Acne.

Evaluation and Management

The diagnosis of psoriasis is often made clinically; however, skin biopsy can be performed in cases that are more complex. In patients with extensive disease, testing may include fasting blood glucose, hemoglobin A1c, fasting lipids, body mass index, and blood pressures. In erythrodermic or pustular psoriasis, evaluation of CBC, comprehensive metabolic panel, human chorionic gonadotropin, total protein, and cardiac monitoring are indicated. If there are concurrent bowel complaints, a colonoscopy (CS) to look for inflammatory bowel disease is prudent, and if signs/symptoms of lymphoma are present, a chest X-ray (CXR) or CT can be obtained. Patients with limited disease can be treated with topical corticosteroids, vitamin D analogs, PDE4 inhibitors, or JAKi. Patients with greater than 5%–10% body surface area involvement and/or psoriatic arthritis may require phototherapy or systemic treatment such as methotrexate, acitretin, cyclosporine, and newer biologic agents (see **Table 3.2**). Enhancing therapeutic modalities with early diagnosis, holistic patient assessment of functional impairment from the patient's perspective, management of comorbidities, and counseling for smoking cessation and increased exercise should be considered.

TABLE 3.2

Biologic Therapy for Psoriasis and Psoriatic Arthritis

Anti-TNF
- Adalimumab
- Infliximab
- Etanercept
- Certolizumab

Anti-IL12/23
- Ustekinumab

Anti-IL17A
- Secukinumab
- Ixekizumab
- Brodalumab
- Bimekizumab

Anti-IL23
- Guselkumab
- Tildrakizumab
- Risankizumab

Anti-IL36R
- Spesolimab

JAK inhibitor
- Tofacitinib

TYK2 inhibitor
- Deucravacitinib

Phosphodiesterase 4 inhibitor
- Apremilast

BIBLIOGRAPHY

Coate LC, Bukhari M, Chan A, et al. Enhancing current guidance for psoriatic arthritis and its comorbidities: Recommendations from expert consensus panel. Rheumatol (Oxford) 2024;64(2):561–573.

Elmets CA, Leonardi CL, Davis DMR, et al. Joint AAD-NPF guidelines of care for the management and treatment of psoriasis with awareness and attention to comorbidities. J Am Acad Dermatol 2019;80(4):1073–1113.

Singh JA, Guyatt G, Ogdie A, et al. Special article: 2018 American College of Rheumatology/National Psoriasis Foundation guideline for the treatment of psoriatic arthritis. Arthritis Rheumatol 2019;71(1):5–32.

Relapsing Polychondritis

Etiopathogenesis

The exact etiology of relapsing polychondritis (RPC) is unclear. Autoantibodies to Type II collagen and matrilin 1 are elevated. Immune complex deposition with CD4+ T-helper cells and B-cell lymphocytes against cartilage proteoglycans in patients with HLA DRB1*16:02, DQB1*05:02 and B*67:01 alleles is observed. There are new associations of RPC with VEXAS (Vacuoles, E1 enzyme [initiates ubiquitylation], X-linked, Autoinflammatory, Somatic) syndrome from UAB1 gene mutations and immune-checkpoint inhibitors (nivolumab) used in cancer therapies.

Clinical Manifestations

Patients present with swollen, painful, and erythematous helices (auricular chondritis) with sparing of the ear lobules (**Figure 3.36**). Chronic disease may produce secondary chondromalacia

(**Figure 3.37**). Nasal pain and epistaxis are suggestive of nasal chondritis and may lead to saddle nose (**Figures 3.38** and **3.39**). Nonspecific associated skin diseases are erythema nodosum, livedo reticularis, superficial thrombophlebitis, purpura, dermal hypersensitivity reactions (**Figure 3.40**), urticarial, and angioedema.

Systemic Manifestations

Hoarseness, stridor, nonproductive cough, and dyspnea are seen with laryngotracheal involvement, which is the leading cause of morbidity and mortality for RPC. Tracheal collapse and pulmonary infections are the most common causes of death. Valvular heart disease and arrhythmia from cardiovascular involvement are the second leading cause of death. Additional findings include conductive/sensory hearing loss, scleritis, episcleritis, conjunctivitis, headaches, seizures, glomerulonephritis, and nonerosive arthritis. Up to 35% of RPC cases have an associated additional autoimmune disease (systemic lupus erythematosus, Sjögren's syndrome, rheumatoid arthritis, antiphospholipid antibody syndrome, Behcet's syndrome [BS], Crohn's disease, spondyloarthritis) or hematologic malignancy (myelodysplastic syndrome [no-UBA1 mutations], lymphoma, leukemia). Concurrent systemic inflammation can cause leukocytoclastic vasculitis (LCV) manifesting from skin purpura to thoracic/aortic aneurysms. VEXAS syndrome-RPC group occurs in older patients (>60) with new-onset chondritis, ocular, pulmonary, heart, cutaneous involvement, and myelodysplastic syndrome. The distinct RPC phenotypes are summarized in **Table 3.3**.

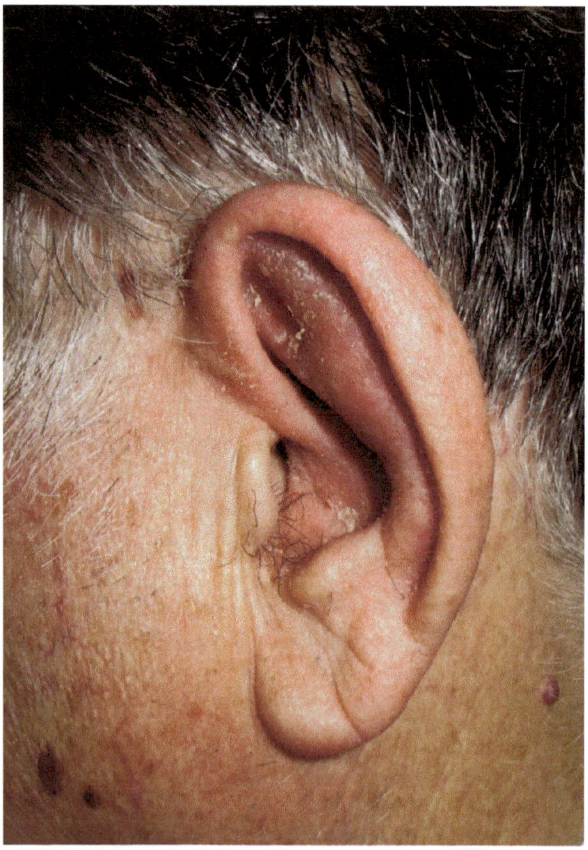

FIGURE 3.36 Relapsing polychondritis: Acute.

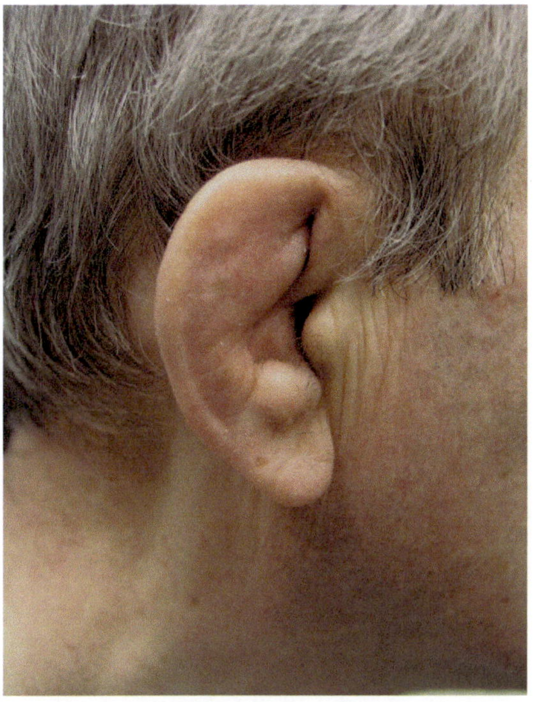

FIGURE 3.37 Relapsing polychondritis: Chronic.

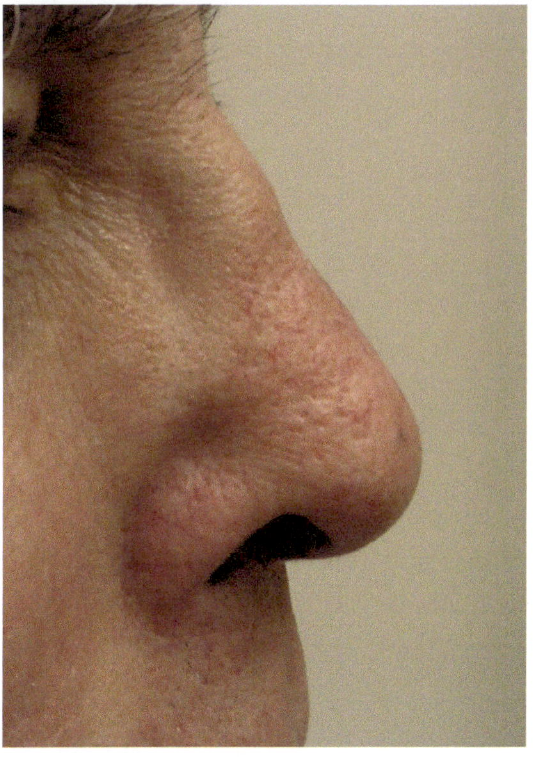

FIGURE 3.38 Relapsing polychondritis: Early saddle nose.

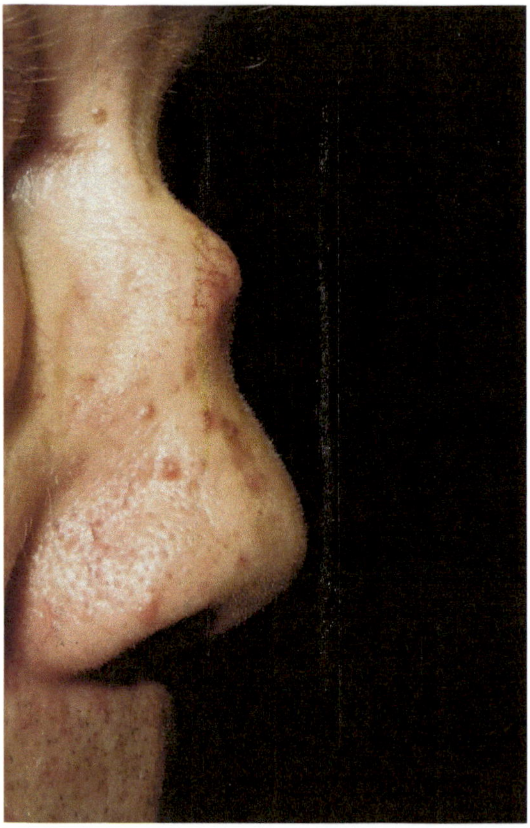

FIGURE 3.39 Relapsing polychondritis: Late saddle nose.

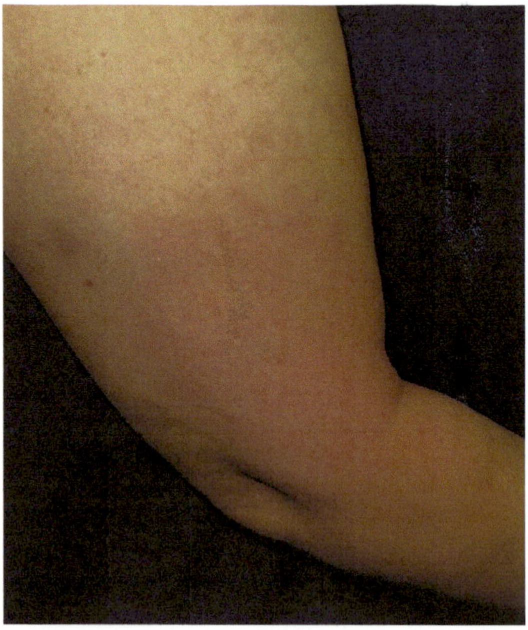

FIGURE 3.40 Relapsing polychondritis: Dermal hypersensitivity reaction.

Evaluation and Management

RPC is diagnosed by correlating the myriad historical and physical manifestations. A biopsy of the ear cartilage often reveals cartilage inflammation. Laboratory testing is nondiagnostic because anti-type II cartilage antibodies are nonspecific, but titers can correlate with disease activity. The same is true for erythrocyte sedimentation rate (ESR), C-reactive protein (CRP), CBC, and serum protein electrophoresis/urine protein electrophoresis (SPEP/UPEP). CT scan or magnetic resonance imaging (MRI) of the laryngotracheal tree may identify areas affected. PFT may help determine the nature of the airway obstruction. Consultation with otolaryngology, cardiology, pulmonology, ophthalmology, and rheumatology is indicated. Testing for UAB1 gene mutations is indicated, especially in males >60 years of age. Treatment of RPC ranges from nonsteroidal anti-inflammatory drugs such as dapsone, colchicine, oral and inhaled corticosteroids, methotrexate, azathioprine, cyclosporine, and cyclophosphamide. The biologic agents abatacept, tocilizumab, and anti-TNFα inhibitors may be superior to methotrexate.

TABLE 3.3

Phenotypes of Relapsing Polychondritis

	First (65%)	Second (25%)	Third (10%)
Chondritis	+	+	+
Lung	+/–	++	+
Cardiac	+/–	–	+
Myelodysplasia	+/–	++	+++
VEXAS	–	–	++
ICU care	–	+	++
Mortality	–	+	+

BIBLIOGRAPHY

Bica BERG, de Souza AWS, Pereira IA. Unveiling the clinical spectrum of relapsing polychondritis: Insights into its pathogenesis, novel monogenic causes and therapeutic strategies. Adv Rheumatol 2024;64(1):29.

Mertz P, Costedoat-Chalumeau N, Ferrada MA, et al. Relapsing polychondritis: Clinical updates and new differential diagnoses. Nat Rev Rheumatol 2024;20(6):347–360.

Mertz P, Sparks J, Kobrin D, et al. Relapsing polychondritis: Best practice & clinical rheumatology. Best Pract Res Clin Rheumatol 2023;37(1):101867.

Rheumatoid Arthritis

Etiopathogenesis

Rheumatoid arthritis (RA) is a systemic autoimmune disorder whose exact etiology appears to be multifactorial. RA occurs in genetically susceptible individuals (HLA DRB1, PTPN22 alleles) who have a tendency to overproduce rheumatoid factor (RF) and anticitrullinated peptide antibodies as well as TNF-α from lymphocytes, synovial-like fibroblasts, and macrophages. This culminates in bone destruction and other systemic diseases. Smoking and other air pollutants are linked to developing RA.

Clinical Manifestations

Patients present with pain, fatigue, and significant articular damage shown on radiographs. General skin changes related to joint disease include skin fragility and atrophic to translucent changes over the joints (**Figure 3.41**). Hand and nail findings include palmar erythema, periungual erythema, onychorrhexis, onycholysis, red lunula, pterygium inversum, splinter hemorrhages, and nail-fold thrombosis (Bywater's lesions). Specific cutaneous manifestations of RA include rheumatoid nodules, rheumatoid vasculitis (purpura to ulcerations [**Figures 3.42** and **3.43**]), pyoderma gangrenosum, noninfectious granulomatous disease (interstitial granulomatous disease, palisaded neutrophilic and granulomatous disorders, reactive granulomatous dermatitis), and rheumatoid neutrophilic dermatitis. Classic cutaneous rheumatoid nodules (RF positive) are the most common extra-articular manifestation (**Figure 3.44**), but may also develop internally (i.e., pulmonary rheumatoid nodules). Accelerated rheumatoid nodulosis is a drug reaction most commonly to methotrexate, which causes painful acral nodules (**Figure 3.45**) in the setting of well-controlled RA. Felty's syndrome includes rheumatoid nodules, hyperpigmentation, and leg ulcers with RA, leukopenia, and splenomegaly.

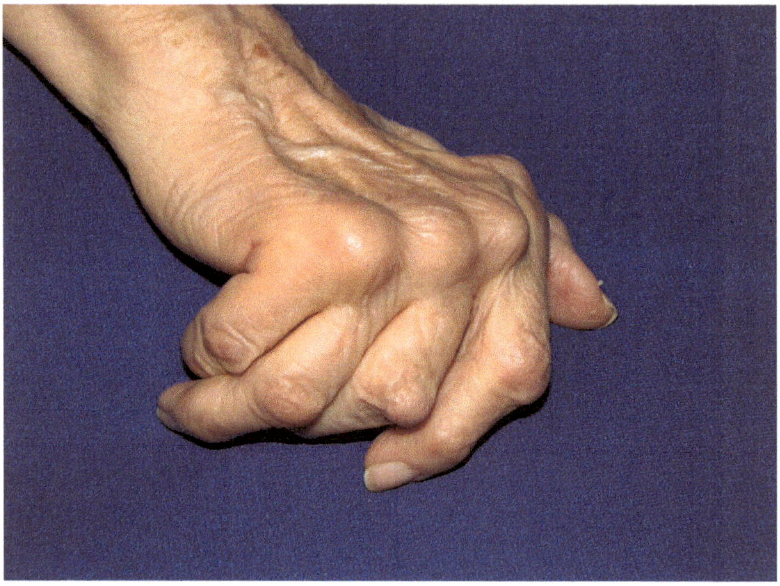

FIGURE 3.41 Rheumatoid arthritis: Atrophic fragile skin.

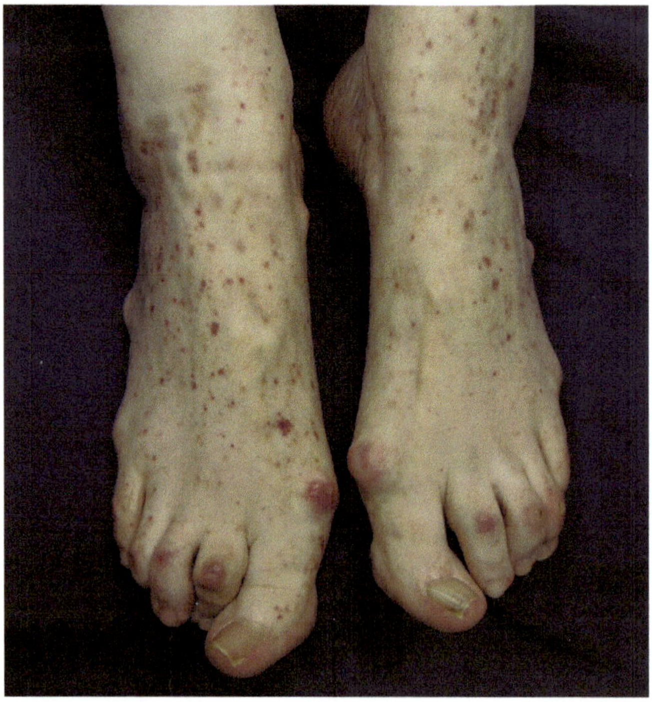

FIGURE 3.42 Rheumatoid vasculitis: Purpuric form with nodules.

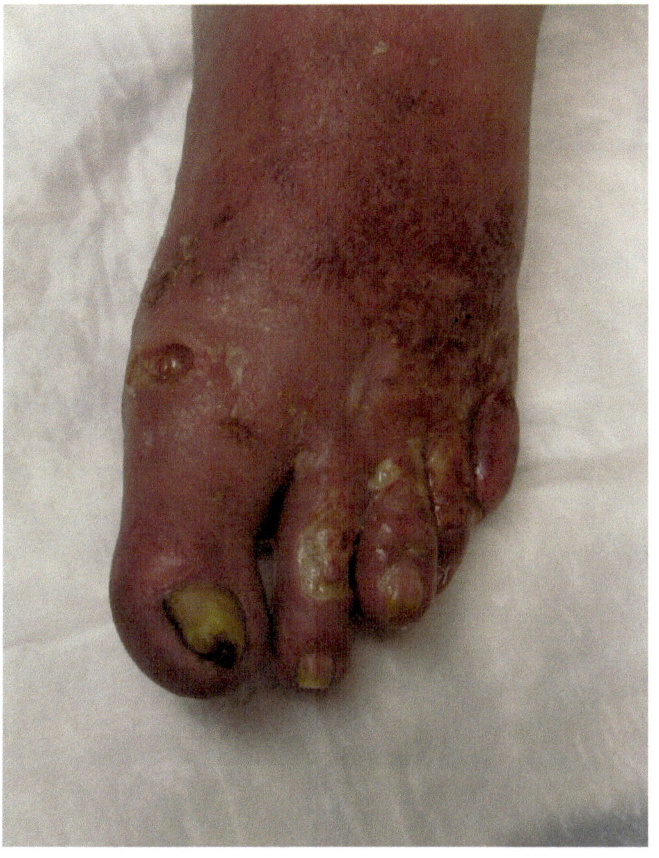

FIGURE 3.43 Rheumatoid vasculitis: Ulcerative form.

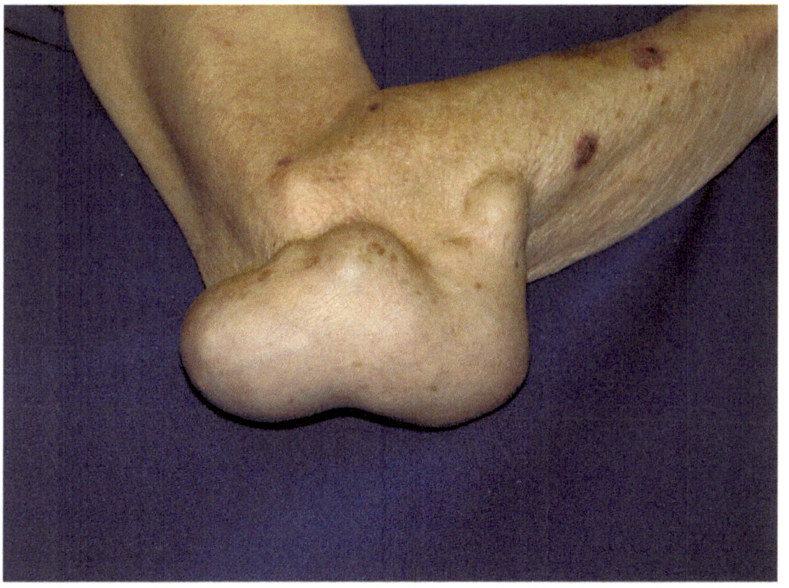

FIGURE 3.44 Rheumatoid nodule: Classic.

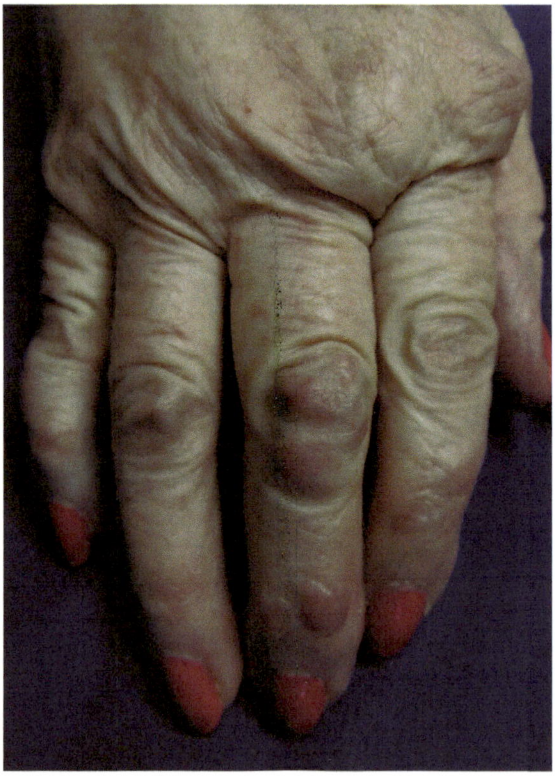

FIGURE 3.45 Rheumatoid nodule: Accelerated rheumatoid nodulosis.

Systemic Manifestations

Besides joint and skin disease, extra-articular manifestations and comorbidities may also be significant. Patients may experience pulmonary fibrosis, scleritis, pericarditis, conduction defects, peripheral neuropathy, mononeuritis multiplex, and develop amyloidosis. Significant comorbidities include myocardial infarction, stroke, life-threatening infections, lymphoproliferative disorders, anemia, and depression.

Evaluation and Management

If cutaneous findings warrant, evaluation for RA investigation should include radiographic studies of joints and lungs (if symptomatic), CBC, iron panel with ferritin (IRON), ESR, CRP, RF, and anticyclic citrullinated protein (anti-CCP) antibodies. Referral to rheumatology with additional subspecialties (cardiology, ophthalmology, neurology) as needed is indicated. Treatment of RA is most commonly methotrexate, anti-TNFα, and JAK inhibitors. The latter have had a profound impact on decreasing the mean incidence. Other immunosuppressant agents (hydroxychloroquine, mycophenolate mofetil, azathioprine) are often used for skin manifestations. Most rheumatoid nodules should be left alone, but surgical removal may be needed if fistula formation develops.

BIBLIOGRAPHY

Mertz P, Wollenschalaeger C, Chasset F, et al. Rheumatoid vasculitis in 2023: Changes and challenges since the biologic era. Autoimmun Rev 2023;22(9):103391.

Radu AF, Bungau SG. Management of rheumatoid arthritis: An overview. Cells 2021;10(11):2857.

Sayah A, English JC III. Rheumatoid arthritis: A review of the cutaneous manifestations. J Am Acad Dermatol 2005;53(2):191–209.

Tilstra JS, Lienesch DW. Rheumatoid nodules. Dermatol Clin 2015;33(3):361–371.

Scleroderma

Etiopathogenesis

Systemic scleroderma is the progressive deposition of collagen in tissues by presumed genetic, epigenetic, and environmental factors causing vasculopathy, and inflammation resulting in inappropriate fibrosis with organ dysfunction. It occurs most commonly in women and has the highest mortality rates among connective tissue diseases. Poor outcomes have been associated with late-onset in men with diffuse systemic sclerosis, digital ulcers, and joint involvement.

Clinical Manifestations

The development of thickened, pale, and indurated skin is the classic presentation of scleroderma. Localized and generalized scleroderma (Morphea) is typically limited to skin on acral areas and face, or disseminated lesions involving the trunk, respectively. Scleroderma with systemic manifestations is referred to as limited systemic sclerosis (LSS) or diffuse systemic sclerosis (DSS). LSS has skin thickening limited distally from the elbow and knees, whereas DSS includes involvement of more proximally located skin and torso (**Figure 3.46**). In systemic scleroderma, skin findings may include features of calcinosis, Raynaud's phenomenon (**Figure 3.47**), acrocyanosis, sclerodactyly, puffy fingers (**Figure 3.48**), telangiectasia (**Figure 3.49**), nailfold-dilated tortuous capillaries, and dyschromia (**Figures 3.50** and **3.51**).

Systemic Manifestations

LSS and DSS (**Table 3.4**) may have esophageal dysmotility, diarrhea or symptoms of intestinal obstruction, ILD, and pulmonary arterial hypertension. DSS is distinguished from LSS based on the presence of renal and cardiac involvement. Renal crisis of scleroderma involves rapid development of hypertension and progressive renal insufficiency. Cardiac involvement can be varied; however, pericarditis with or without effusion, arrhythmia, cardiomyopathy, and heart failure have been reported. Anti-RNA polymerase III positivity correlates with increased risk of breast, hematologic, and GI/genitourinary (GU) malignancy.

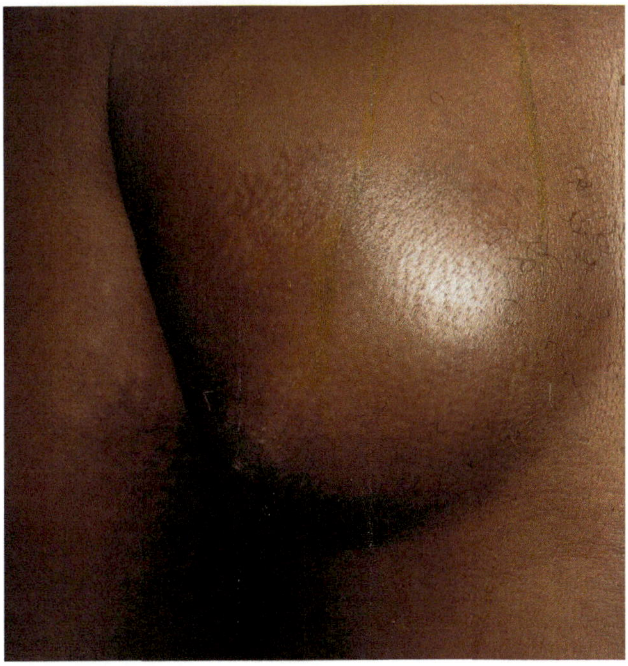

FIGURE 3.46 Diffuse systemic sclerosis: Scleroderma.

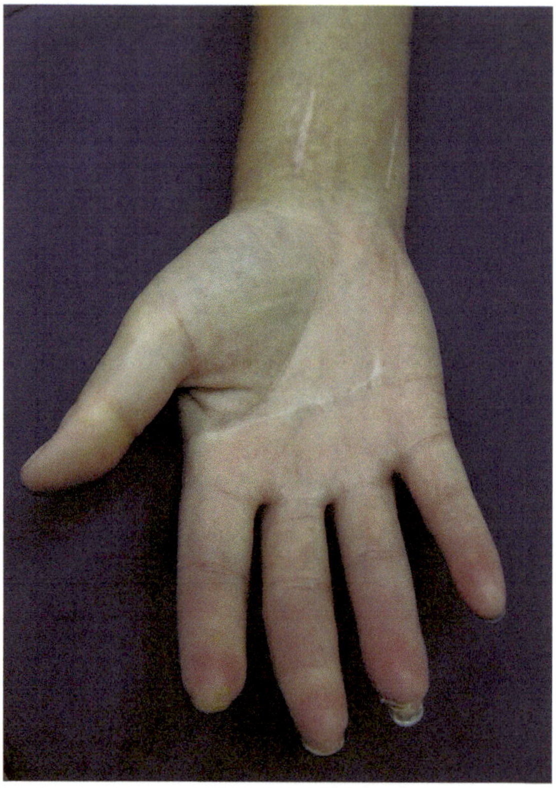

FIGURE 3.47 Limited systemic sclerosis: Sympathectomy scars for Raynaud's phenomenon.

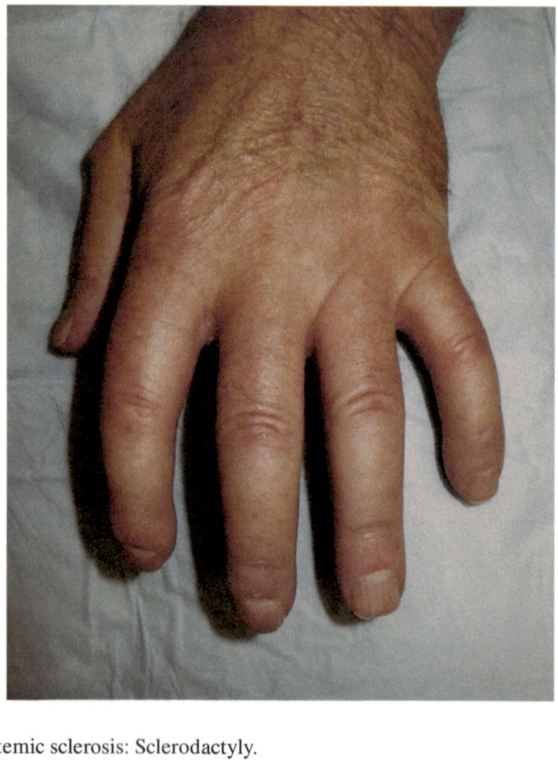

FIGURE 3.48 Limited systemic sclerosis: Sclerodactyly.

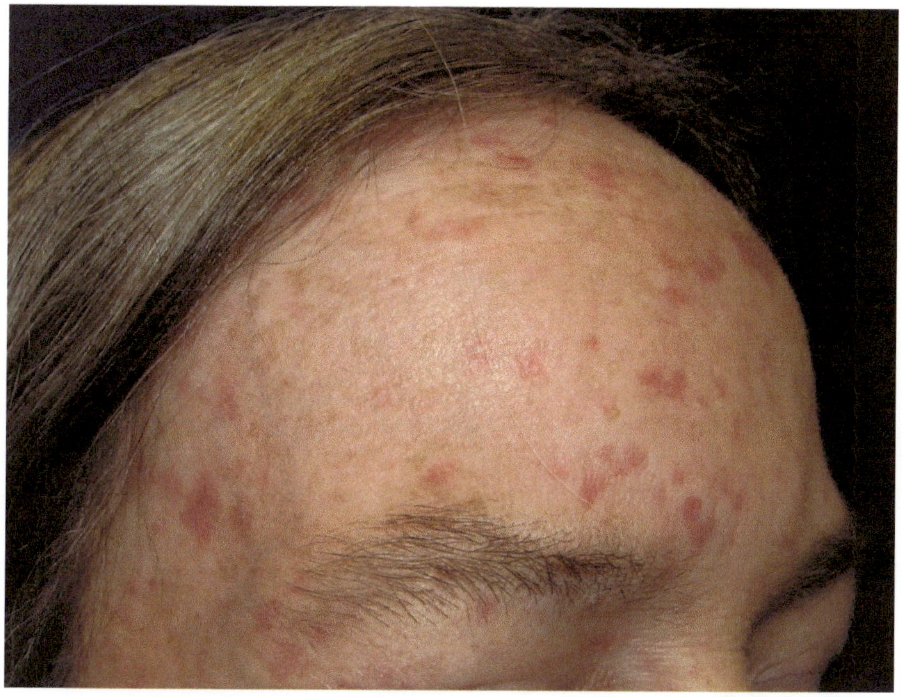

FIGURE 3.49 Limited systemic sclerosis: Telangiectatic mats.

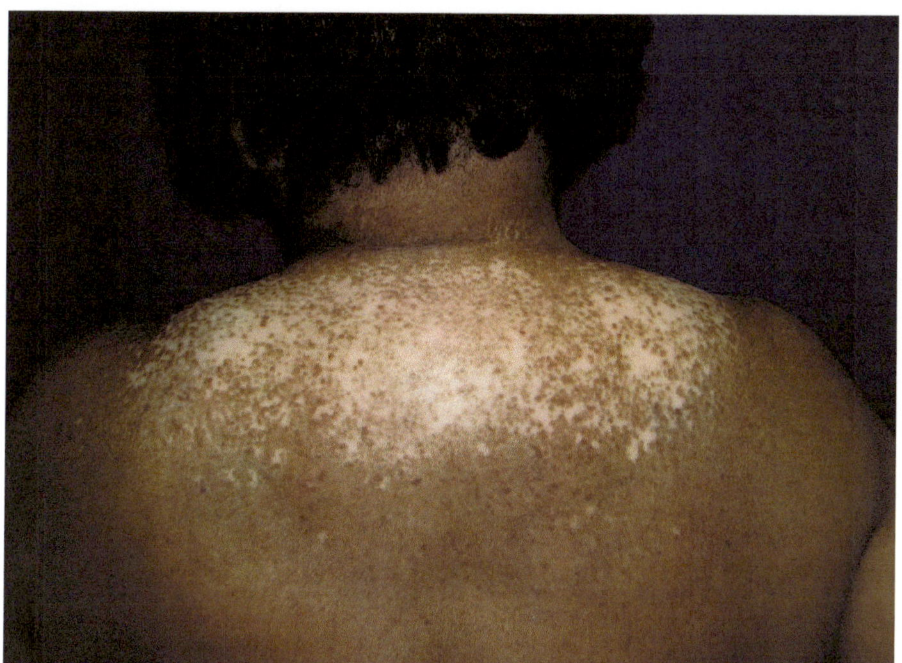

FIGURE 3.50 Diffuse systemic sclerosis: Dyschromia.

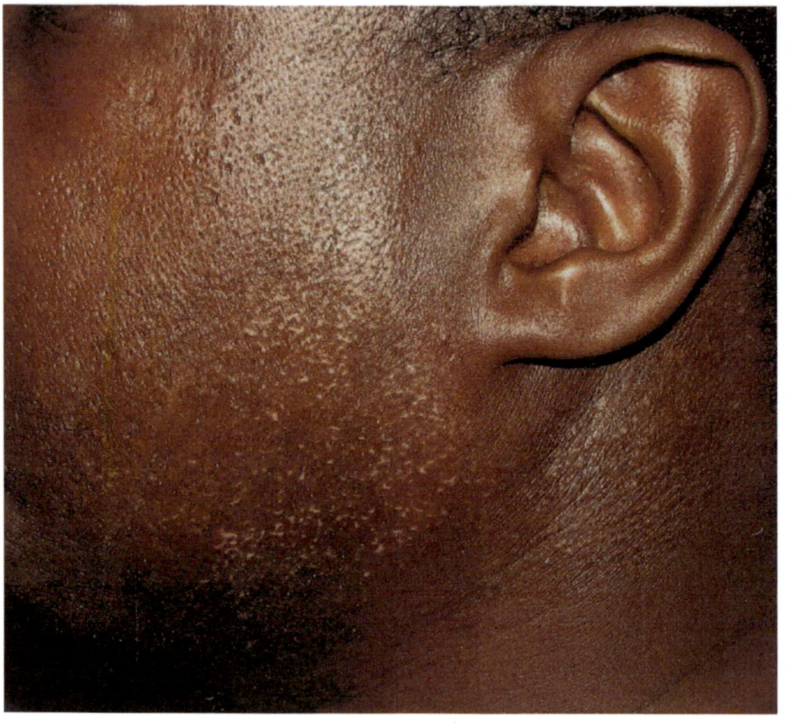

FIGURE 3.51 Diffuse systemic sclerosis: Dyschromia.

Evaluation and Management

A thorough physical exam and review of systems is the key to the diagnosis of scleroderma variants and uncovering of extracutaneous disease. A battery of antibody serologies includes ANA, anti-scl 70 (topoisomerase) antibodies (Scl-70), anticentromere antibodies (ACA), anti-U1/3 nuclear ribonucleoprotein antibodies (U1RNP, U3RNP), and anti-RNA polymerase III antibodies (RNAP III) (if positive, needs cancer screening). Given the presence of appropriate symptoms, consider GI motility testing (barium follow-through, esophagogastroduodenoscopy [EGD]), CXR, PFT, electrocardiogram [EKG], RFT, and UA. Treatment of systemic sclerodermas is complex and typically involves immunomodulation or immunosuppressive therapies depending on the organ system involved. Therapy may range from methotrexate to anti-B-cell therapies to hematopoietic stem cell transplantation. The treatment of pulmonary, vascular, and renal manifestations often includes prostacyclin analogs, phosphodiesterase type-5 inhibitors, and endothelin antagonists. Proton pump inhibitors and pro-motility agents are used for esophageal dysmotility. Raynaud's and digital ulcerations can be treated with calcium channel blockers, angiotensin II receptor antagonists, and intravenous iloprost.

TABLE 3.4

Limited vs. Diffuse Systemic Sclerosis

Type	Scleroderma	Raynaud's	Esophageal	Pulmonary	Renal	Cardiac
Limited (Anti-centromere)	Knee/elbow	>10 yr prior	+	+	-	-
Diffuse (Anti-topoisomerase)	Past knee/elbow	At onset	+	+	+	+

Manifestation	Limited SS	Diffuse SS
Sclerodactyly	+	+
Scleroderma	Extremities	Torso & extremities
Raynaud's	>10 yr prior	At onset

(Continued)

TABLE 3.4 (*Continued*)

Limited vs. Diffuse Systemic Sclerosis

Type	Scleroderma	Raynaud's	Esophageal	Pulmonary	Renal	Cardiac
Gastrointestinal	+		+			
Respiratory	+		+			
Cardiac	-		+			
Renal	-		+			
Urogenital	-		+			
Malignancy	-		+			
Anti-centromere	+		-			
Anti-topoisomerase	-		+			
Anti-U1/3 ribonucleoprotein	-		+ (Lung, Cardiac)			
Anti-RNA polymerase III	-		+ (Renal/Malignancy)			

BIBLIOGRAPHY

Calderon LM, Pope JE. Scleroderma epidemiology update. Curr Opin Rheumatol 2021;33(2):122–127.

Jergen R, Nikpour M, Krieg T, et al. Systemic sclerosis in adults. Part I: Clinical features and pathogenesis. J Am Acad Dermatol 2022;87(5):937–954.

Jergen R, Nikpour M, Krieg T, et al. Systemic sclerosis in adults. Part II: Management and therapeutics. J Am Acad Dermatol 2022;87(5):957–978.

Zhao M, Wu J, Wu H, et al. Clinical options in scleroderma: Recommendations and comprehensive review. Clin Rev Allergy Immunol 2022;62(2):273–291.

Sjögren Syndrome

Etiopathogenesis

Sjögren syndrome (SS) is an autoimmune connective tissue disease that typically features symptoms of xerostomia, xerophthalmia (sicca symptoms), fatigue, and pain due to destruction of these exocrine glands. Current research notes SS patients demonstrate overexpression of a novel long non-coding RNA (LINC01871), interferon γ, and circulating B-cell clones. It is more common in women, but is more aggressive in male patients. Secondary SS is associated with overlap with other connective tissue diseases, including systemic LE, RA, and scleroderma.

Clinical Manifestations

Skin manifestations of SS consist of xerosis cutis, pruritus, Raynaud's phenomenon, livedo racemosa, perniosis, subacute and chronic cutaneous lupus eruptions, urticaria (**Figure 3.52**), urticarial vasculitis, and purpura from LCV (**Figure 3.53**) have been described. The most commonly described symptoms of Sjögren syndrome include xerostomia (dry mouth) and xerophthalmia (dry eye). Mucosal ulceration and disease, including mucocutaneous candidiasis, periodontitis, angular cheilitis, and stomatitis, have been described.

Systemic Manifestations

Autoimmune phenomenon in Sjögren syndrome can involve several organ systems, including musculoskeletal (arthralgia/arthritis), central/peripheral nervous system (meningitis, mononeuritis multiplex), endocrine (autoimmune thyroiditis, parotitis), immune (adenopathy), pulmonary (pneumonitis, pulmonary hypertension), renal (interstitial nephritis), cardiac (pericarditis, cardiomyopathy), hematologic (neutropenia, thrombosis or embolic phenomenon due to pro-coagulation, hypocomplementemia, hypergammaglobulinemia, and cryoglobulinemia), and ocular (xerophthalmia, iritis/uveitis, blepharitis). SS is associated with lymphoma (10- to 44-fold), parotitis, melanoma, lung cancer (men), breast and thyroid cancer (women).

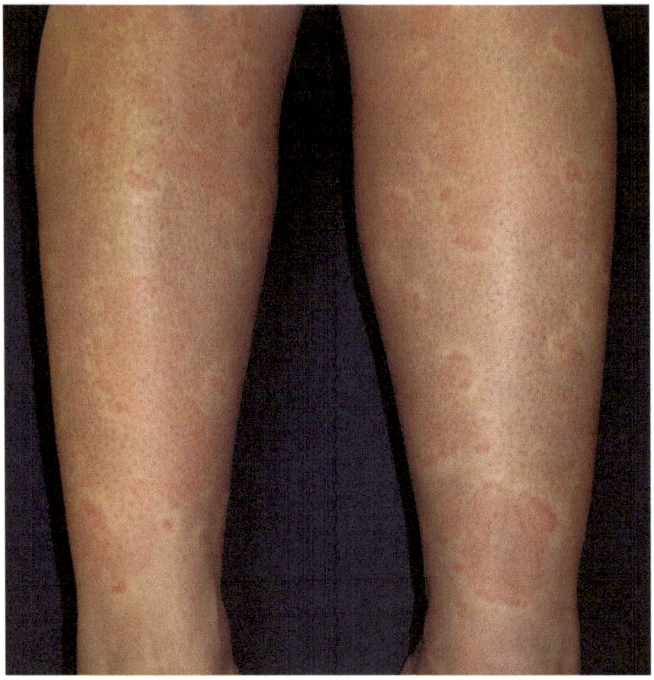

FIGURE 3.52 Sjögren syndrome: Urticaria.

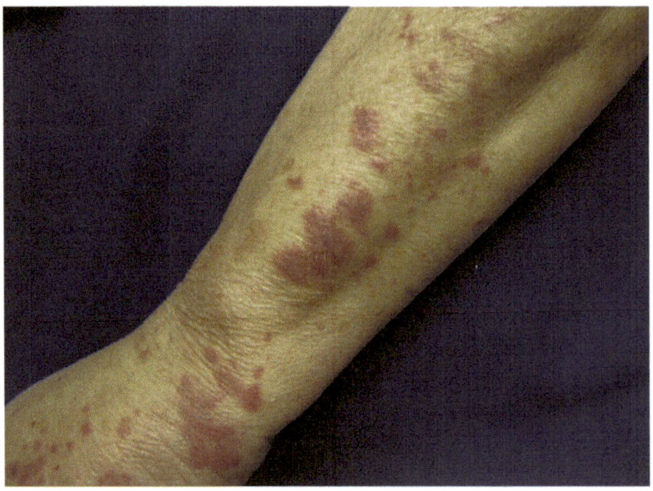

FIGURE 3.53 Sjögren syndrome: Leukocytoclastic vasculitis.

Evaluation and Management

A detailed history and physical examination to evaluate complaints of xerostomia and xerophthalmia are required. ANA and Ro/La are helpful because the presence of these antibodies is highly correlated with Sjögren syndrome (100% and 70%, respectively). Systemic function testing, including the following, can be helpful in evaluating extraglandular and extracutaneous involvement: RFT,

LFT, C3/4, cryoglobulin (CRYO), lupus anticoagulant (LAC), antiphospholipid antibodies (APLA), Schirmer or Rose–Bengal testing of lacrimal glands, major salivary gland shear wave elastography and ultrasound-guided core needle biopsy of major salivary glands or incisional biopsy of labial salivary glands. Oral glucocorticoid therapy is considered if extracutaneous manifestations are present or if purpura/vasculitis is present. For steroid sparing effects, drugs such as mycophenolate mofetil, belimumab, rituximab, abatacept, and JAK inhibitors have also been used. Ocular/oral symptoms are treated symptomatically with saline or other lacrimal/oral lubricants or with local immunosuppression with topical cyclosporine or tacrolimus.

BIBLIOGRAPHY

Andre F, Bockle BC. Sjögren's syndrome. J Dtsch Dermatol Ges 2022;20(7):980–1002.

Longhino S, Chatzis LG, Dal Pozzolo R, et al. Sjögren's syndrome: One year in review 2023. Clin Exp Rheumatol 2023;41(12):2343–2356.

Mihau A, Caruntu C, Jurcut C, et al. The spectrum of extraglandular manifestations in primary Sjögren's syndrome. J Pers Med 2023;13(6):961.

Vasculitis

Etiopathogenesis

Vasculitis refers to inflammation of the vasculature; the causes and manifestations have incredible variability. Key to the pathogenesis of vasculitis is inflammation caused by direct antibody attack on vessels, immune complex deposition, or in some cases, a pauci-inflammatory reaction associated with antineutrophilic cytoplasmic antibodies (ANCA).

Clinical Manifestations

The most notable dermatologic manifestation of vasculitis is purpura (**Figure 3.54**). Although the lesions will often begin as small erythematous macules or even urticaria-like wheals, these often become papular and even pustular (**Figures 3.55** and **3.56**). If blood flow is compromised, local tissue necrosis results in bullae or even ulceration (**Figure 3.57**). These lesions can present as a single acute eruption with resolution, a relapsing and remitting disease, or as a non-remitting, chronic disorder.

Systemic Manifestations

The development of vasculitis in the skin may be associated with similar inflammation in any organ system throughout the body. Renal involvement (glomerulonephritis, renal failure) is the most common sequela of systemic involvement. In broad categories, vasculitis can result from hypersensitivity reactions (idiopathic), autoimmune disorders (**Figure 3.58**), infections (**Figure 3.59**), drug exposures (**Figure 3.60**), or malignancies (**Figure 3.61**). Vasculitis has been associated with autoimmune disorders (lupus, RA, DMM scleroderma, Sjögren syndrome), IgA vasculitis [**Figure 3.62**]), and Type II/III mixed cryoglobulinemia (hepatitis C associated [**Figure 3.63**]). Infectious causes most commonly come from bacterial and fungal sepsis. If inflammation becomes granulomatous/necrotizing vasculitis ± ANCA positivity with lung, cardiac, or renal involvement disorders, such as granulomatosis with polyangiitis (**Figure 3.64**), eosinophilic granulomatosis with polyangiitis, microscopic polyangiitis, and polyarteritis nodosa (**Figure 3.65**), can be considered. Most cutaneous LCV are self-limited. Relapses can be seen in 20% of cases especially with peripheral neuropathy, hepatitis, or extensive skin involvement.

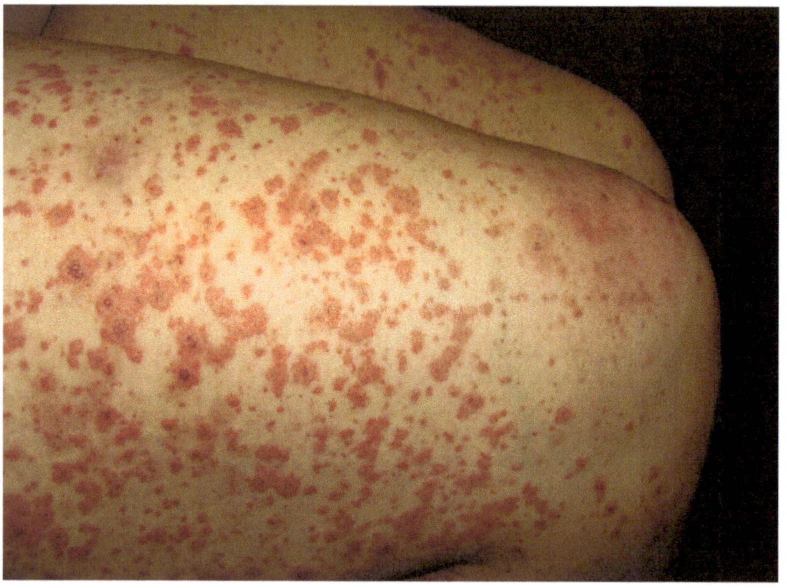

FIGURE 3.54 Cutaneous vasculitis: Hypersensitivity (idiopathic).

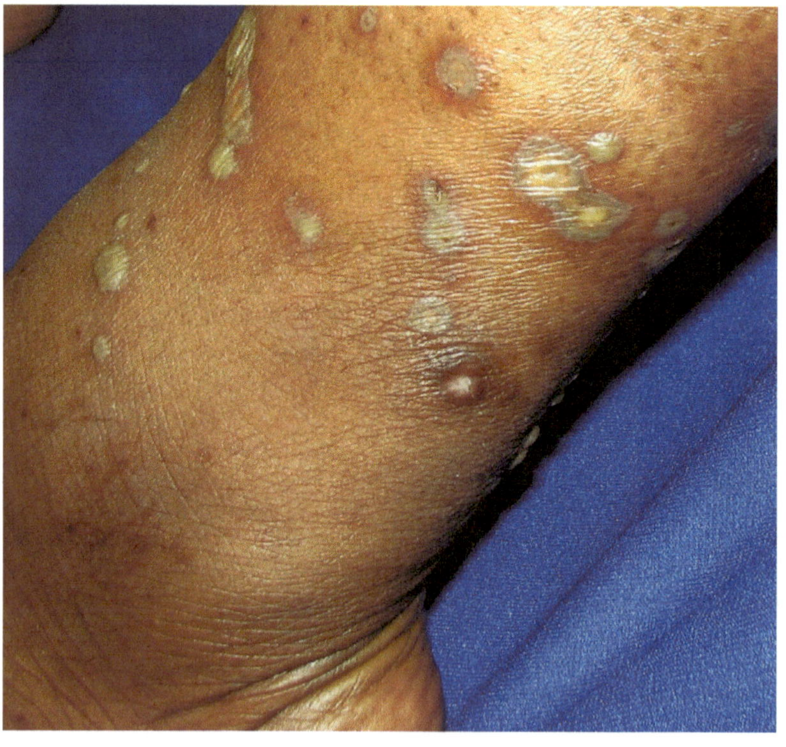

FIGURE 3.55 Cutaneous vasculitis: Pustular.

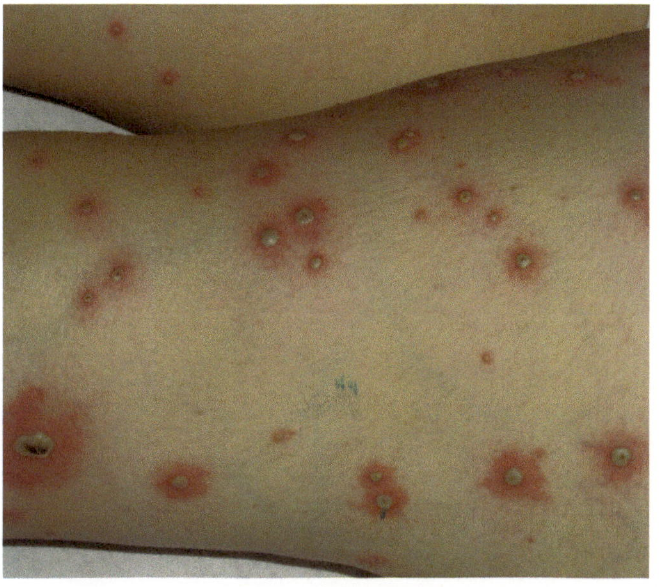

FIGURE 3.56 Cutaneous vasculitis: Pustular.

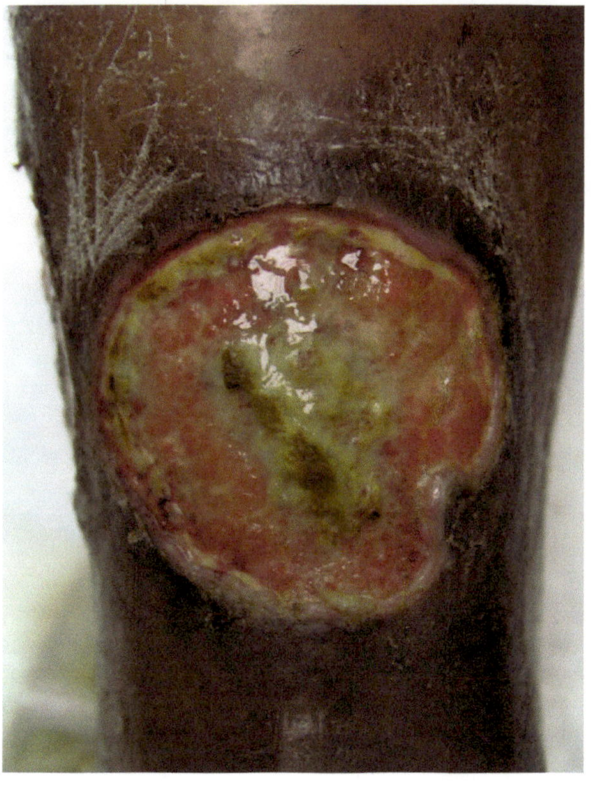

FIGURE 3.57 Cutaneous vasculitis: Ulcerative.

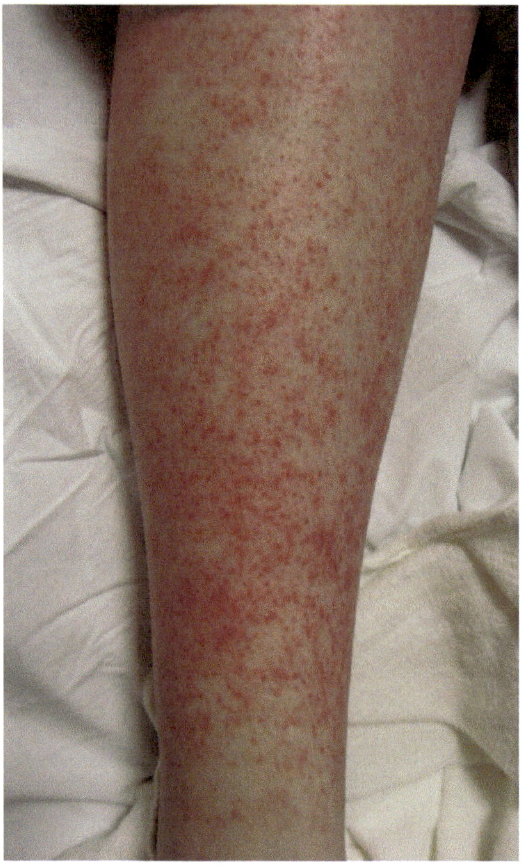

FIGURE 3.58 Cutaneous vasculitis: Lupus.

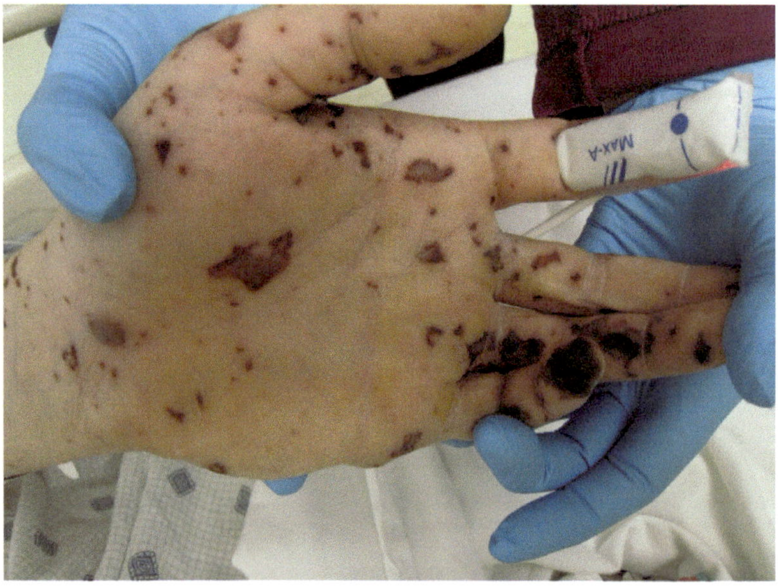

FIGURE 3.59 Infectious vasculitis: Meningococcemia.

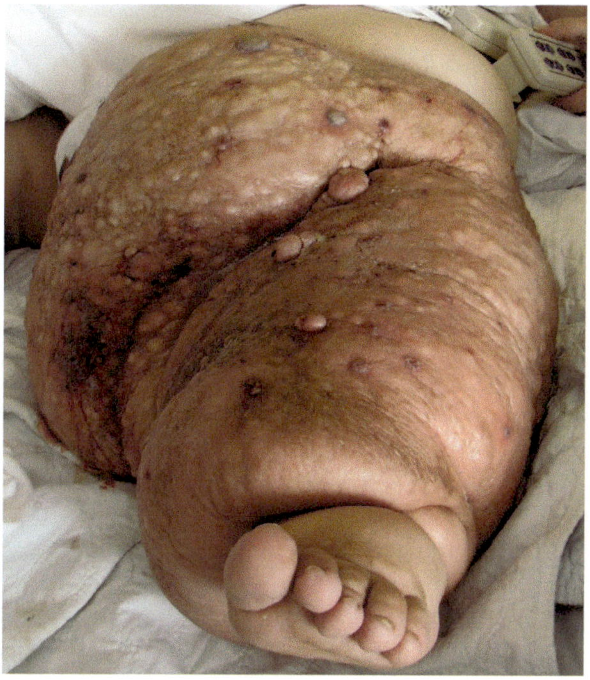

FIGURE 3.60 Drug-induced vasculitis: Antibiotic.

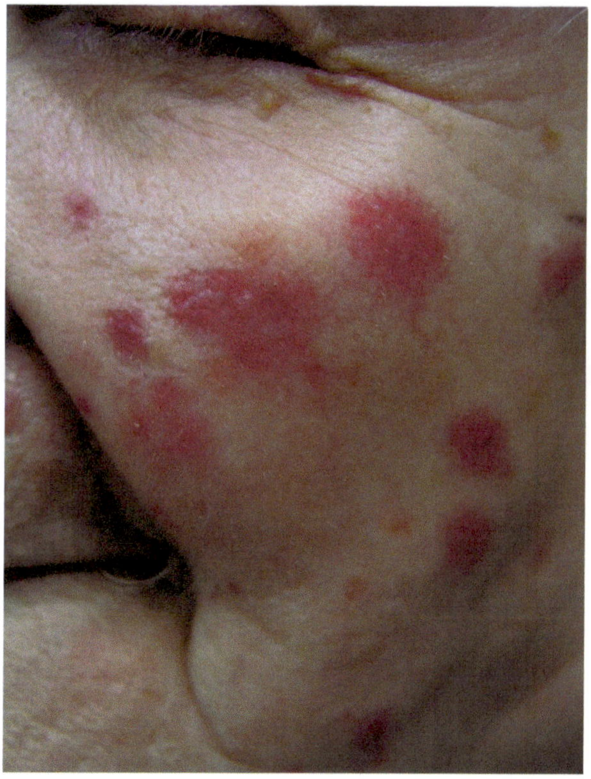

FIGURE 3.61 Malignancy associated vasculitis: Lymphoma.

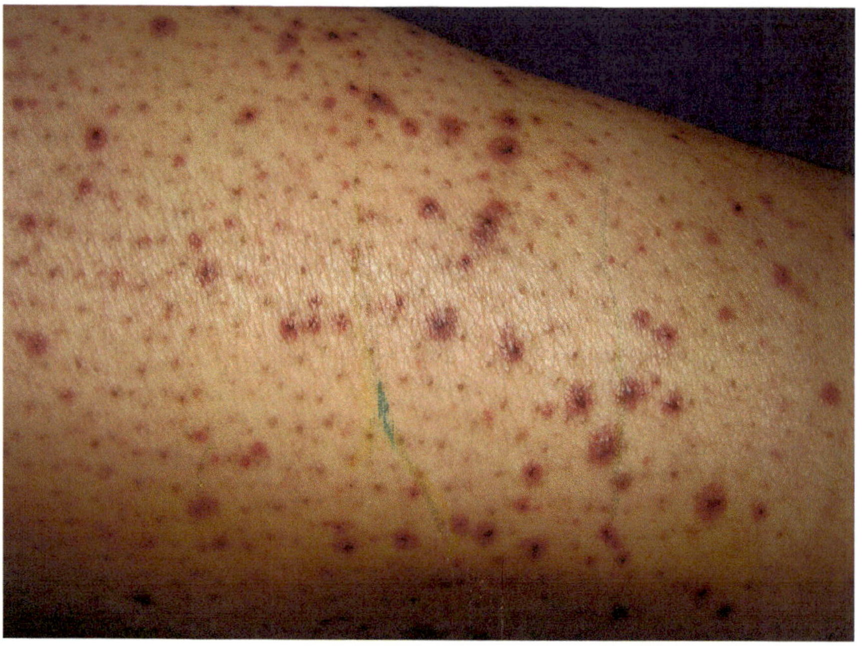

FIGURE 3.62 Cutaneous vasculitis: IgA vasculitis.

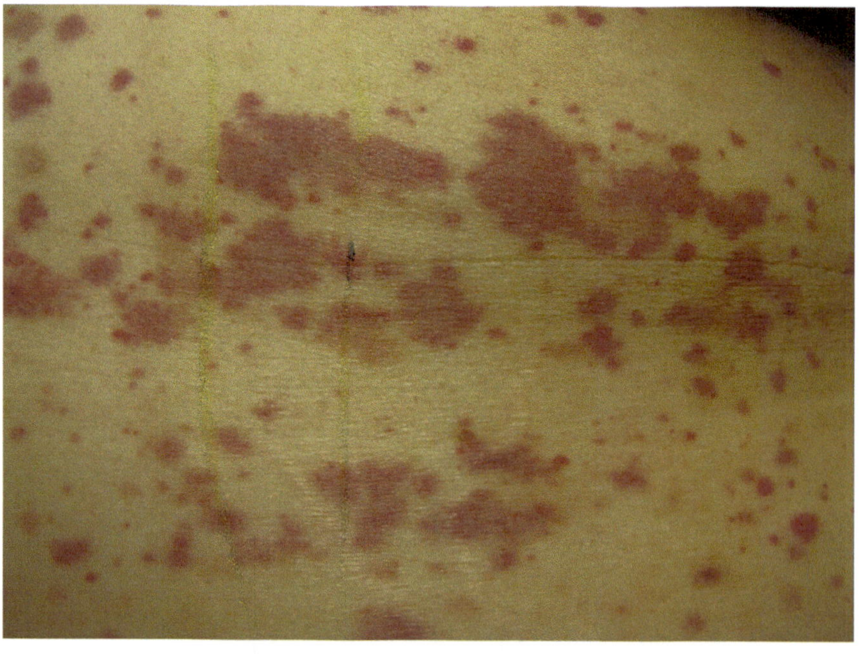

FIGURE 3.63 Cutaneous vasculitis: Type II mixed cryoglobulinemia from hepatitis C.

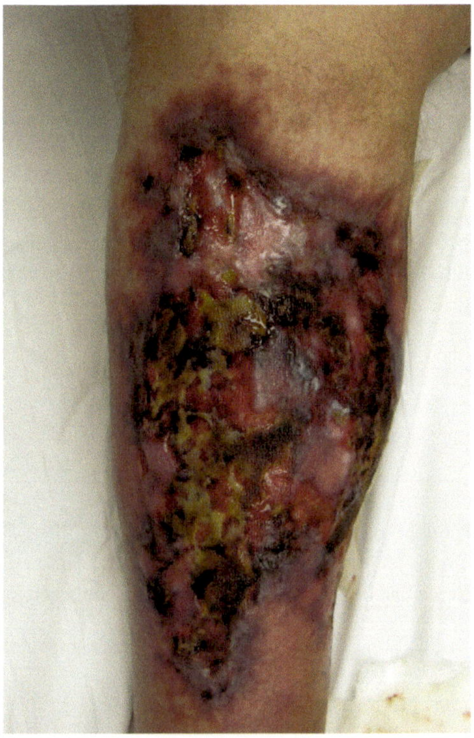

FIGURE 3.64 Necrotizing granulomatous vasculitis: Granulomatosis with polyangiitis.

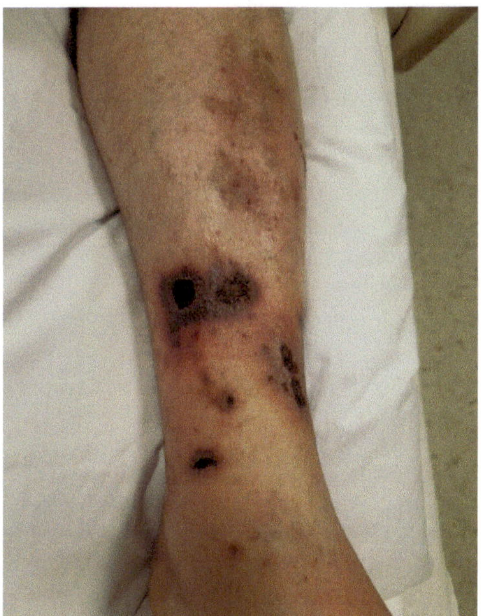

FIGURE 3.65 Necrotizing granulomatous vasculitis: Polyarteritis nodosa.

Evaluation and Management

A thorough history, physical examination, medication review, and review of systems should be undertaken to seek symptoms suggesting systemic involvement. Skin biopsy can be used to verify the presence of vessel damage due to inflammation (leukocytoclasis) with fibrinoid necrosis, as well as invasive infectious bacteria or fungi. Additional tissue should be sent for direct immunofluorescence to evaluate for IgA vasculitis. Laboratory evaluation is summarized in **Table 3.5**. Treatment of vasculitis is variable, depending on the underlying cause. Once an infectious etiology has been ruled out, often nonsteroidal immunosuppression with dapsone or colchicine can be attempted. In severe cases, immunosuppression with mycophenolate mofetil, methotrexate, azathioprine, or cyclophosphamide or biologics can be considered.

TABLE 3.5

Vasculitis Workup

Biopsy

- Pathology and direct immunofluorescence

Labs & other

- Complete blood count with platelets and differential (peripheral eosinophilia may suggest drug-induced vasculitis)
- Liver function tests
- Renal function tests and urinalysis
- Complement 3/4
- Anti-nuclear antibody
- Anti-double stranded DNA antibody
- Anti-Smith antibody
- Anti-Ro/La antibody
- Anti-topoisomerase antibody
- Rheumatoid factor and anti-cyclic citrullinated antibody
- Anti- neutrophilic cytoplasmic antibodies
- Serum protein electrophoresis/Serum immunofixation electrophoresis/Serum free light
- 24-hour Urine protein electrophoresis/Urine immunofixation electrophoresis
- Cryoglobulins and hepatitis C antibodies
- Bacterial/Fungal cultures
- *Viral serology*: cytomegalovirus (CMV), Epstein–Barr virus (EBV), human immunodeficiency virus (HIV), Hep B/C, Parvovirus B19, COVID-19
- Hemoccult testing
- Age-appropriate cancer screening should be completed
- Review of medications

BIBLIOGRAPHY

Fracticelli P, Benfaremo D, Gabrielli A. Diagnosis and management of leukocytoclastic vasculitis. Intern Emerg Med 2021;16(4):831–841.

Frumholtz L, Laurent-Roussel S, Lipsker D, et al. Cutaneous vasculitis: Review on diagnosis and clinicopathologic correlations. Clin Rev Allergy Immunol 2021;61(2):181–193.

Moretti M, Treppo E, Monti S, et al, Systemic vasculitis: One year in review. Clin Exp Rheum 2023;41(4):765–773.

4

Genetic Paraneoplastic Disorders

Basal Cell Nevus Syndrome

Etiopathogenesis

Basal cell nevus syndrome (BCNS), also known as Gorlin syndrome or Gorlin–Goltz syndrome, is a rare, autosomal dominant disorder characterized by the development of multiple basal cell carcinomas (BCCs), odontogenic keratocysts, and skeletal abnormalities. The genetic basis of BCNS has been linked to mutations in the PTCH1, PTCH 2, and SUFU tumor suppressor genes on chromosome 9. These genes are all members of the sonic hedgehog signaling pathway. Dysregulation of this pathway leads to unregulated stimulation and downstream activation of oncogenes such as the glioma-associated oncogene family, ultimately causing abnormal proliferation and cancer development.

Clinical Manifestations

The major and minor criteria are summarized in **Table 4.1**. The cutaneous manifestations of BCNS include BCCs (several to thousands [**Figures 4.1** and **4.2**]), palmar plantar pits (**Figures 4.3** and **4.4**), and milia around the eyes or on the forehead. The BCCs in BCNS tend to appear early, with reports in patients as young as 3 years; the mean age of onset is approximately 20 years. In general, the BCCs of BCNS affect similar areas as those seen in sporadic BCCs. There is controversy as to whether the biological behavior of the BCCs in BCNS is more aggressive than standard BCCs. The rate of metastasis for BCC in general is quite low (under 1%). Additional clinical manifestations include oral findings (odontogenic keratocysts, cleft lip/palate, bilateral hyperplasia of the mandibular coronoid processes), skeletal abnormalities (increased height, prominent frontal bossing, wide-set eyes, rib abnormalities, scoliosis, finger deformities, spina bifida), ocular and auditory findings, genitourinary findings (bilateral ovarian cysts, fibromas, renal abnormalities), and cardiovascular findings, such as cardiac fibromas in the left anterior ventricular wall.

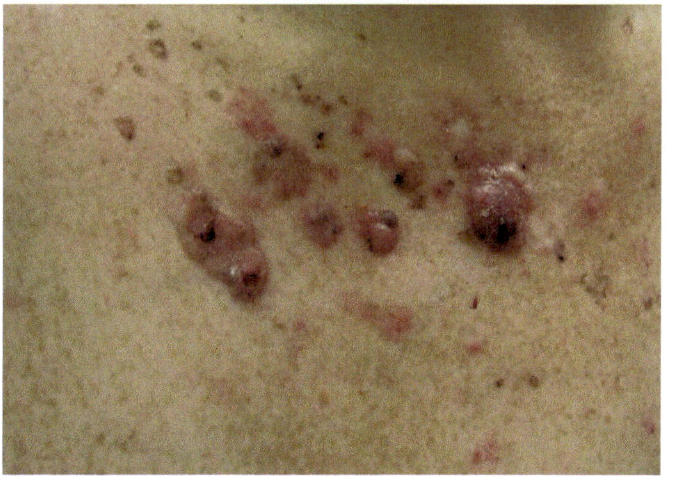

FIGURE 4.1 Basal cell nevus syndrome: Multiple basal cell carcinoma.

DOI: 10.1201/9781003492665-4

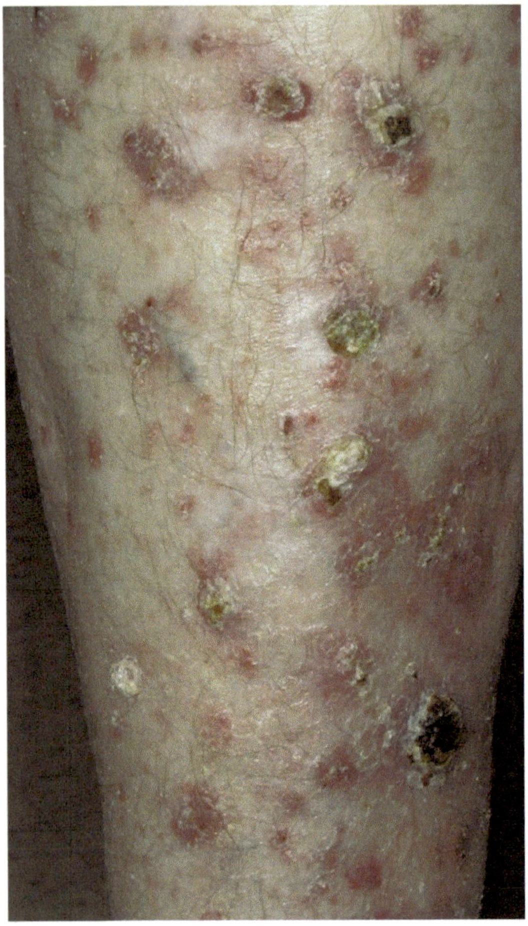

FIGURE 4.2 Basal cell nevus syndrome: Multiple basal cell carcinoma.

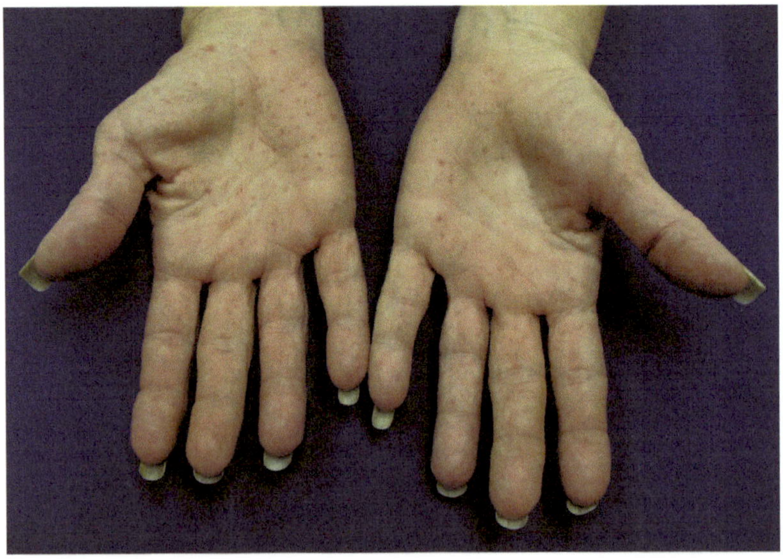

FIGURE 4.3 Basal cell nevus syndrome: Palmar pitting.

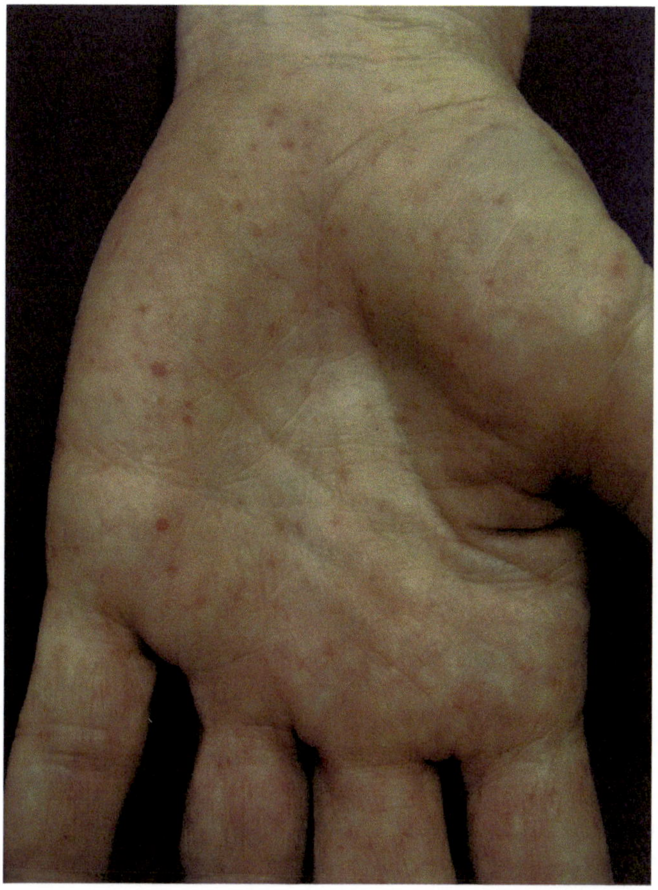

FIGURE 4.4 Basal cell nevus syndrome: Palmar pitting.

Systemic Manifestations

Patients with BCNS need to be monitored for the development of underlying malignancy. In particular, medulloblastomas have been reported at a very young age, more commonly in SUFU mutations. Multiple other malignancies, including Hodgkin and non-Hodgkin lymphoma, leiomyosarcoma, and rhabdomyosarcoma, have been reported.

Evaluation and Management

The First International Colloquium on BCNS suggested that the clinical criteria for diagnosis are quite comprehensive, and genetic testing is not required in all cases. However, in borderline cases or in prenatal testing, a referral to a geneticist/genetic counselor is recommended. Key recommendations include a baseline magnetic resonance imaging (MRI) of the brain with contrast and epilepsy protocol, a full skin examination by a dermatologist every 4 months, digital panoramic X-ray of the jaw annually, genetic counseling at baseline, psychological evaluation, neurology evaluation annually, obstetrics and gynecologic evaluation annually, nutritional assessment, and education regarding minimizing exposure to ionizing radiation. Vismodegib, an oral hedgehog pathway inhibitor, may be used for suppressing BCC growth/development for tumors that cause dysfunction or are cosmetically disfiguring and may shrink odontogenic keratocysts. Intermittent dosing helps make side effects of alopecia and dysgeusia more tolerable.

TABLE 4.1

Major and Minor Criteria for BCNS

Major	
1.	Greater than 5 BCCs or one under the age of 30
2.	Lamellar calcification of the falx
3.	Odontogenic keratocysts of the jaw
4.	Palmar pits (2 or more)
5.	First-degree relative with BCNS
Minor	
1.	Childhood medulloblastoma
2.	Lymphomesenteric or pleural cysts
3.	Macrocephaly
4.	Cleft lip or palate
5.	Bifid ribs or vertebrae
6.	Polydactyly
7.	Fibromas (ovarian or cardiac)
8.	Pigmented changes of the retinal epithelium

BIBLIOGRAPHY

Fernandez LT, Ocampo-Garza SS, Elizondo-Riojas G. Basal cell nevus syndrome: An update on clinical findings. Int J Dermatol 2022;61:1047–1055.

Lukowiak TM, Cahn B, Samie F, et al. Developing expert consensus for the use of hedgehog inhibitors in basal cell nevus syndrome. Arch Dermatol Res 2024;316(7):453.

Palmeiro AG, Carvalho M, Goncalves Costro C, et al. Vismodegib in Gorlin-Goltz syndrome: A systematic review. Australas J Dermatol 2024;65(6):e123–e133.

Birt–Hogg–Dubé Syndrome

Etiopathogenesis

Birt–Hogg–Dubé (BHD) syndrome is a rare, autosomal dominant disorder characterized by cutaneous lesions (fibrofolliculomas, trichodiscomas, perifollicular fibromas, acrochordons), lung cysts, spontaneous pneumothoraxes, and renal cancers (oncocytomas, chromophobe renal carcinoma, papillary carcinoma, clear cell carcinoma). Diagnostic criteria are summarized in **Table 4.2**. BHD is linked to mutations in the FLCN (*folliculin*) gene on chromosome 17. The function of the gene product, folliculin, is not entirely clear, but appears to have a tumor suppressor function and may be involved in the mammalian target of rapamycin (mTOR) pathway, which is also implicated in the development of tuberous sclerosis.

Clinical Manifestations

The classic cutaneous manifestations of BHD include fibrofolliculomas, trichodiscomas, and acrochordons (**Figures 4.5–4.8**). Fibrofolliculomas are dome-shaped, white-to-flesh-colored papules commonly found on the face, neck, and upper trunk; they are indistinguishable clinically from trichodiscomas. More recent evidence suggests that the classic lesions of BHD may actually be a spectrum of presentation of fibrofolliculomas (pedunculated fibrofolliculomas identified clinically as acrochordons). Although many of these lesions can be seen in the normal population, multiple lesions within the same patient should prompt further investigation.

Systemic Manifestations

Patients with BHD need to be evaluated for underlying malignancy. The most commonly reported cancer in these patients is renal cancer (mixed chromophobe and oncocytic renal tumors), which often begins quite early. There is a sevenfold increase in the risk of renal cancer for BHD patients. The age of diagnosis of renal cancer is 31–74 years, with a mean age of 50.4 years. Pulmonary examination is consistent with multiple lung cysts, most often in the basal lung regions. Despite the cysts, lung function is usually unaffected. The prevalence of pneumothorax in these patients has been reported to be as high as 24%, with first occurrence at 38 years (range 22–71). Recurrent pneumothorax is common in this population.

Evaluation and Management

Recent recommendations from the European BHD Guideline Group suggest that all patients suspected of having BHD should be offered genetic testing for an underlying *folliculin* mutation and referral to a geneticist/genetic counselor. Management guidelines for patients with BHD continue to evolve, but include annual physical exams and an annual renal MRI beginning at age 20 (the roles of computed tomography [CT] and ultrasound [US] have not been fully investigated). Dermatologic management of the fibrofolliculomas includes electrodesiccation of the lesions or laser ablation (Erbium:YAG or CO_2 laser). Patient education regarding smoking cessation to prevent pneumothorax should be performed, and early pleurodesis can prevent recurrent disease. Because general anesthesia can also provoke pneumothorax in these patients, evaluation with a pulmonologist is advised prior to surgical procedures.

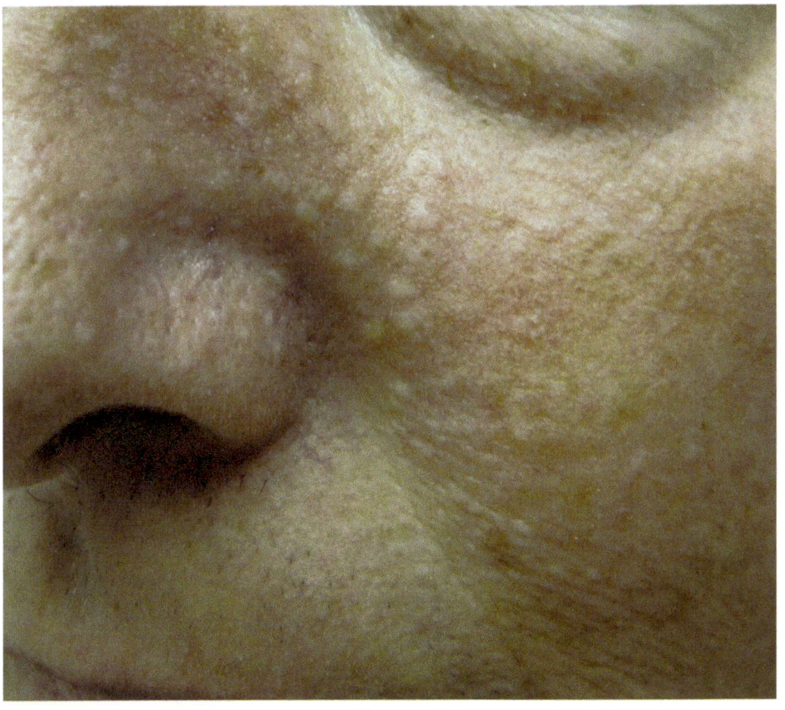

FIGURE 4.5 Birt–Hogg–Dubé syndrome: Fibrofolliculomas.

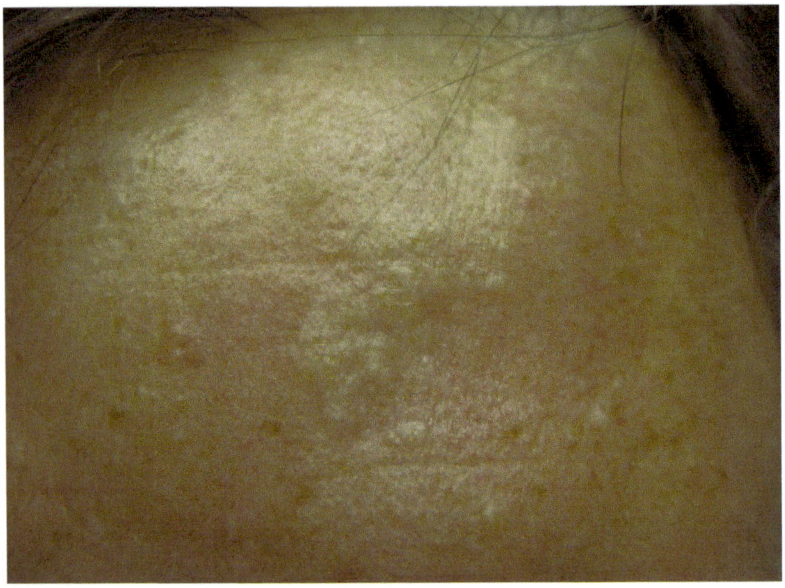

FIGURE 4.6 Birt–Hogg–Dubé syndrome: Fibrofolliculomas (forehead).

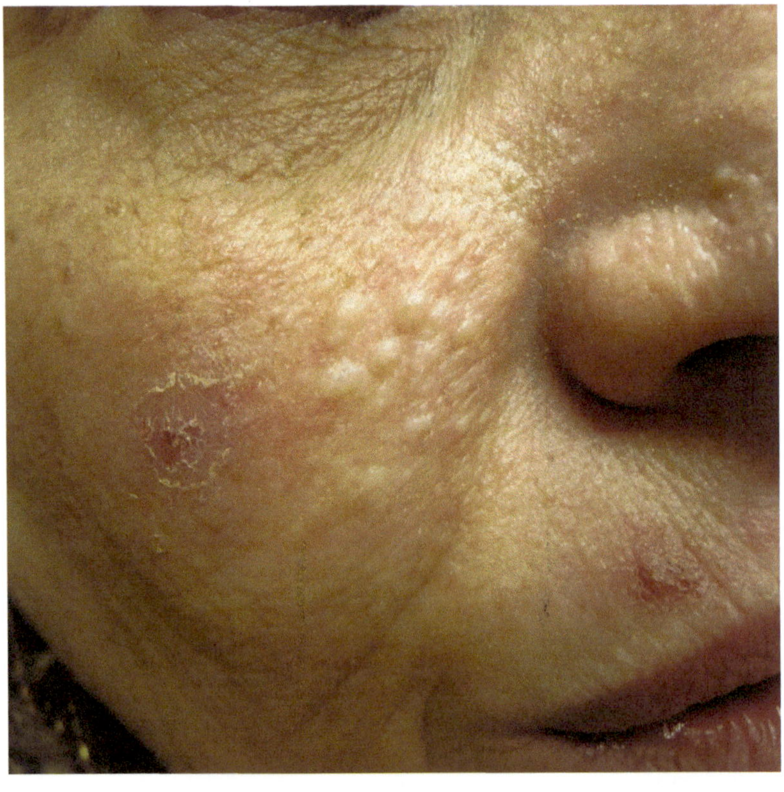

FIGURE 4.7 Birt–Hogg–Dubé syndrome: Fibrofolliculomas.

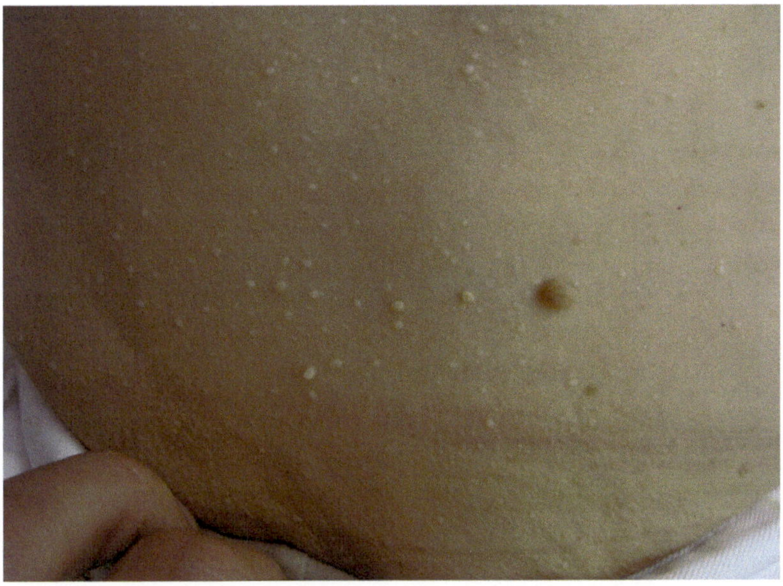

FIGURE 4.8 Birt–Hogg–Dubé syndrome: Acrochordon-like fibrofolliculomas.

TABLE 4.2

Diagnostic Criteria for BHD Syndrome

Major criteria (one)
• A least 5 fibrofolliculomas or trichodiscomas of adult onset
• FLCN germline mutation
Minor criteria (two)
• Multiple lung cysts +/- spontaneous pneumothorax
• Early onset renal cancer (<50 years old)
• First-degree relative with BHD syndrome

BIBLIOGRAPHY

Bruinsma FJ, Dowty JG, Win AK, et al. Update of penetrance estimates in Birt-Hogg-Dube syndrome. J Med Gnet 2023;60(4):317–326.

Daccord C, Good JM, Morren MA, et al. Birt-Hogg-Dube syndrome. Eur Respir Rev 2020;29(157):200042.

Geilswijk M, Genuardi M, Woodward R, et al. ERN GENTURIS clinical guidelines for the diagnosis, surveillance and management of people with Birt-Hogg-Dube syndrome. Eur J Hum Genet 2024;32(12):1542–1550.

Tong Y, Schneider JA, Coda AB, et al. Birt-Hogg-Dube syndrome: A review of dermatologic manifestations and other manifestations. Am J Clin Dermatol 2018;19(1):87–101.

Cowden Syndrome

Etiopathogenesis

Cowden syndrome (CS), or phosphatase and tensin homolog (PTEN) hamartoma tumor syndrome, is an autosomal dominant disorder linked to mutations in the PTEN tumor suppressor gene on chromosome 10 causing dysregulation of the P13K/AKT/mTOR signaling pathway. The prevalence of CS has been estimated to be 1 in 200,000 to 1 in 250,000. When mutated, there is enhanced cell migration and prolonged cell survival. Consequently, PTEN mutations are associated with an increased risk of breast, thyroid, renal, colorectal, melanoma, and endometrial cancers, in addition to hamartomatous growth of the skin, colon, brain (Lhermite–Duclos disease), and other tissues.

Clinical Manifestations

CS presents with a wide array of mucocutaneous lesions, including multiple trichilemmomas (**Figures 4.9** and **4.10**) of the face and neck (>3), oral papillomas (>3) (**Figures 4.11** and **4.12**), acral keratoses (>3), neuromas, sclerotic fibromas, macular pigmentation of the glans penis, lipomas, and arteriovenous malformations. Although many of these lesions can be seen in the normal population, multiple lesions within the same patient should prompt further investigation.

Systemic Manifestations

The systemic manifestations of CS are protean and commonly include macrocephaly, breast lesions (fibrocystic breast disease, intraductal papillomas, fibroadenomas), gastrointestinal disease (hamartomatous colonic polyps, ganglioneuromas), and thyroid disease (follicular adenomas, thyroiditis), but also nervous system, renal, and vascular disorders. Patients with Cowden syndrome need to be evaluated for underlying malignancy. The most commonly reported cancers in these patients are breast cancer (25%–50%) and non-medullary thyroid cancer (3%–10%). The average age of breast cancer diagnosis in this population is 38–46 years. No histopathologic differences were noted in the type of breast cancer in CS patients when compared to the general population. The average age of thyroid cancer diagnosis is unclear but has been reported to occur in childhood. Thyroid cancer in this population is exclusively of follicular or papillary histology.

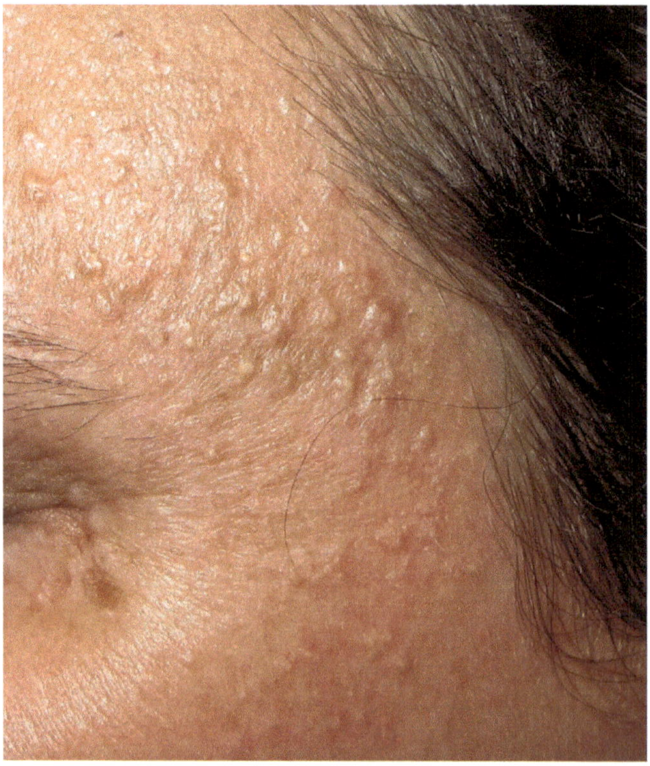

FIGURE 4.9 Cowden syndrome: Trichilemmomas.

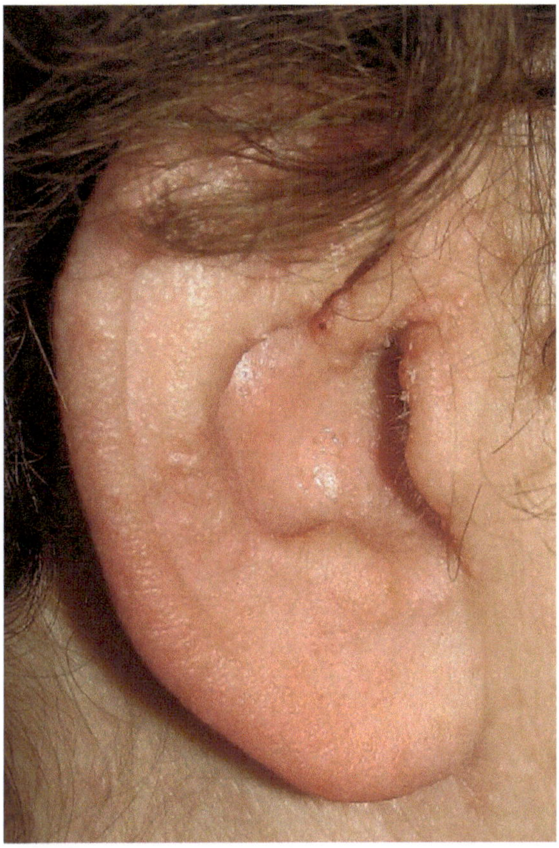

FIGURE 4.10 Cowden syndrome: Trichilemmomas.

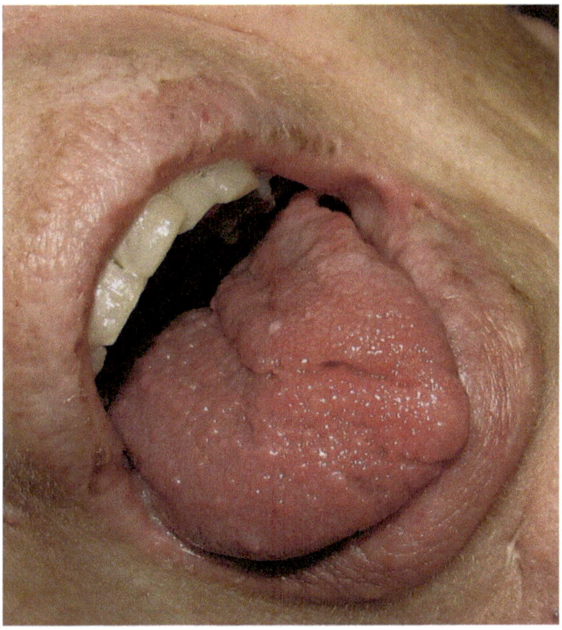

FIGURE 4.11 Cowden syndrome: Oral papillomas.

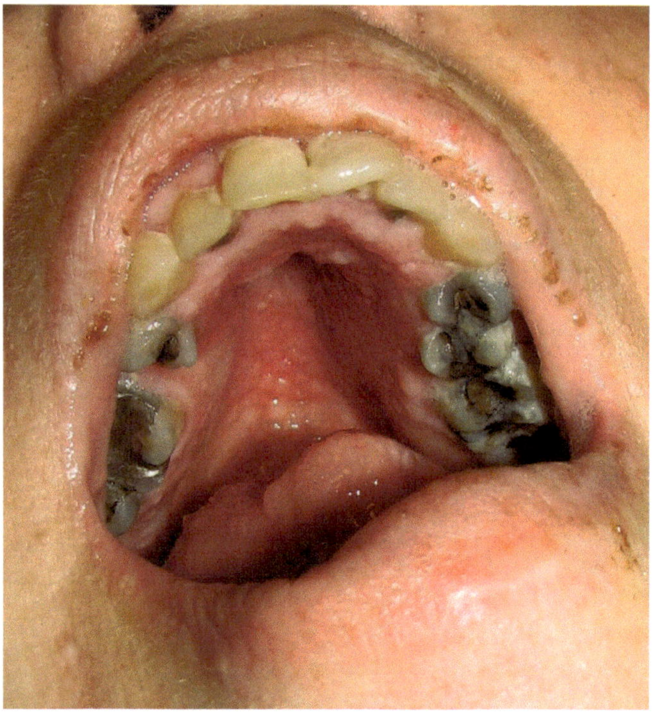

FIGURE 4.12 Cowden syndrome: Oral papillomas.

Evaluation and Management

Given the wide variability in presentation, it can be difficult to determine which patients may require PTEN gene analysis. Referral to a geneticist with knowledge and experience in PTEN-opathies is recommended. Management guidelines for patients with CS have been adopted by the National Comprehensive Cancer Network (NCCN), and cancer screening recommendations are summarized in **Table 4.3**.

TABLE 4.3

Cancer Screening Recommendations for Cowden Syndrome

Cancer	Method	Interval	Starting Age
Breast	MRI/MMGX	Yearly	30–35
Thyroid	US	Yearly	7
Renal	US	Every 1–2 years	40
Colorectal	Colonoscopy	Every 5 years	35
Melanoma	Skin exam	Yearly	30
Endometrial	Transvaginal US	Physician discretion	Post-menopausal

BIBLIOGRAPHY

Dragoo DD, Taher A, Wong VK, et al. PTEN Hamartoma tumor syndrome/Cowden syndrome: Genomics, oncogenesis and imaging review of associated lesions and malignancy. Cancers (Basel) 2021;13(13):3120.

Pirlog LM, Patrascanu AA, Militaru MS, et al. Insights into clinical disorders in Cowden syndrome: A comprehensive review. Medicina (Kaunas) 2024;60(5):767.

Takayama T, Muguruma N, Igarashi M, et al. Clinical guidelines for diagnosis and management of Cowden syndrome/PTEN hamartoma tumor syndrome in children and adults-secondary publication. J Anus Rectum Colon 2023;7(4):284–300.

Fabry Disease

Etiopathogenesis

Fabry disease (FD), or Anderson–Fabry disease, is an X-linked, recessive disorder caused by a deficiency in the activity of the α-galactosidase A enzyme. This enzyme deficiency leads to the accumulation of neutral glycosphingolipids (globotriaosylceramide) in the lysosomes of cells throughout the body, with a predilection for vascular endothelium and vascular smooth muscle cells. This causes fibrotic thickening, endothelial dysfunction, hypercontractility, vasospasm, and a pro-thrombotic phenotype that leads to ischemia and infarction (kidney, brain, and heart); also organomegaly and multiorgan dysfunction. FD is the second-most common lysosomal storage disease in humans and is estimated to occur once in every 117,000 live Caucasian births.

Clinical Manifestations

Cutaneous angiokeratomas (**Figures 4.13** and **4.14**) are the hallmark clinical presentation of FD and usually appear in adolescence. Although angiokeratomas can be seen in the general population, numerous angiokeratomas (angiokeratoma corporis diffusum) involving the genitals, lumbosacral area, gluteal cleft, trunk, periungual areas, and palms are pathognomonic for FD. They are present in 66% of male patients and 36% of female patients with FD. Facial dysmorphism, or *Fabry facies*, is typical and includes a recessed forehead, prominent supraorbital ridges, widened nasal bridge, and bulbous nasal tip. Telangiectasias, hypohidrosis, xerophthalmia, decreased saliva production, corneal opacities, Fabry cataract, and retinal and conjunctival vascular aneurismal dilatations have also been reported.

Systemic Manifestations

Systemic manifestations can begin in childhood, including gastrointestinal (GI) disturbances and chronic, severely limiting acral paresthesias in the hands and feet. In later life, cardiovascular, renal, and central nervous system dysfunction are most prominent, such as left ventricular hypertrophy, valvular and conduction system abnormalities, proteinuria (characteristic birefringent Maltese cross appearance on polarization microscopy), end-stage renal disease, and ischemic strokes.

Evaluation and Management

FD can be difficult to diagnose, given its wide-ranging signs and symptoms. In the absence of a known family history, the diagnosis is often made later, when the patient is faced with end-organ dysfunction. Diagnosis is based on detection of low α-galactosidase A enzyme activity in dried blood spots, leukocytes, and cultured skin fibroblasts. Mutational analyses can be performed; however, the defect that causes FD is heterogeneous, and isolating specific mutations may be challenging. Management of these patients requires a multidisciplinary approach—including involvement of the dermatologist, ophthalmologist, cardiologist, neurologist, nephrologist, and genetic counselor, among others. The skin manifestations of FD are treated according to their symptomatology. Angiokeratomas and telangiectasias can be treated with electrodesiccation or laser treatment. Prior to the development of recombinant α-galactosidase A enzyme replacement therapy, the average life expectancy was 50–55 (men) and 70 (women). With regular infusions, disease progression has halted for many of the patients, and life expectancy has increased.

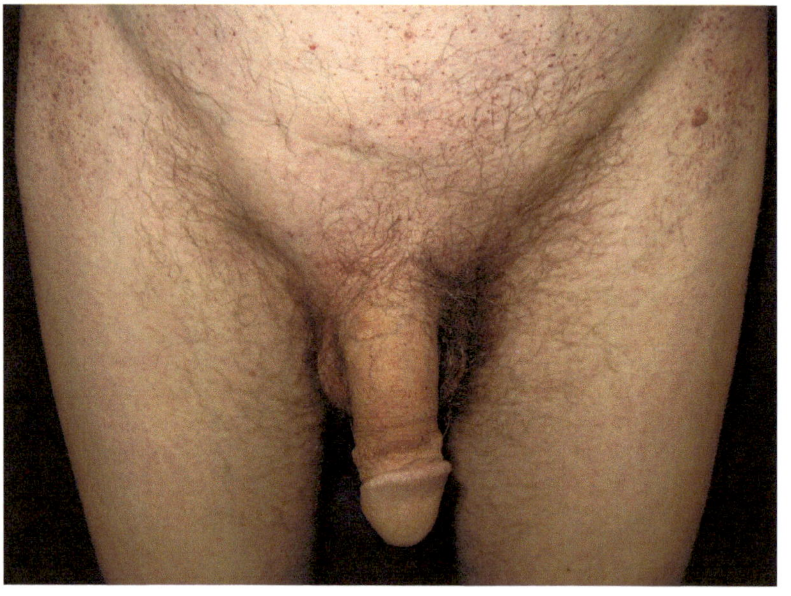

FIGURE 4.13 Fabry disease: Penile shaft angiokeratomas.

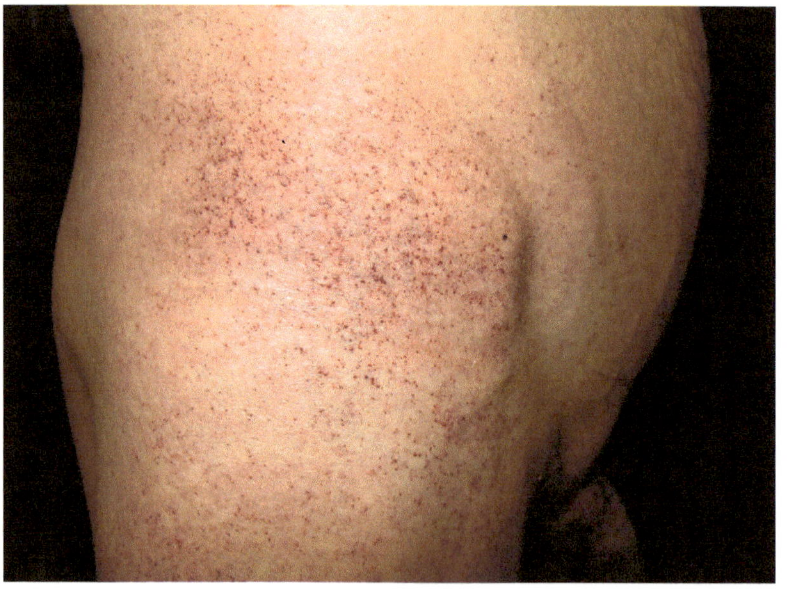

FIGURE 4.14 Fabry disease.

BIBLIOGRAPHY

Faro DC, Di Pino FL, Monte IP. Inflammation, oxidative stress, and endothelial dysfunction in the pathogenesis of vascular damage: Unraveling novel cardiovascular risk factors in Fabry disease. Int J Mol Sci 2024;25(15):8273.

Kok K, Zwiers KC, Boot RG, et al. Fabry disease: Molecular basis, pathophysiology, diagnostics and potential therapeutic directions. Biomolecules 2021;11(2):271.
Michaud M, Mauhin W, Belmatoug N, et al. When and how to diagnosis Fabry disease in clinical practice. AM J Med Sci 2020;360(6):641–649.

Gardner Syndrome

Etiopathogenesis

Gardner syndrome (GS), a phenotypic variant of familial adenomatous polyposis (FAP) syndrome, is an autosomal dominant disorder linked to mutations in the adenomatous polyposis coli (APC) gene (chromosome 5). Mutations in the APC gene predispose patients to colon cancer through the development of hundreds to thousands of precancerous colonic polyps that begin at an early age. GS is characterized by colonic polyposis typical of FAP together with extracolonic manifestations. Differences in the phenotypic presentations of these entities may be related to the location of the mutation within the APC gene. The prevalence of all the APC-associated polyposis conditions is reported to be approximately 2.29–3.2 per 100,000 individuals.

Clinical Manifestations

Clinically, patients with GS present with extracolonic manifestations, which may precede the development of colon polyps. These include osteomas of the mandible and skull, dental abnormalities (unerupted teeth, congenital absence of one or more teeth, supernumerary teeth, odontomas), multiple epidermal cysts (often in atypical locations such as the face, neck, and axilla [**Figure 4.15**]), fibromas, other nonspecific skin tumors and cysts, desmoid tumors, and ocular abnormalities, including congenital hypertrophy of the retinal pigment epithelium (CHRPE).

Systemic Manifestations

Although it is imperative that a patient with GS can be evaluated for underlying colorectal cancer, there is also an increased risk of other neoplasms, including papillary/follicular thyroid cancer, hepatoblastoma, as well as gastric, duodenal, and ampulla of Vater adenocarcinoma. The risk of colon cancer cannot be overstated. By the age of 35, 95% of individuals with FAP have polyps, and without colectomy, colon cancer is inevitable.

Evaluation and Management

Molecular genetic testing of suspected individuals should be performed. Full gene sequencing of the APC gene is available and appears to be the most accurate clinical test available. Management of these patients requires a multidisciplinary approach—including involvement of the dermatologist, the gastroenterologist, and/or colorectal surgeon, dentist/oral surgeon, ophthalmologist, and genetic counselor, among others. Practice guidelines from the NCCN have been developed for FAP patients (**Table 4.4**), and although no specific guidelines exist for Gardner syndrome patients, it is recommended that FAP guidelines are applied. The skin manifestations of GS are treated according to their symptomatology. A regular complete dermatologic exam is advised. Epidermal cysts can be surgically excised, or, if they are inflamed, the patient may be given intralesional injections of corticosteroids, which may minimize the cysts' size. Other benign skin tumors can be treated with surgical removal or electrodesiccation.

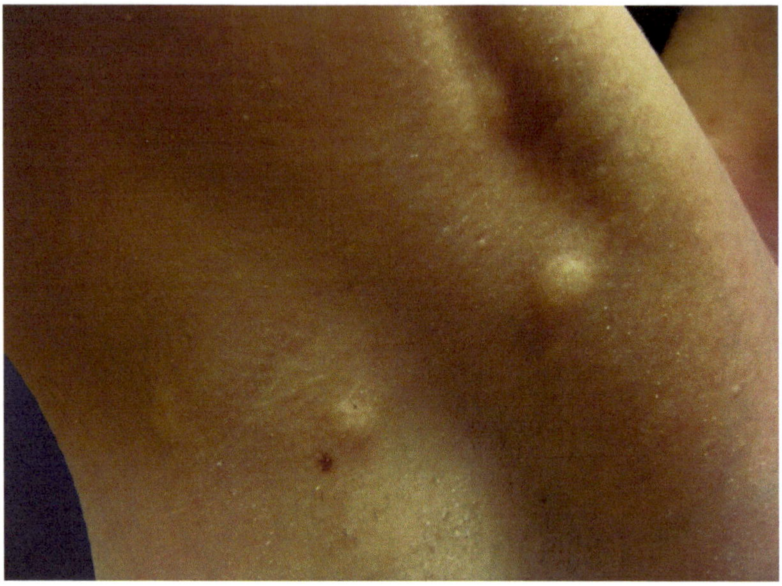

FIGURE 4.15 Gardner syndrome.

TABLE 4.4

Familial Adenomatous Polyposis Screening Guidelines

Procedure	Duration	Age
Colonoscopy	Annual	10–15
Endoscopy	Annual	20–25
Thyroid US	Annual	Late teens
Abdominal palpation	Annual	At diagnosis

BIBLIOGRAPHY

Ladd R, Davis M, Dyer JA. Genodermatoses with malignant potential. Clin Dermatol 2020;28(4): 432–454.

Menon G, Carr S, Kasi A. Familial adenomatous polyposis. In: StatPEarls {Internet]. Treasure Island (FL): StatPearls Publishing; 2024.

Takao A, Koizumi K, Takao M, et al. Upper gastrointestinal tumors are unrelated to the APC genotype in APC-associated polyposis. Jpn J Clin Oncol 2022;52(6):554–561.

Muir–Torre Syndrome

Etiopathogenesis

Muir–Torre syndrome (MTS) is a phenotypic variant of hereditary nonpolyposis colorectal cancer (Lynch syndrome) characterized by multiple cutaneous sebaceous neoplasms, keratoacanthomas, and internal malignancies. MTS is inherited in an autosomal dominant pattern with 80% penetrance (chromosomes

2 and 3). Mutations in DNA mismatch repair genes MSH2, MLH1, MSH6, and PMS2 have all been identified. These mutations lead to errors in DNA replication and microsatellite instability, which is a hallmark of this syndrome.

Clinical Manifestations

The cutaneous manifestations of MTS can precede (27%), develop after (57%), or develop concomitantly with the first internal malignancy (10%). The clinical manifestations of MTS include sebaceous adenomas (**Figure 4.16**), sebaceomas, sebaceous carcinomas (**Figures 4.17** and **4.18**), keratoacanthomas (**Figure 4.19**), and BCC with sebaceous differentiation. Sebaceous adenomas and sebaceomas (sebaceous epitheliomas) are yellowish to flesh-colored nodules usually located on the face. Both are clinically very similar and only vary histologically in the ratio of cells present. Sebaceous carcinoma is a malignant lesion with metastatic potential and most commonly occurs on the eyelid. Classic sebaceous hyperplasia is not considered part of MTS. Keratoacanthomas are well-differentiated squamous cell carcinomas that present as a nodule with a central keratinaceous core, and in MTS they demonstrate sebaceous differentiation (seboacanthoma).

Systemic Manifestations

Patients with lesions suggestive of MTS need to be evaluated for underlying malignancy. The most commonly reported cancer in MTS patients is colorectal carcinoma, followed by genitourinary cancers, breast carcinomas, and hematologic disorders. This varies slightly from the malignancies noted in classical Lynch syndrome (colorectal, endometrial, ureter, renal pelvis, small bowel). The age at presentation of first malignancy ranges from 23 to 89 years, with a median of 53 years, and greater than 50% of MTS patients have two or more visceral malignancies.

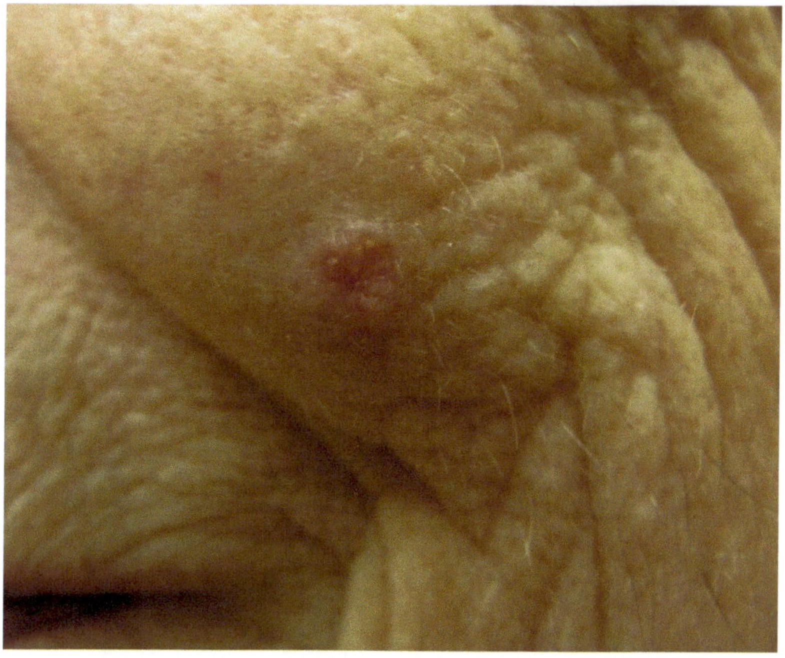

FIGURE 4.16 Muir–Torre syndrome: Sebaceous adenoma.

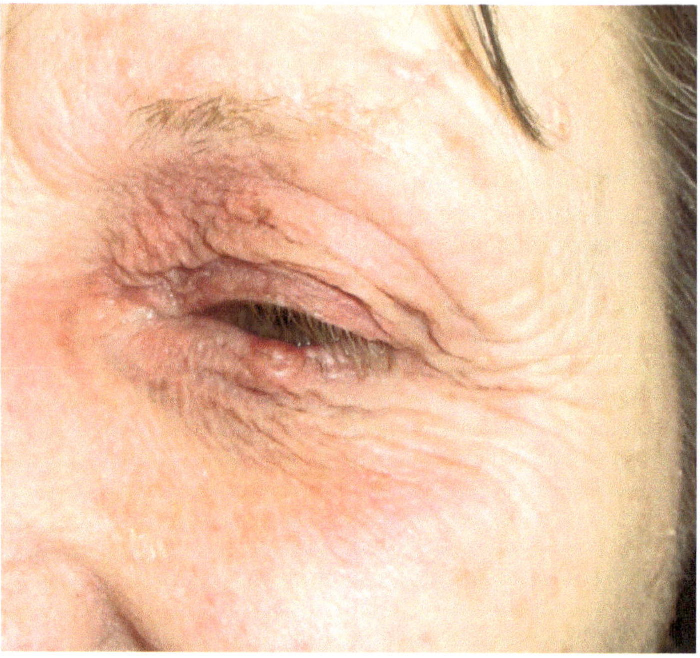

FIGURE 4.17 Muir–Torre syndrome: Sebaceous carcinoma lower eyelid.

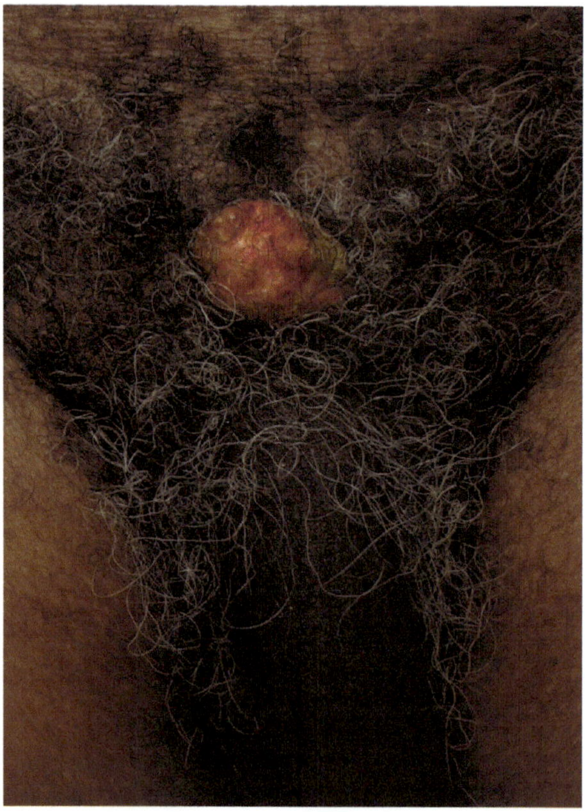

FIGURE 4.18 Muir-Torre syndrome: Sebaceous carcinoma atypical pubic location.

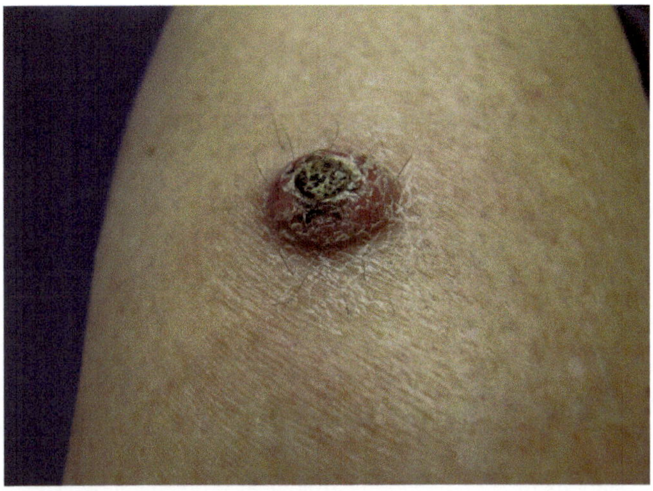

FIGURE 4.19 Muir–Torre syndrome: Keratoacanthoma.

Evaluation and Management

Skin biopsy and histologic evaluation for microsatellite instability analysis and immunohistochemistry for mismatch repair genes in suspected skin tumors are prudent. Completion of a colonoscopy and other age-appropriate cancer screening is advisable. Additional testing, including CT, Mammography (MMGX), transvaginal US, endometrial biopsy, and esophagogastroduodenoscopy (EGD), may be focused based on patient- or family-specific risk factors. Referral to a geneticist/genetic counselor is recommended because unaffected family members may need testing for the presence of germ-line mutations. Once the diagnosis of MTS has been confirmed, screening recommendations as suggested by the collaborative group of the European experts in hereditary GI cancer should be followed. Treatment of the skin and visceral lesions is primarily surgical; however, chemoprevention of the cutaneous neoplasms using systemic retinoids (acitretin or isotretinoin) appears promising.

BIBLIOGRAPHY

Cook S, Petick J, Hollestein L, et al. Sebaceous carcinoma epidemiology, associated malignancies and Lynch/Muir-Torre syndrome screening in England from 2008–2018. J Am Acad Dermatol 2023;89(6):1129–1135.

Gay JT, Troxell T, Gross GP. Muir-Torre Syndrome. In: StatPearls[Internet]. Treasure Island (FL): StatPearls Publishing; 2023.

Shah RR, Allman P, Schwartz RA. Muir-Torre Syndrome: A cutaneous finding amidst broader malignancies. Am J Clin Dermatol 2023;24(3):375–380.

Neurofibromatosis Type 1

Etiopathogenesis

Neurofibromatosis type 1 (NF1) is a highly penetrant, autosomal dominant disorder with variable phenotypic expression that often develops from spontaneous mutations. The birth incidence of NF1 is 1 in 3000. Loss of neurofibromin (NF gene 1, chromosome 17) appears to dysregulate the normal Ras-GTP signaling pathway, leading to uncontrolled cell proliferation. Up to 50% of cases are sporadic or due to de novo mutation.

Clinical Manifestations

The diagnostic criteria of NF1 include café-au-lait macules (six or more, >0.5 cm in children and >1.5 cm in adults [**Figure 4.20**]), two or more cutaneous neurofibromas or one plexiform neurofibroma (**Figures 4.21–4.23**), axillary or groin freckling, optic glioma, two or more Lisch nodules (iris hamartomas), bony dysplasia, and a first-degree relative with NF1. Axillary or groin freckling (Crowe sign) is the most specific of the NF1 diagnostic criteria. Cutaneous neurofibromas (**Figure 4.24**) are soft, flesh-colored, rounded, protuberant nodules that can appear anywhere on the body. Plexiform neurofibromas are usually congenital, often diffuse, and classically have a *bag of worms* texture.

Systemic Manifestations

The systemic manifestations of NF1 are protean, and 8%–13% of NF1 patients develop malignant peripheral nerve sheath tumors (MPNSTs). MPNSTs often occur in preexisting plexiform neurofibromas and can metastasize widely. Orthopedic issues include bowing of the long bones, pseudoarthrosis, scoliosis, and spontaneous fractures. Eye abnormalities, including optic gliomas, may impair visual acuity. Other systemic manifestations of NF1 include neurological problems (cognitive problems, behavioral difficulty, neurologic tumors and malformations, cerebrovascular disease), congenital heart disease (pulmonary stenosis and hypertension), GI problems (GI neurofibromas, GI stromal tumors), and fertility issues. Of note, classical NF1 complications are infrequent in patients with segmental NF1, and the rate of recurrence in offspring is low.

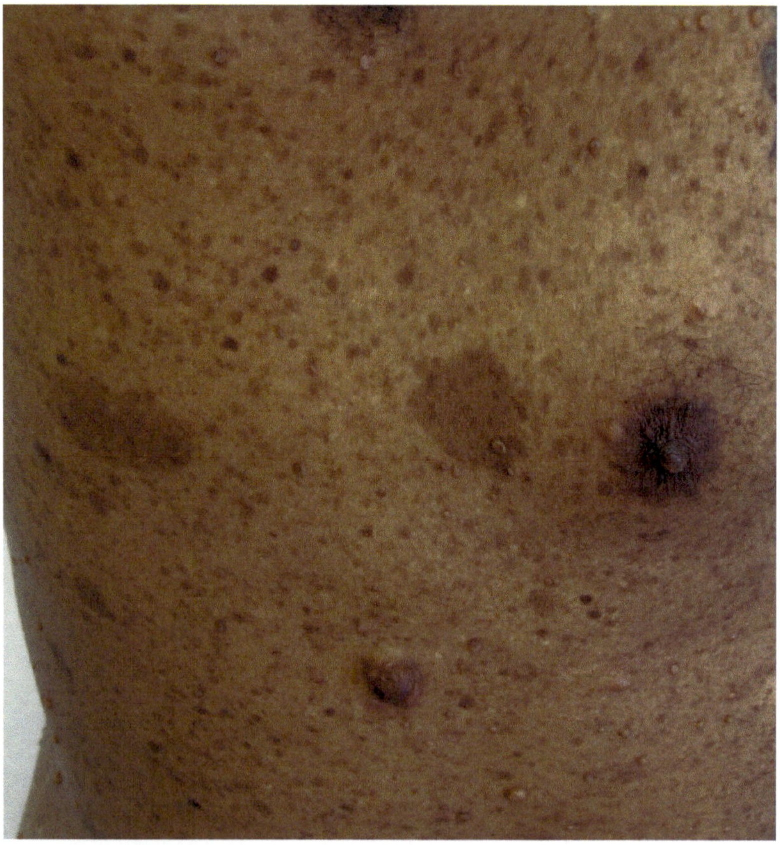

FIGURE 4.20 Neurofibromatosis: Freckling and café-au-lait macules.

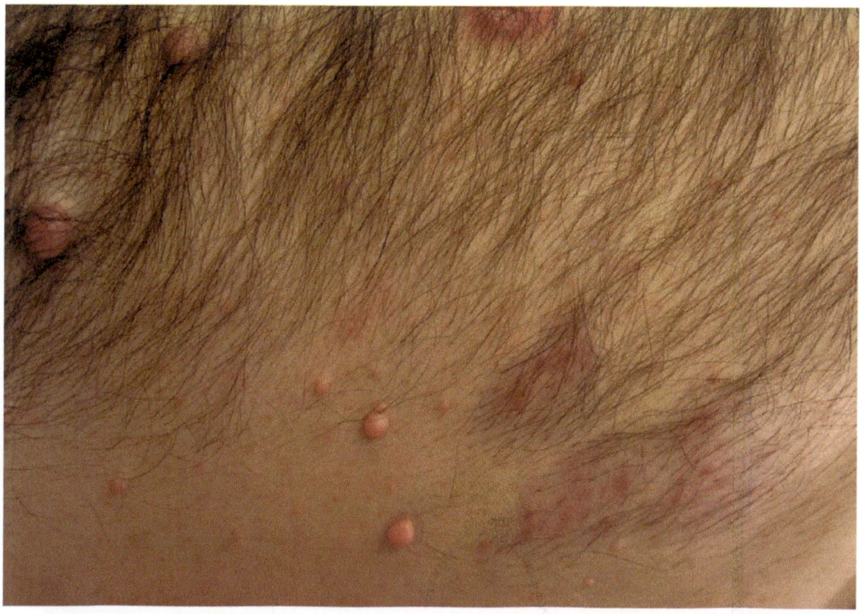

FIGURE 4.21 Neurofibromatosis: Neurofibromas and early plexiform neurofibromas.

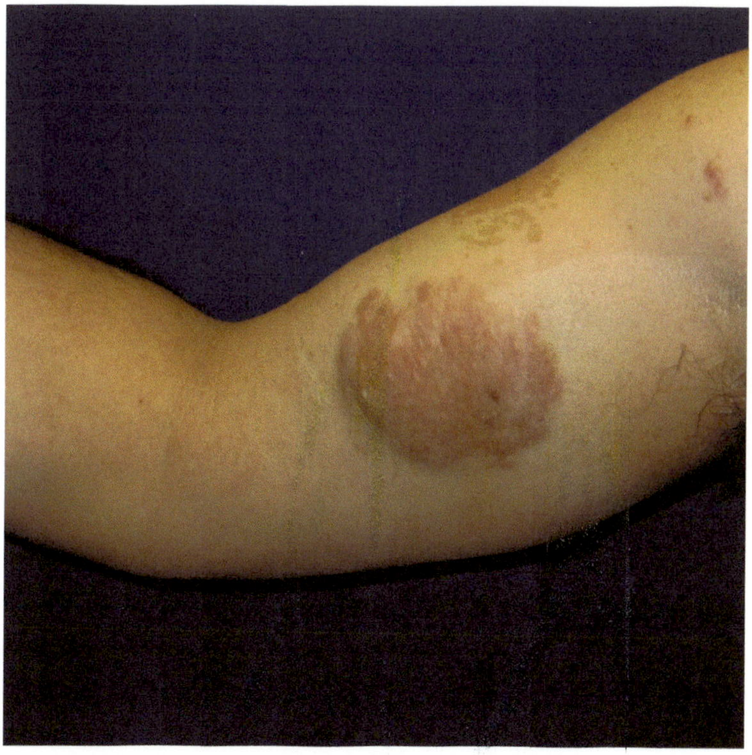

FIGURE 4.22 Neurofibromatosis: Plexiform neurofibroma and café-au-lait macule.

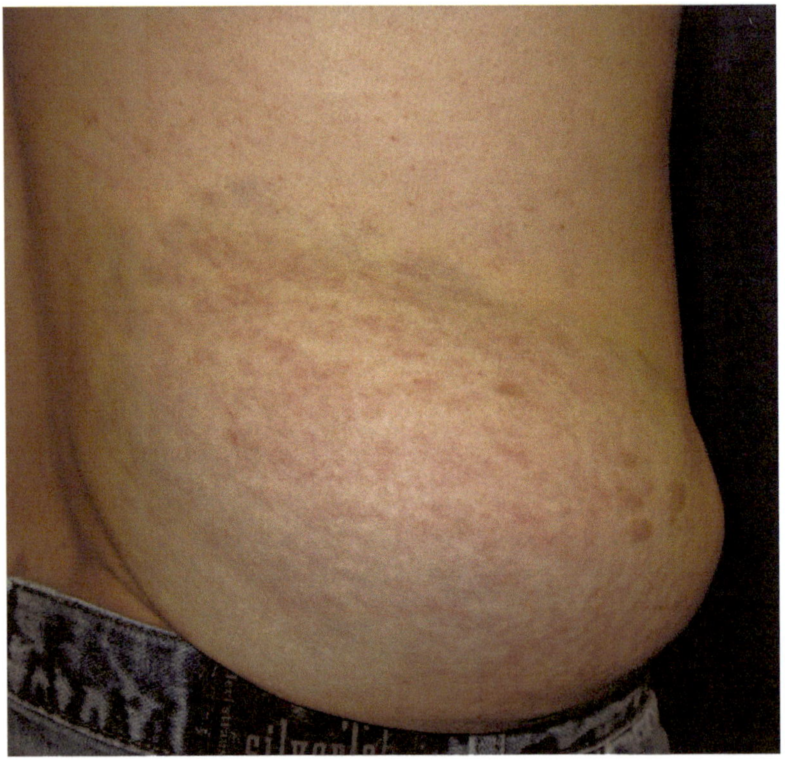

FIGURE 4.23 Neurofibromatosis: Massive plexiform neurofibroma.

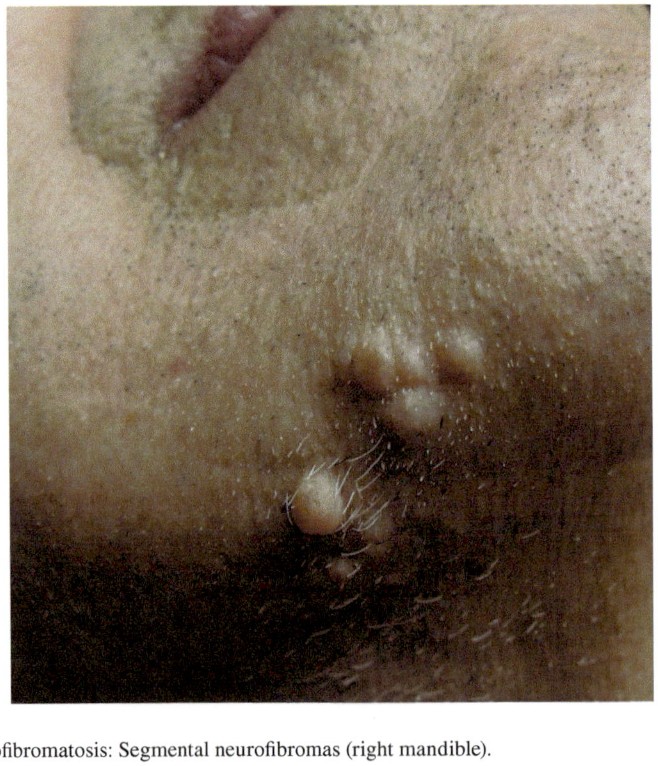

FIGURE 4.24 Neurofibromatosis: Segmental neurofibromas (right mandible).

Evaluation and Management

Genetic and molecular testing is available for NF1. Patients with NF1 need to be managed by a multidisciplinary team (dermatologist, neurologist, ophthalmologist, geneticist) with expertise in NF1. Age-specific monitoring of disease manifestations and patient education are imperative. From a treatment standpoint, cutaneous neurofibromas can be surgically excised if bothersome. Surgical removal of plexiform neurofibromas can be challenging and requires a surgeon with expertise in the removal of soft tissue tumors. MEK 1/2 inhibitors and selumetinib are appropriate in inoperable pediatric cases. MPNSTs may be noted secondary to textural change in the plexiform neurofibroma, an increase in pain, or an increase in size. MPNSTs require complete surgical excision, with adjuvant radiotherapy or chemotherapy as indicated. Annual neurological assessment is an absolute requirement to adequately evaluate for the variety of neurological problems noted previously.

BIBLIOGRAPHY

Armstrong AE, Belzberg AJ, Crawford JR, et al. Treatment decisions and the use of MEK inhibitors for children with neurofibromatosis type 1 – Related plexiform neurofibromas. BMC Cancer 2023;23(1):553.

Bayat M, Bayat A. Neurologic manifestation of neurofibromatosis: A review. Neurol Sci 2020;41(10):2685–2690.

Saleh M, Dib A, Beaini S, Saad C, et al. Neurofibromatosis type 1 system-based manifestations and treatment: A review. Neurol Sci 2023;44(6):1931–1947.

Reed Syndrome

Etiopathogenesis

Reed syndrome, or hereditary leiomyomatosis and renal cell cancer (HLRCC), is a highly penetrant, autosomal dominant tumor syndrome characterized by painful cutaneous pilar leiomyomas, uterine leiomyomas, and renal cancers. HLRCC is linked to germ-line mutations in the fumarate hydratase (FH) gene on chromosome 1. The gene product of FH, an enzyme in the tricarboxylic acid (TCA) cycle, is integral in cellular metabolism, but also has a role as a tumor suppressor.

Clinical Manifestations

The cutaneous manifestations of HLRCC include multiple painful cutaneous leiomyomas (CLMs) (**Figures 4.25–4.27**). CLMs arise from the hair follicle arrector pili muscle and are usually located on the trunk, limbs, and face. They are flesh-colored to reddish-brown papules, usually grouped together, ranging in size from about 2 to 20 mm. They are almost uniformly painful, especially to touch and changes in temperature.

Systemic Manifestations

Uterine leiomyomas in HLRCC are numerous and large, and tend to occur at an earlier age than sporadic uterine leiomyomas. They are frequently symptomatic, causing menorrhagia, pain, and fertility issues. The risk of development of uterine leiomyosarcoma in these patients is reported to be quite rare. Patients with HLRCC need to be evaluated for underlying malignancy. The most commonly reported cancer in these patients is renal cancer (renal papillary type II cancer, renal collecting duct cancer, clear cell carcinoma), which often begins quite early and metastasizes when the primary tumor is small. The median age of renal cancer diagnosis is 43 years. Several other tumors (breast cancer, bladder cancer, Leydig cell tumors) have been reported in patients with FH mutations; however, the significance of these findings has not been shown.

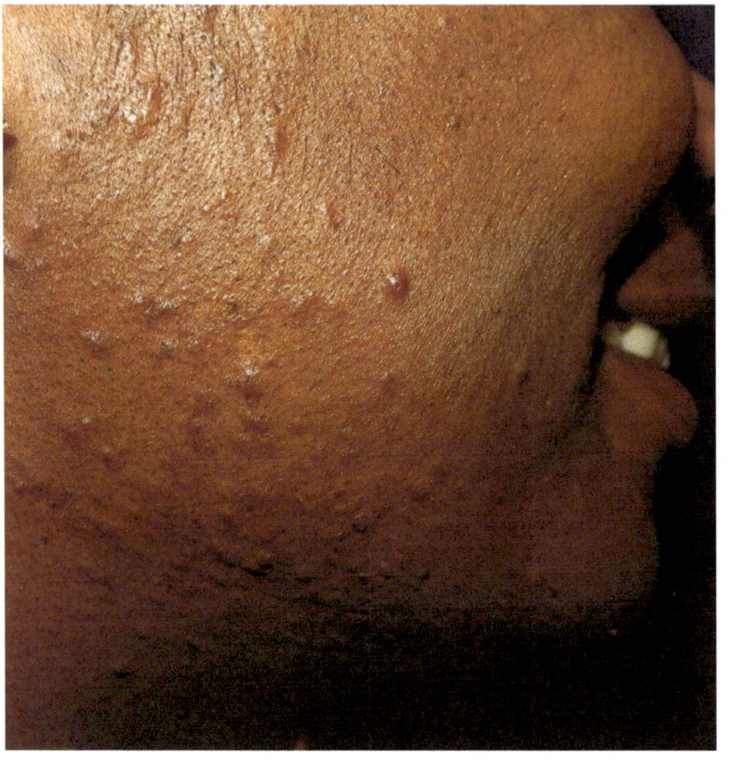

FIGURE 4.25 Reed syndrome: Leiomyomas.

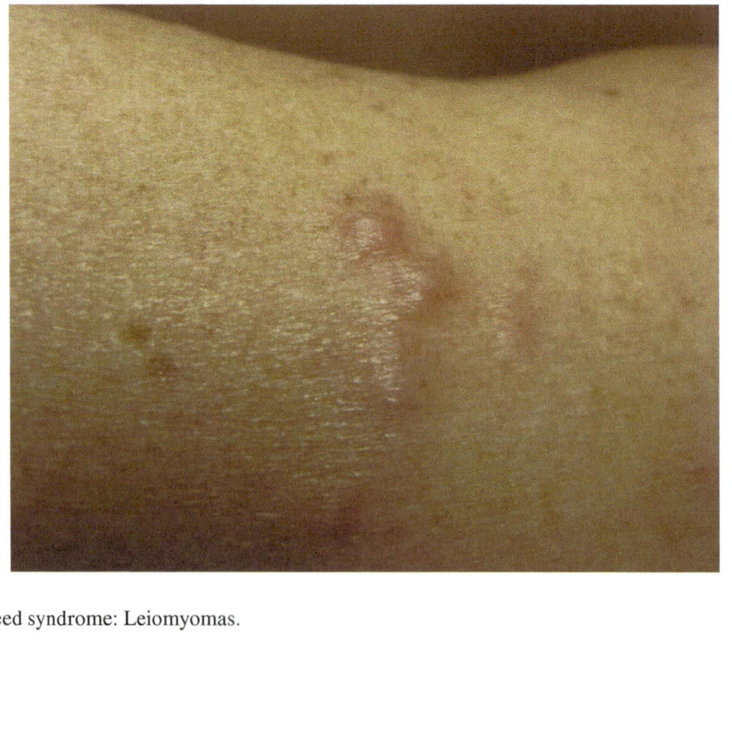

FIGURE 4.26 Reed syndrome: Leiomyomas.

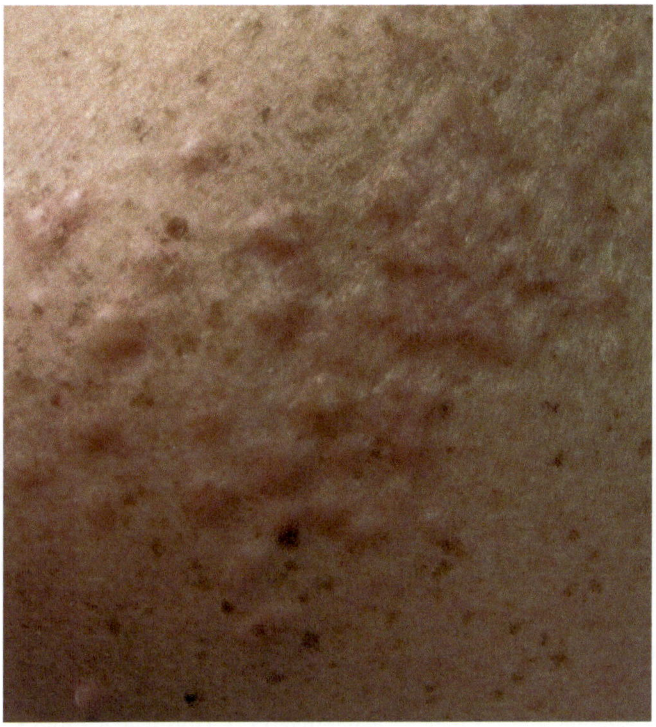

FIGURE 4.27 Reed syndrome: Leiomyomas.

Evaluation and Management

CLMs are often the initial presenting sign of this tumor syndrome. Therefore, providers need to maintain a high level of suspicion when a patient presents with painful flesh-colored to reddish-brown papules. Skin biopsy and histologic evaluation of the lesions are recommended. Treatment of the cosmetic- and pain-related complications of CLMs includes surgical excision, laser ablation, cryotherapy, topical anesthetics, and lesional botulinum toxin injection. Uterine leiomyomas can be severely symptomatic, and referral to an obstetrician/gynecologist is recommended. Treatment may be surgical (hysterectomy, myomectomy) or medical (gonadotropin-releasing hormone agonist, progesterone-releasing intrauterine device [IUD]). Renal carcinoma screening recommendations have been a challenge, given their aggressive nature. Guidelines from various sources suggest contrast-enhanced MRI every year to every other year. It has been suggested to start at 18–20 years; however, given the reported cases of juvenile renal carcinomas, starting surveillance earlier has been discussed. Once discovered, immediate surgical removal of the renal cell carcinomas is advised. The efficacy of vascular endothelial growth factor (VEGF) inhibitors, epidermal growth factor receptor (EGFR) inhibitors, and Anti-PD1limmunotherapies on these tumors are in current clinical trials. Referral to a medical geneticist for FH gene testing is also indicated.

BIBLIOGRAPHY

Gao F, Gu D, Zhang H, et al. Case report: Response to immunotherapy and association with the fh gene in hereditary leiomyomatosis and renal cell cancer-associated renal cell cancer. BMC Med Genomics 2024;17(1):215.

Ooi A. Advances in hereditary leiomyomatosis and renal cell carcinoma (HLRCC) research. Semin Cancer Biol 2020;61:158–166.

Zhang C, Li L, Zhang Y, et al. Hereditary leiomyomatosis and renal cell cancer: Recent insights to mechanisms and systemic treatment. Front Oncol 2021;11:686556.

5

Granulomatous Disorders

Granuloma Annulare

Etiopathogenesis

Granuloma annulare (GA) is a noninfectious granulomatous disorder characterized by palisading granuloma formation in the dermis. The exact etiology is unknown; however, the upregulation of the Th1/2/17/22 axes and the Janus kinase-signal transducer of activation (JAK-STAT) pathways inducing cytokines (tumor necrosis factor-α [TNF-α]; interleukin [IL]-1β; interferon-γ; IL12/23, IL-4, and IL- 31), and M1/M2 macrophage expression play a part in granuloma formation. Drug-induced GA is reported as well.

Clinical Manifestations

GA is polymorphic and can present as localized or generalized disease. The clinical presentations of GA associated with systemic disease include generalized GA (**Figures 5.1** and **5.2**), disseminated GA (**Figures 5.3** and **5.4**), and atypical GA (**Figures 5.5–5.7**). Generalized GA consists of classic erythematous dermal annular lesions that are widespread on the torso and extremities. Disseminated GA consists of reddish-brown dermal papules that are found diffusely on the torso and extremities. Atypical GA is often combinations of annular, arcuate, papular, and plaque-like lesions in random distributions.

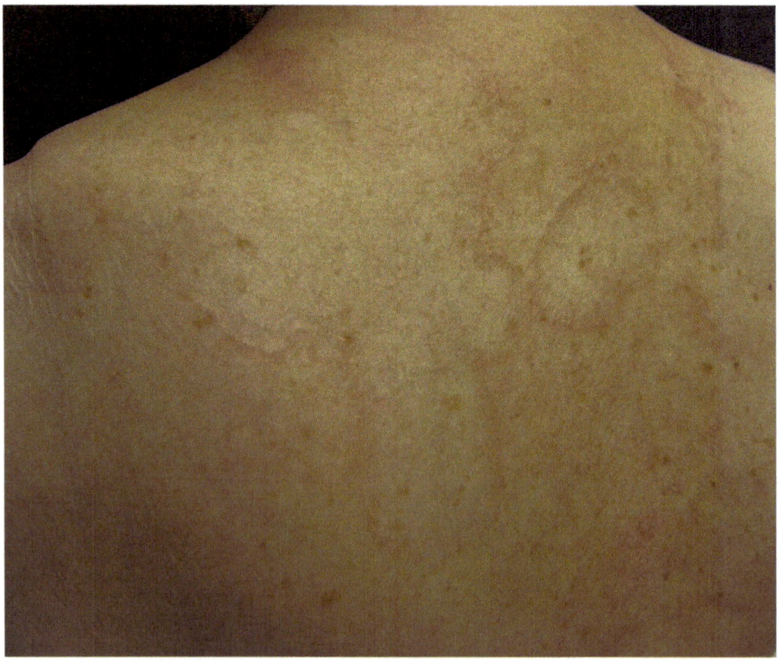

FIGURE 5.1 Granuloma annular: Generalized.

DOI: 10.1201/9781003492665-5

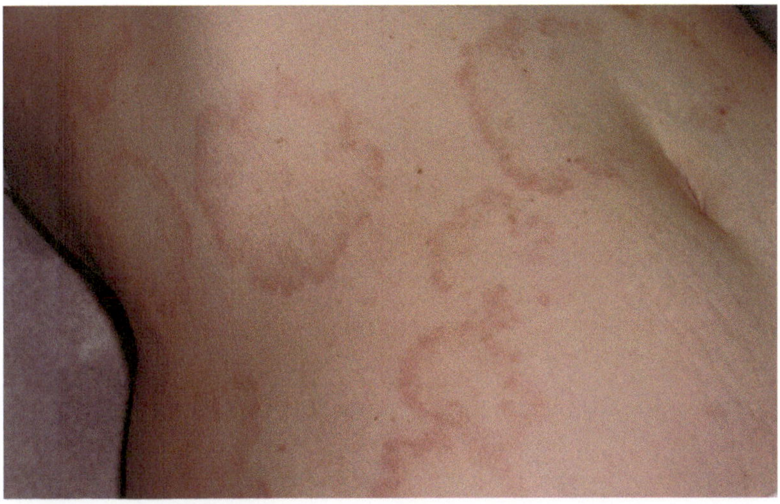

FIGURE 5.2 Granuloma annulare: Generalized.

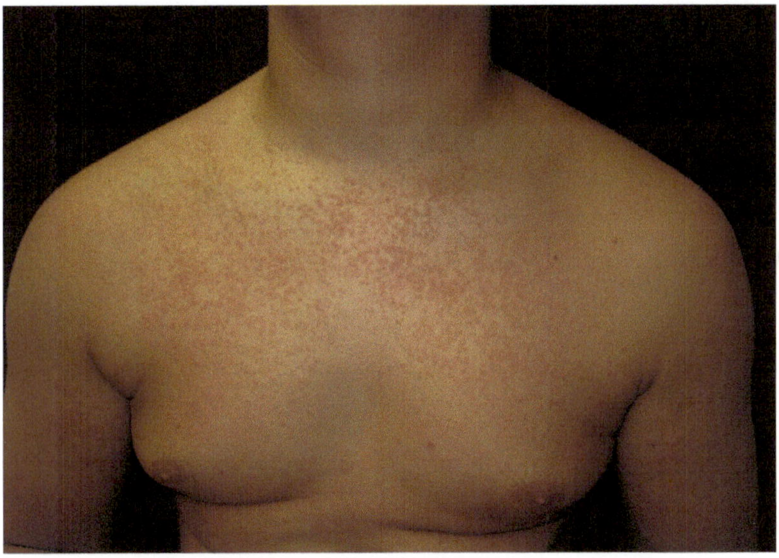

FIGURE 5.3 Granuloma annulare: Disseminated.

Systemic Manifestations

Generalized, disseminated, and atypical GA, especially in older patients (>60), are most frequently associated with systemic disease. The associations reported include diabetes mellitus, autoimmune thyroiditis, hyperlipidemia, human immunodeficiency virus (HIV), viral hepatitis, drug reactions, autoimmune disease (systemic lupus erythematosus and rheumatoid arthritis), as well as hematologic, lymphoproliferative, and solid malignancies. Although no causal relationship between malignancy and GA has been determined at present, there is evidence that GA may present in older patients with cancer.

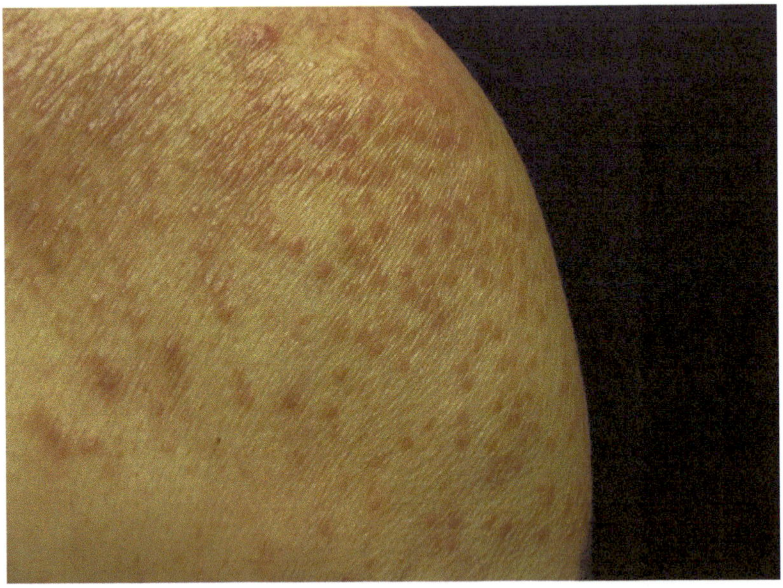

FIGURE 5.4 Granuloma annulare: Disseminated.

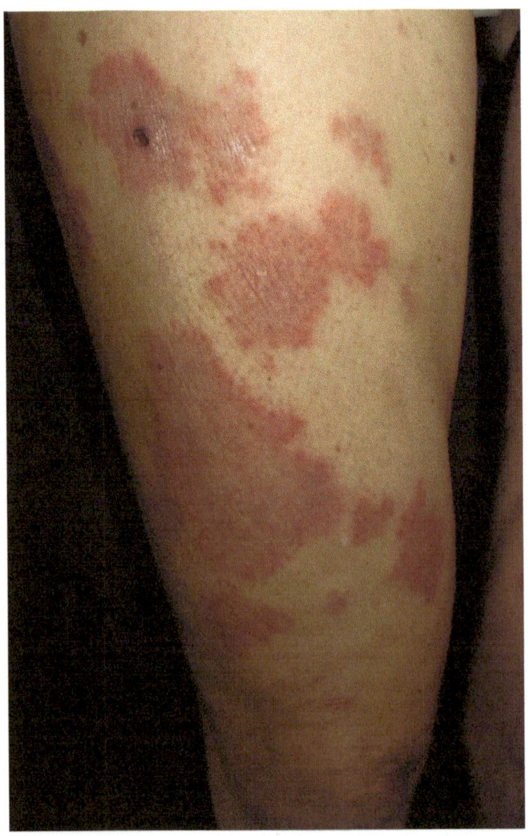

FIGURE 5.5 Granuloma annulare: Atypical.

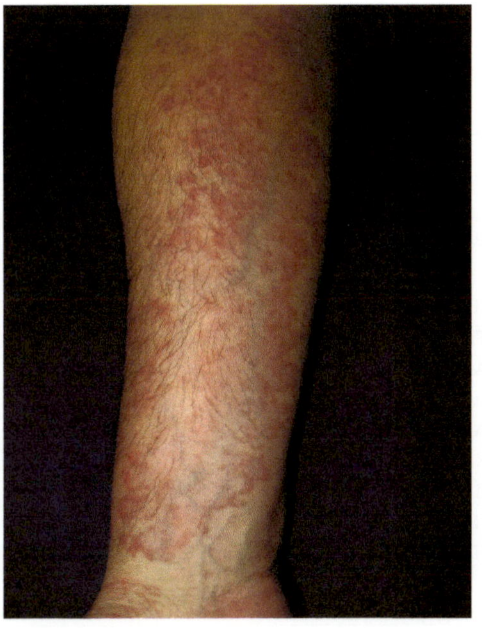

FIGURE 5.6 Granuloma annulare: Atypical.

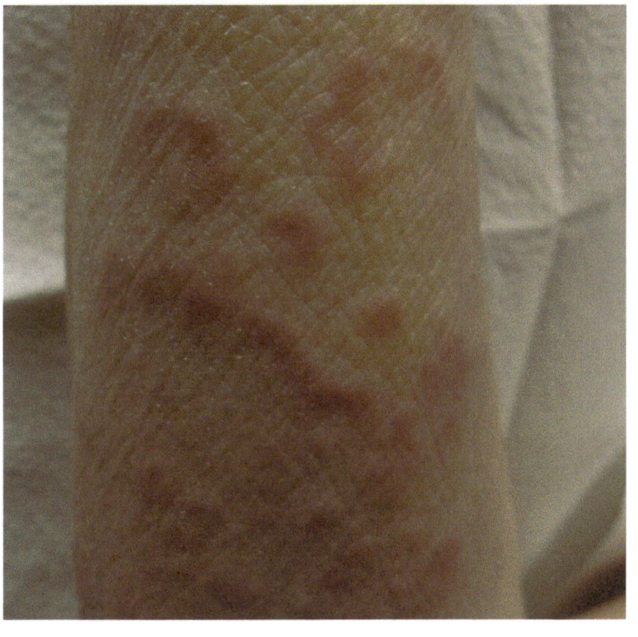

FIGURE 5.7 Granuloma annulare: Atypical.

Evaluation and Management

Because of clinical overlap with other noninfectious granulomatous diseases (sarcoidosis, necrobiosis lipoidica [NL]), a biopsy is recommended. Histologically, lesions are lymphohistiocytic palisaded or interstitial granuloma with necrobiosis and significant mucin deposition. If a clinical variant associated with systemic disease presents, a focused review-of-systems physical exam (lymph nodes), labs, and imaging studies can be performed (**Table 5.1**).

Therapeutic options to resolve skin lesions range from topical/intralesional steroids, phototherapy, doxycycline, hydroxychloroquine, dapsone, methotrexate, biologics, phosphodiasterase-4, and JAK inhibitors.

TABLE 5.1

Evaluation of Generalized, Disseminated, and Atypical GA

Labs
• Fasting blood glucose
• Fasting lipid
• Hemoglobin A1c
• Thyroid function test
• Anti-thyroglobulin antibody
• Anti-thyroid peroxidase antibody
• Anti-nuclear antibody
• Rheumatoid factor
• Anti-cyclic citrullinated protein antibody
• HIV
• Hepatitis B and Hepatitis C serology
• Complete blood count
• Serum protein immunofixation and Serum free light chains
Imaging (if new onset > 60 years old)
• Age-appropriate cancer screening
• Chest X-ray (CXR)
Pan computed tomography (CT)

BIBLIOGRAPHY

Garate D, Thang CJ, Damsky W, et al. Granuloma annulare is associated with an increased risk of hematologic malignancies: A multicenter cohort study using TriNetX. J Am Acad Dermatol 2024;90(4):862–864.

Hawang E, Abdelghaffar M, Shields BE, et al. Molecular targeted therapies for inflammatory granulomatous disorders: A review of the evidence and implications for understanding disease pathogenesis. JID Innov 2023;3(5):100220.

Joshi TP, Duvic M. Granuloma annulare: An updated review of epidemiology, pathogenesis and treatment options. Am J Clin Dermatol 2022;23:37–50.

Metastatic Crohn's Disease

Etiopathogenesis

Metastatic or noncontiguous cutaneous Crohn's disease (MCD) is a noninfectious granulomatous disorder of unknown etiology that occurs in the skin distant from gastrointestinal (GI) inflammation. Circulating immune complexes and a T-helper cell (Th1)-mediated delayed hypersensitivity reaction generated by intestinal disease may lead to similar granulomatous inflammation in the skin.

Clinical Manifestations

MCD granulomatous inflammation presents as erythematous papules to nodules that may ulcerate most commonly in adults on the extremities, knife-cut fissuring in skin folds or genital erythema, and edema (**Figures 5.8–5.11**). This presentation is opposite that of MCD in children, which presents most commonly with genital findings. MCD does not include direct GI tract disease in the perianal or peristomal areas (fissures, abscesses, and fistulas [**Figure 5.12**]), oral mucosa (pyostomatitis vegetans), or the cutaneous reactive diseases (erythema nodosum and pyoderma gangrenosum), which are often seen in patients with Crohn's disease (CD).

Systemic Manifestations

Patients with skin findings consistent with MCD should be evaluated for CD. Although most patients with MCD have active disease or well-controlled CD, up to 20% of patients may lack the characteristic GI complaints of CD at the time of initial skin diagnosis. Additional systemic diseases may be associated with CD, which include sacroiliitis, peripheral arthritis, nonalcoholic steatohepatitis, cholelithiasis, uveitis, osteoporosis, anemia, nephrolithiasis, and nutritional deficiencies.

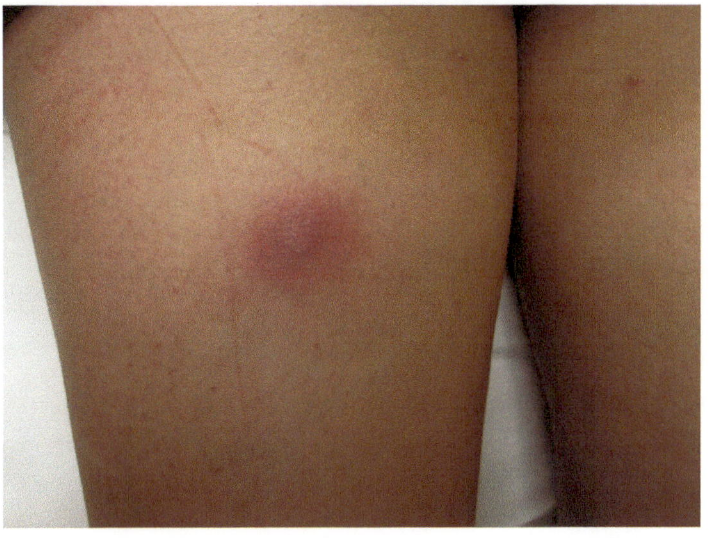

FIGURE 5.8 Metastatic Crohn's disease: Posterior thigh.

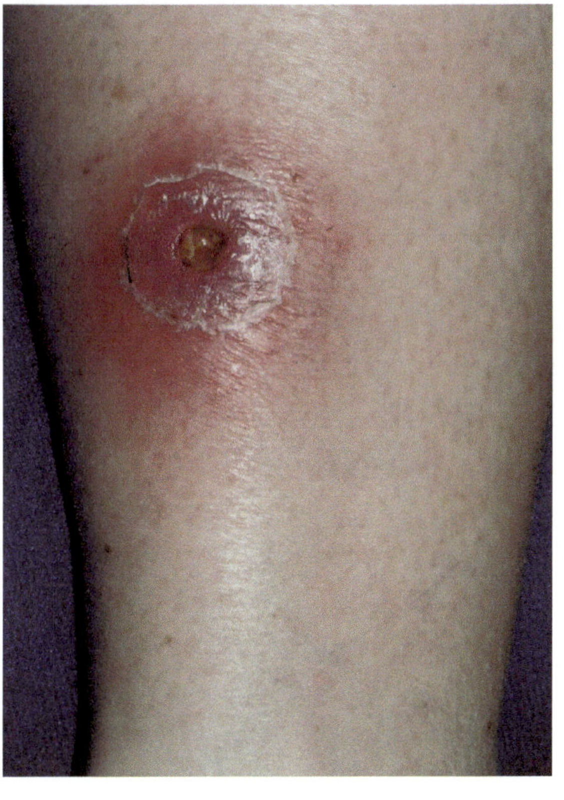

FIGURE 5.9 Metastatic Crohn's disease: Lower leg.

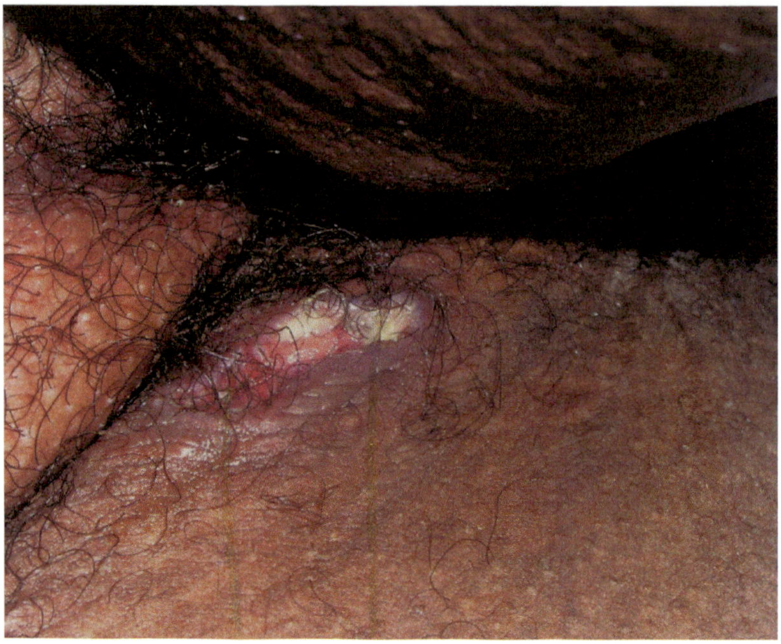

FIGURE 5.10 Metastatic Crohn's disease: Groin area.

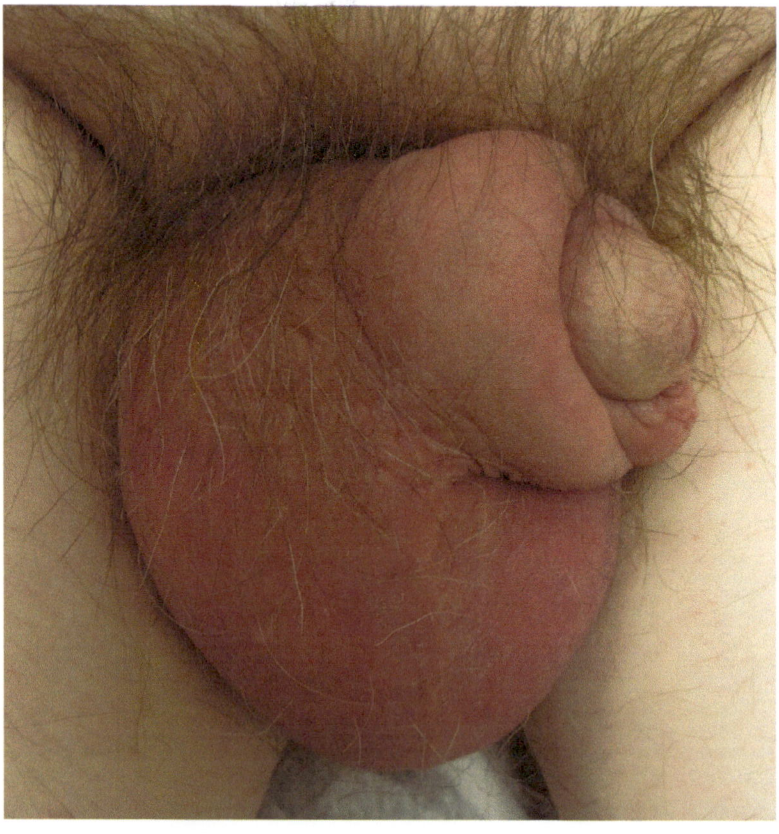

FIGURE 5.11 Metastatic Crohn's disease: Genital erythema and edema.

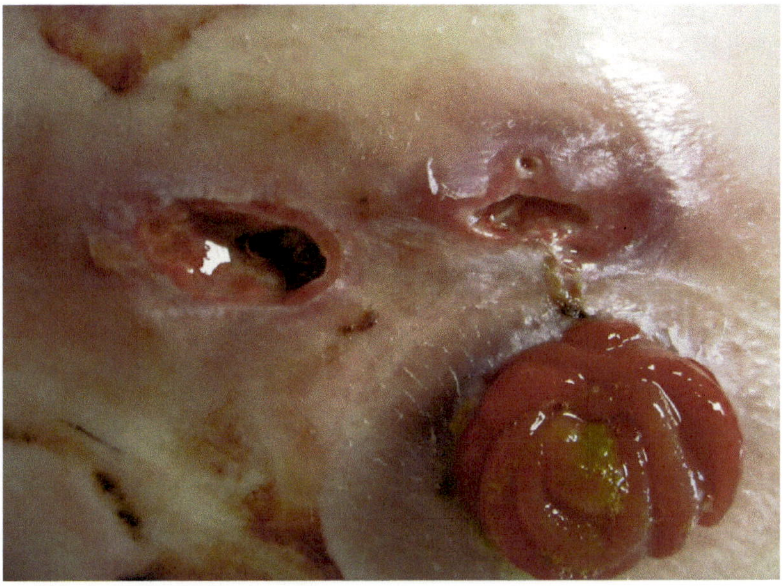

FIGURE 5.12 Cutaneous Crohn's disease: Enterocutaneous fistula.

Evaluation and Management

A biopsy of MCD reveals the characteristic non-epithelioid granulomas, with spare peripheral lymphocytes similar to GI pathology. Laboratory testing may include complete blood count (CBC), liver function test (LFT), urinalysis (UA), erythrocyte sedimentation rate (ESR), C-reactive protein (CRP), vitamin D, zinc, and B vitamins levels. Consultation with gastroenterology is essential, and with ophthalmology if indicated. Spontaneous remission is rare, and most patients require treatment. Therapy for MCD consists of oral metronidazole, oral/topical steroids, topical tacrolimus, azathioprine, cyclosporine, sulfasalazine, adalimumab, infliximab, ustekinumab, ixekizumab, or guselkumab. Removal of diseased bowel does not affect the course of MCD.

BIBLIOGRAPHY

Aberumand B, Howard J, Howard J. Metastatic Crohn's disease: An approach to an uncommon but important cutaneous disorder. Biomed Res Int 2017:8192150.

Beysens S, Wellens J, De Hertogh G, et al. Managing metastatic Crohn's disease: A single center experience, review of the current evidence, and treatment algorithm. Scand J Gastroenterol 2023;58(10):1122–1130.

Ickrath F, Stoevesandt J, Schulmeyer L, et al. Metastatic Crohn's disease: An underestimated entity. J Dtsch Dermatol Ges 2021;19(7):973–982.

Necrobiosis Lipoidica

Etiopathogenesis

NL is an idiopathic noninfectious granulomatous disorder, characteristically known for its association with diabetes mellitus (11%–65%). Although the pathophysiologic relationship between these entities is unknown, microangiopathy, metabolic alterations, trauma, abnormal collagen alteration, and aberrant immunity (TNF, interferon gamma [IFN-γ], JAK-STAT pathways) are considered as forces that lead to the development of this disease. Familial NL cases have been reported, but a gene locus has not been identified to date.

Clinical Manifestations

NL occurs most commonly (85%) on the lower extremities (**Figures 5.13–5.18**), but may occur anywhere on the skin surface (face, scalp, extremities, abdomen). The early-stage lesions present as erythematous plaque. Subsequently, the plaques turn reddish brown, often with a central yellowish hue (middle stage), and in the late stage, sclerotic shiny atrophic plaques with predominant vasculature (telangiectasia to veins) develop. Lesions are very susceptible to trauma and develop isomorphic responses. Up to 35% of cases develop painful ulcerations. Biopsy is required to differentiate from granuloma annulare, sarcoidosis, and xanthogranulomas.

Systemic Manifestations

NL has also been reported to occur with diabetes mellitus with high insulin requirements, metabolic syndrome, hyperlipidemia, hypertension, celiac disease, and autoimmune thyroiditis.

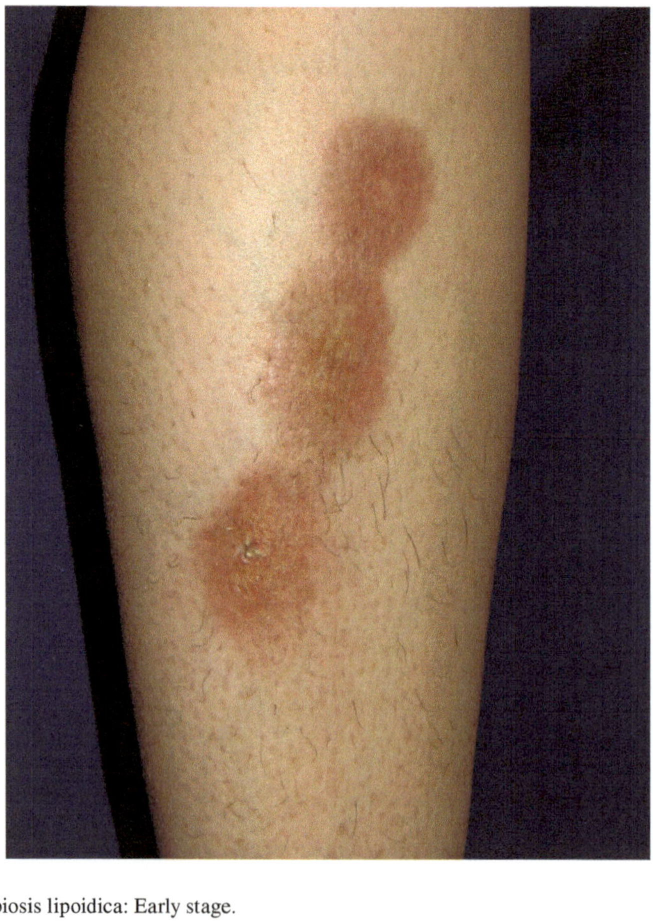

FIGURE 5.13 Necrobiosis lipoidica: Early stage.

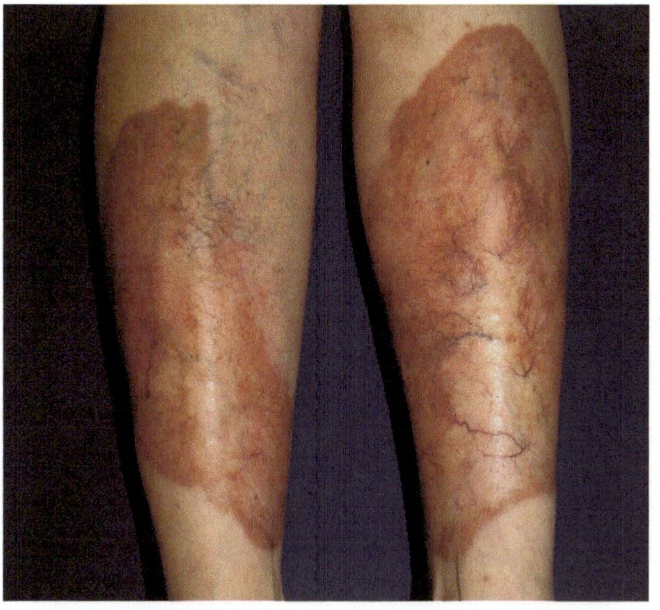

FIGURE 5.14 Necrobiosis lipoidica: Mid stage.

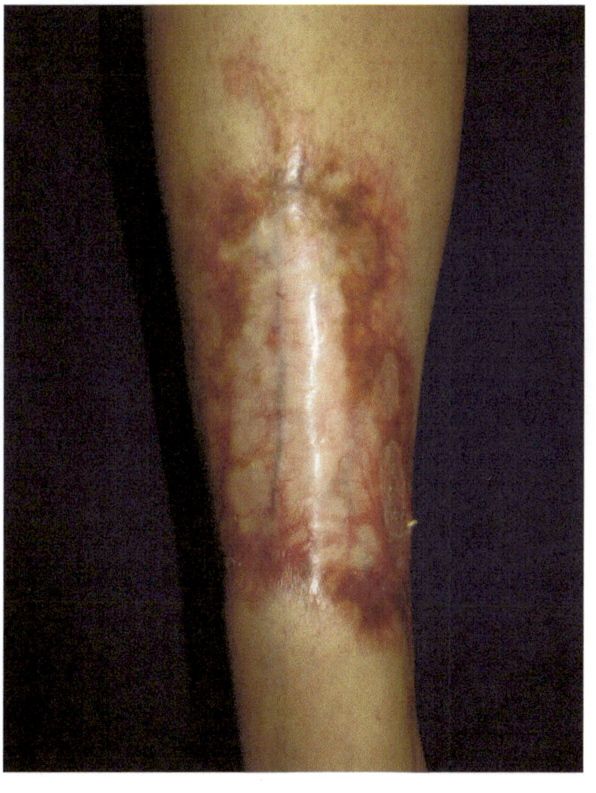

FIGURE 5.15 Necrobiosis lipoidica: Late stage.

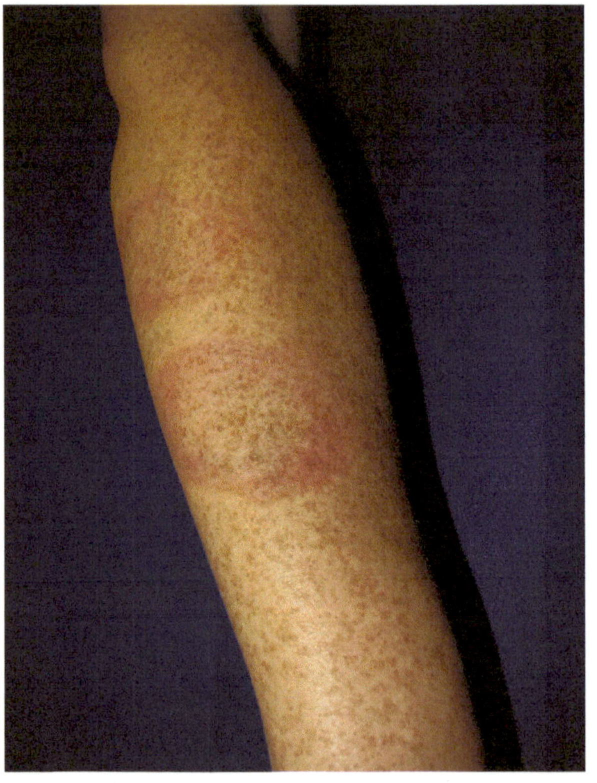

FIGURE 5.16 Necrobiosis lipoidica: Upper extremity.

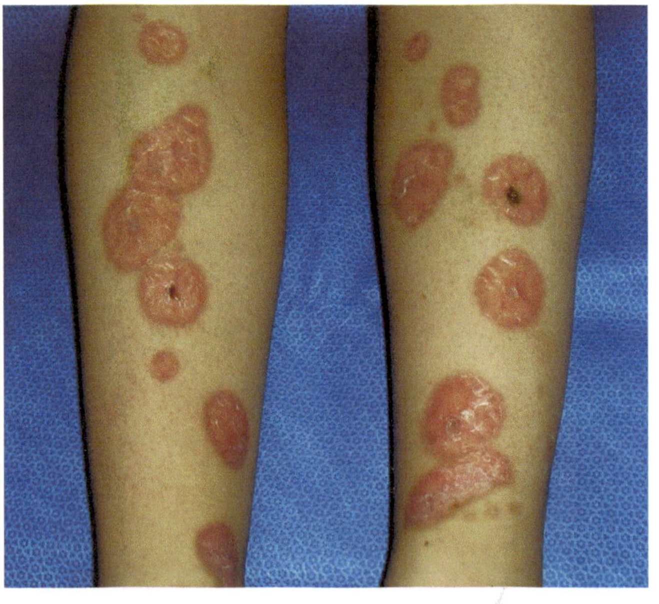

FIGURE 5.17 Necrobiosis lipoidica: Early ulcerative.

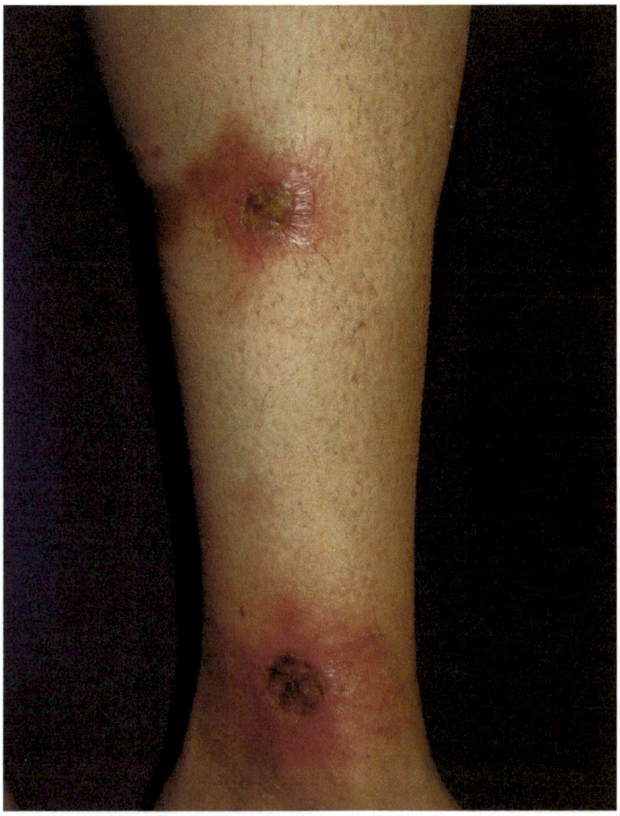

FIGURE 5.18 Necrobiosis lipoidica: Ulcerative.

However, NL may occur in patients with normal glucose tolerance and without underlying diseases. Although NL occurs only in about 1.0% of diabetics, those who develop NL are usually insulin-dependent and are at higher risk for end-organ failure (retinopathy, nephropathy) than those diabetics without NL.

Evaluation and Management

It is reasonable to monitor all patients with NL for glucose intolerance with routine fasting blood glucose (FBG) and hemoglobin A1c (HA1c). Up to 60% develop diabetes after the diagnosis of NL, so educating patients on signs/symptoms of diabetes is indicated. For patients with diabetes-associated NL, routine eye exams and monitoring urine for proteinuria are prudent. For further disease association workup, see **Table 5.2**. Although spontaneous resolution has been reported, treatment of NL consists of steroids (topical, intralesional, and oral), calcineurin inhibitors (topical tacrolimus), pentoxifylline, antimalarials, and phototherapy. Ulcerative NL is often resistant to treatment, requiring oral immunosuppressants such as cyclosporine and mycophenolate mofetil. Biologic agents (infliximab, etanercept, adalimumab, ustekinumab) and JAK inhibitors (ruxolitinib, baricitinib, tofacitinib) have been reported as reasonable therapeutic options for the more complicated ulcerative cases.

TABLE 5.2

Evaluation for Patients with NL

Labs
• Fasting blood glucose
• HA1c
• Urinalysis
• Fasting lipids
• Anti-transglutaminase antibody
• Anti-gliadin antibody
• Thyroid stimulating hormone
• Free T4
• Anti-thyroglobulin antibody
• Anti-thyroid peroxidase antibody
Other
• Blood pressure
• Retinal eye exam

BIBLIOGRAPHY

Hughes AN, Xing L, Lehman JS, et al. Drug repurposing using molecular network analysis identified Jak as targetable driver of necrobiosis lipoidica. JIA Innov 2024;4(6):100296.

Ionescu C, Petca A, Dumitrascu MC, et al. The intersection of dermatologic dilemmas and endocrinological complexities: Understanding necrobiosis-lipoidica-a comprehensive review. Biomedicines 2024;12(2):337.

Lepe K, Riley CA, Hashmi MF, et al. Necrobiosis lipoidica. In: StatPearls[internet]. Treasure Island (FL): StatPearls Publishing; 2024.

Necrobiotic Xanthogranuloma

Etiopathogenesis

Necrobiotic xanthogranuloma (NXG) is a rare, chronic, treatment-resistant, noninfectious, granulomatous, and non-Langerhans cell histiocytosis that is strongly associated with plasma cell dyscrasias. The etiology is unknown but has been hypothesized to be from monoclonal paraproteins eliciting a granulomatous reaction or binding to lipoprotein receptors on monocytes that induce xanthoma formation.

Clinical Manifestations

NXG lesions classically develop in the periorbital area (**Figure 5.19**) but may occur on the torso (**Figure 5.20**) and extremities (**Figure 5.21**). The lesions present as erythematous plaques with a yellowish xanthomatous appearance. Lesions develop telangiectasia and frequently ulcerate. Middle-aged men and women are equally affected. Diagnostic criteria are summarized in **Table 5.3**.

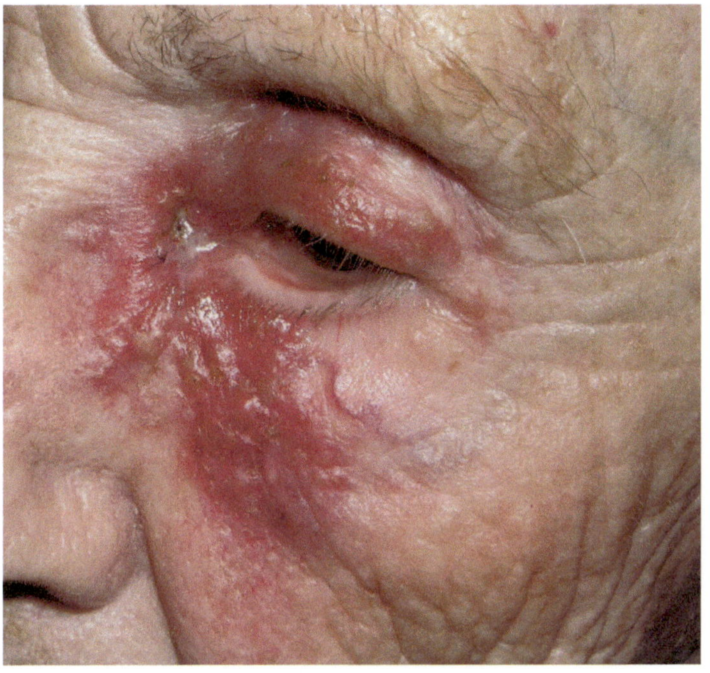

FIGURE 5.19 Necrobiotic xanthogranuloma: Periorbital with blepharitis.

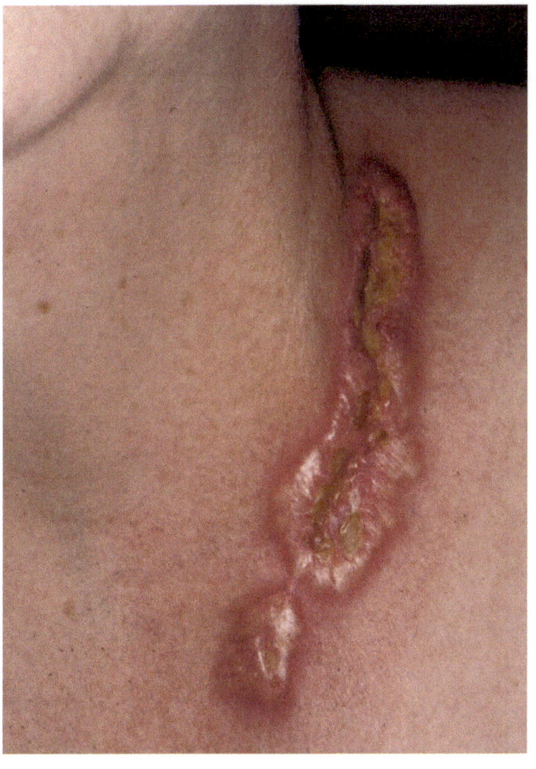

FIGURE 5.20 Necrobiotic xanthogranuloma: Torso.

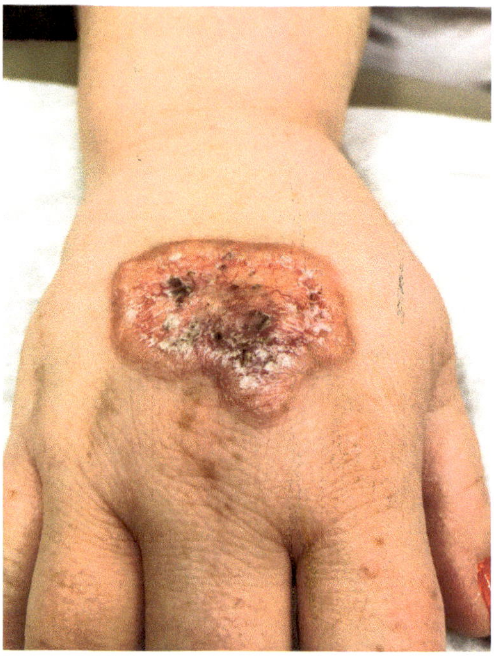

FIGURE 5.21 Necrobiotic xanthogranuloma: Extremity.

Systemic Manifestations

NXG inflammation is not limited to the skin. Ocular involvement can lead to vision changes, blepharitis, episcleritis, iritis, and corneal perforation. Other internal organ dysfunction can occur from myocardial, lung, larynx, kidney, intestine, and skeletal muscle infiltration.

NXG is associated with a serum monoclonal gammopathy (IgG κ>IgG λ>IgA) in up to 90% of cases. Predominately, they are classified as a monoclonal gammopathy of underdetermined significance (MGUS), with 10% developing multiple myeloma (MMy).

Evaluation and Management

Biopsy reveals histologic findings similar to those of necrobiosis lipoidica; however, more extensive necrobiosis, Touton giant cells, lymphoid follicles, and cholesterol clefting can distinguish NXG. Although plasma cell infiltrates in cutaneous NXG are polyclonal, laboratory testing should include serum protein electrophoresis (SPEP), serum immunofixation electrophoresis (SIFE), serum free light chain (SLFC), urine protein electrophoresis (UPEP), and urine immunofixation electrophoresis (UIFE). Because MGUS is a risk factor for developing MMy, consultation with a hematologist/oncologist for further evaluation and bone marrow biopsy is recommended. If MMy is detected, appropriate chemotherapeutic agents can be instituted. If NXG is confirmed, a screening ocular examination and echocardiogram for eye and heart disease, respectively, is suggested. Cutaneous NXG, with or without MMy, is often treatment-resistant. First-line therapies to consider are intravenous immunoglobulin (IVIG), corticosteroids, or a combination of both.

TABLE 5.3

Diagnostic Criteria for NXG

Major (requires 2)
1. Cutaneous papules, plaques and/or nodules, most often yellow-orange
2. Dermatopathologic evidence of palisading granulomas with lymphoplasmacytic infiltrate and necrobiosis
Minor (requires 1)
1. Paraproteinemia (IgG κ), plasma cell dyscrasia, and/or associated lymphoproliferative disorder
2. Periorbital skin lesions

BIBLIOGRAPHY

Bassir F, Valido K, Maciejewski KR, et al. Validation of the Delphi consensus diagnostic criteria for necrobiotic xanthogranuloma. JAMA Dermatol 2024:160 (12): 1361–1362.

Higgins LS, Go RS, Dingli D, et al. Clinical features and treatment outcomes of patient with necrobiotic xanthogranuloma associated with monoclonal gammopathies. Clin Lymphoma Myeloma Leuk 2016;16(8):447–452.

Stienhelfer L, Kuhnel T, Jagel H, et al. Systemic therapy for necrobiotic xanthogranuloma: A systemic review. Orphanet J Rare Dis 2022;17(1):132.

Orofacial Granulomatosis

Etiopathogenesis

Orofacial granulomatosis (OFG) is a granulomatous inflammatory condition of the orofacial region of unclear etiology. There is no distinctive genetic association with this presumed delayed-type hypersensitivity (CD4 + Th1 cell-mediated) reaction to an unknown antigen. OFG has been linked with reactions to food substances/preservatives, dental materials, and infections. However, there are data conflicts concerning the role of *Mycobacteria* species.

Clinical Manifestations

OFG presents most commonly with lower lip enlargement (granulomatous cheilitis [**Figure 5.22**]). However, both lips may be involved. Additional orofacial changes reported include gingival enlargement, fissured tongue (lingua plicata [**Figure 5.23**]), cobblestoning, and aphthous-like to linear deep ulcerations of buccal mucosa, angular cheilitis, lip fissuring, and facial edema with or without swelling (**Figure 5.24**).

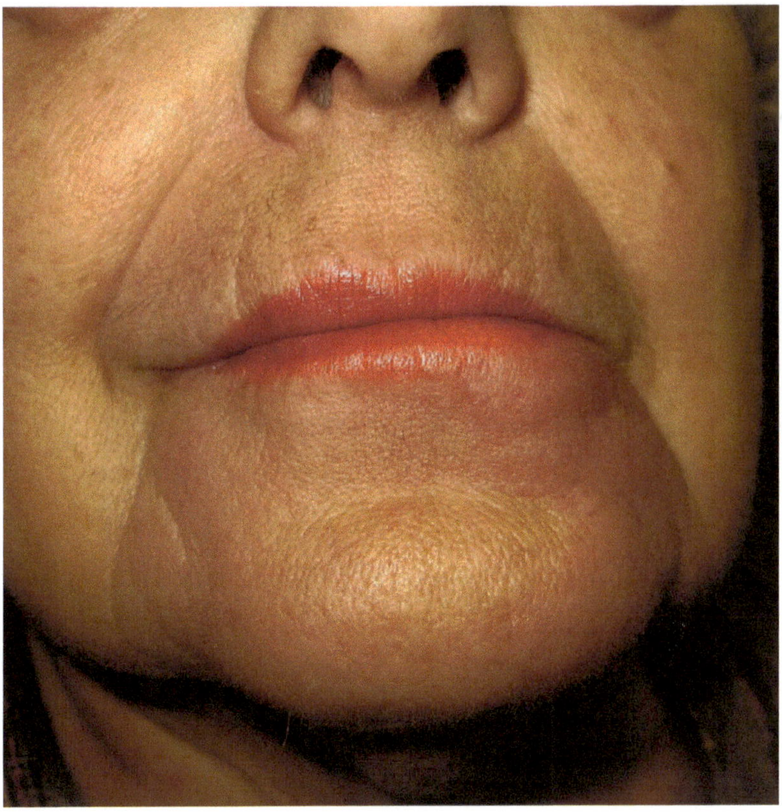

FIGURE 5.22 Orofacial granulomatosis: Lip edema and chin erythema.

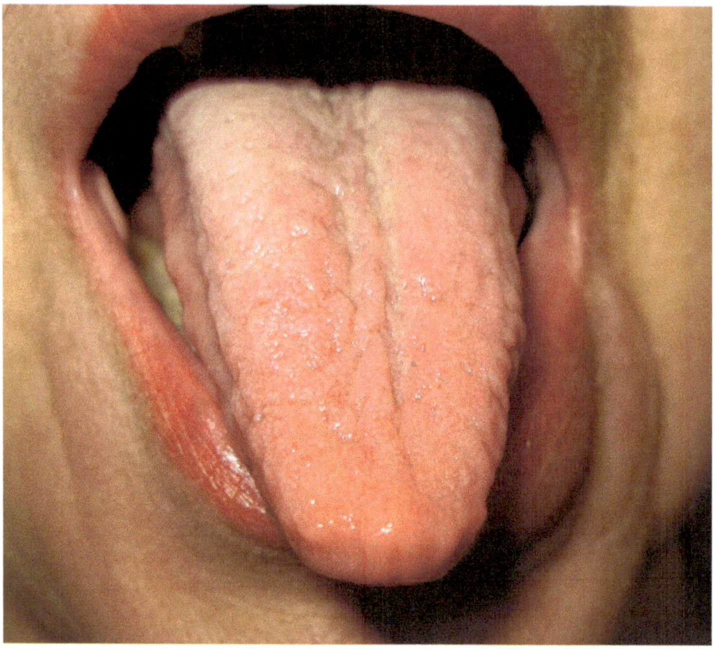

FIGURE 5.23 Orofacial granulomatosis: Lingua plicata.

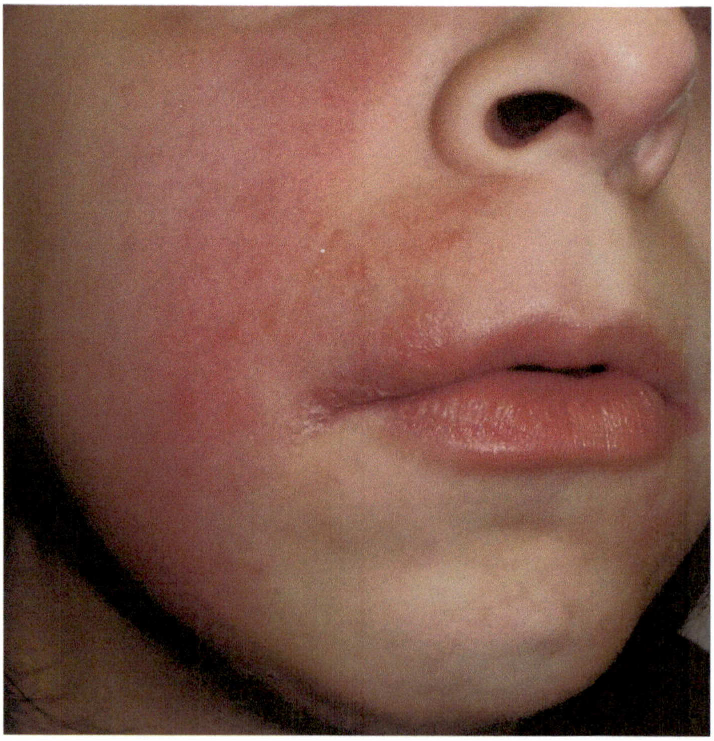

FIGURE 5.24 Orofacial granulomatosis: Lip edema, cheilitis, and facial erythema.

Systemic Manifestations

Although OFG may be limited to mucocutaneous findings, patients may present with cervical lymphadenopathy and facial nerve palsy. The term *Melkersson–Rosenthal syndrome* is used when OFG, lingua plicata, and lower motor neuron facial paralysis occur in combination. The facial nerve palsy may present partially or completely unilateral. It is more common in female patients and has a tendency to develop over many years. In fact, most patients do not start off with facial paralysis. Additional cranial nerve defects such as oral sensory loss, auditory deficits, and pharyngeal abnormalities have been reported. A possible association with psoriasis has also been reported.

Evaluation and Management

Histologic evaluation reveals noncaseating granulomas associated with lymphedema. Therefore, sarcoidosis and CD must be ruled out prior to diagnosing OFG. OFG in adults appears to be a separate entity, but childhood onset of OFG creates a higher risk of developing Crohn's disease. Although OFG and sarcoidosis may develop facial nerve paralysis, OFG will not have abnormalities in other organ systems, as seen with sarcoidosis. OFG patients will not have serologic or other laboratory abnormalities. Systemic antibiotics (doxycycline, azithromycin, metronidazole) and oral or intralesional steroids are therapy mainstays. Addition of immunosuppressants (azathioprine, methotrexate) or biologic agents (infliximab, adalimumab, ustekinumab) may be needed if not steroid responsive. Cinnamon- and benzoate-free diets have been shown to decrease OFG in up to 78% of patients. Up to 23% of patients on this exclusion diet may not require immunosuppressive therapies.

BIBLIOGRAPHY

Galdiero MR, Maio F, Arcoleo F, et al. Orofacial granulomatosis: Clinical and therapeutic features in an Italian cohort and review of the literature. Allergy 2021;76(7):2189–2220.

Gavioli CFB, Florezi GP, Dabronzo MLD, et al. Orofacial granulomatosis and Crohn disease: Coincidence or pattern? A systemic review. Dermatology 2021;237(4):635–640.

Joshi S, Mawdsley J, Hullah E, et al. Management of orofacial granulomatosis. Br J Hosp Med (London) 2023;29(3):1–16.

Reactive Granulomatous Dermatitis

Etiopathogenesis

Reactive granulomatosis dermatitis (RGD) encapsulates three entities with overlapping histologic, clinical, and systemic associations: interstitial granulomatous dermatitis (IGD), palisaded neutrophil granulomatous dermatitis (PNGD), and GA-like eruption (GALE). The etiology of RGD is unknown. Because these skin diseases are reactions to underlying systemic disease, circulating immune complexes that initiate cutaneous granuloma formation have been proposed.

Clinical Manifestations

IGD presents as thin linear erythematous plaques termed as a *rope sign* that occurs on the torso and extremities (**Figure 5.25**). GALE lesions (**Figures 5.26–5.28**) are large annular plaques on the back and abdomen. The peripheral erythema has a feathered appearance, with the inner plaque spreading outward in a diffusing papular pattern. However, erythematous plaques have also been reported. Erythematous papulonodular lesions that may appear crusted and localized on the elbows and knees are characteristic of PNGD (**Figure 5.29**). RGD drug reactions (**Table 5.4**) can also occur in these patterns, and the interstitial granulomatous drug reaction is histologically different with the addition of atypical lymphocytes and interface changes.

Systemic Manifestations

Because of nomenclature confusion, especially in terms of histological and clinical descriptions, systemic associations with these entities have been overlapped. Overall, the systemic diseases include systemic lupus erythematosus, rheumatoid arthritis, scleroderma, Sjögren syndrome, antiphospholipid antibody syndrome, antineutrophilic cytoplasmic antibody (ANCA) vasculitis, mixed cryoglobulinemia, autoimmune thyroiditis, autoimmune hepatitis, and lymphoproliferative disorders (lymphoma and hematologic malignancy).

Evaluation and Management

A skin biopsy for histologic evaluation is important to distinguish from other noninfectious granulomatous disorders, especially GA. IGD and GALE have a sparse but diffuse palisaded interstitial histiocytic and neutrophilic infiltrate with localized necrobiosis without mucin deposition, differentiating it from GA. PNGD has intense neutrophilic inflammation with significant necrobiosis, palisading granuloma, and, at times, a leukocytoclastic vasculitis without mucin deposition. If clinical pathologic correlation suggests an RGD, evaluating the patient for autoimmune and lymphoproliferative disorders is recommended. Laboratory tests are summarized in **Table 5.5**. If concern for lymphoma is present, a screening CXR with appropriate CT follow-up is recommended. RGD drug reactions can also occur in these patterns, but the interstitial granulomatous drug reaction is histologically different with the addition of atypical lymphocytes and interface changes. However, the same medications have been reported to cause both. Discontinuation of medications possibly associated with RGD is recommended. Treatment of the disorder is often disappointing and requires immunosuppressive therapy with hydroxychloroquine, methotrexate, mycophenolate mofetil, or adalimumab and JAK inhibitors.

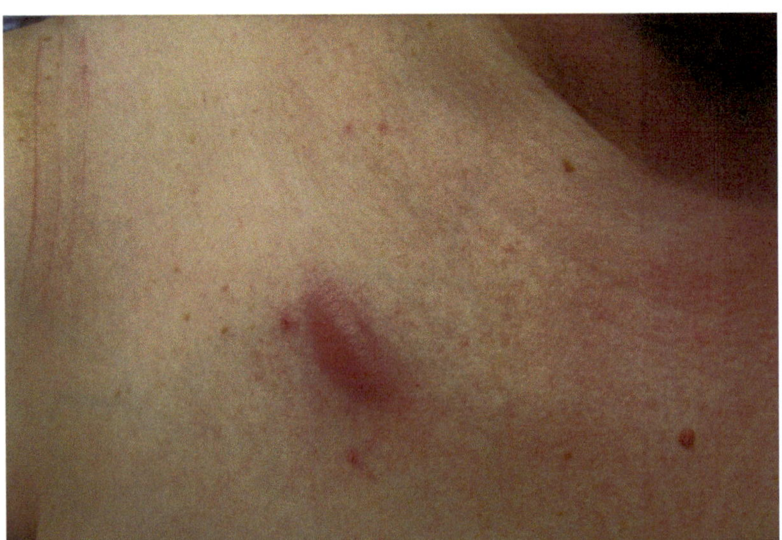

FIGURE 5.25 Reactive granulomatous dermatitis: Interstitial granulomatous dermatitis (rope sign).

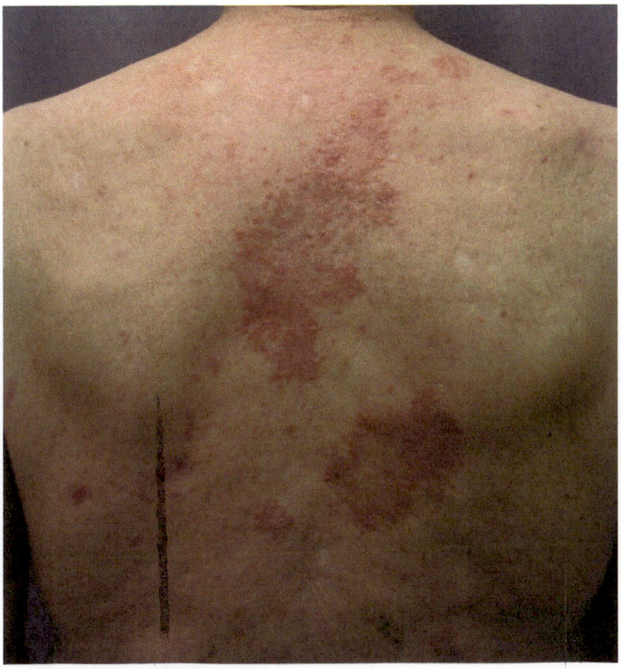

FIGURE 5.26 Reactive granulomatous dermatitis: Granuloma annulare-like.

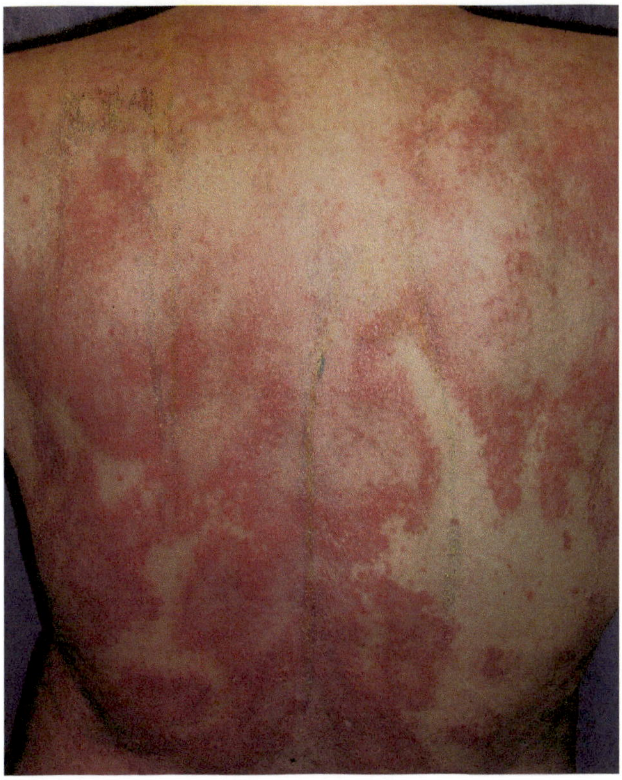

FIGURE 5.27 Reactive granulomatous dermatitis: Granuloma annulare-like.

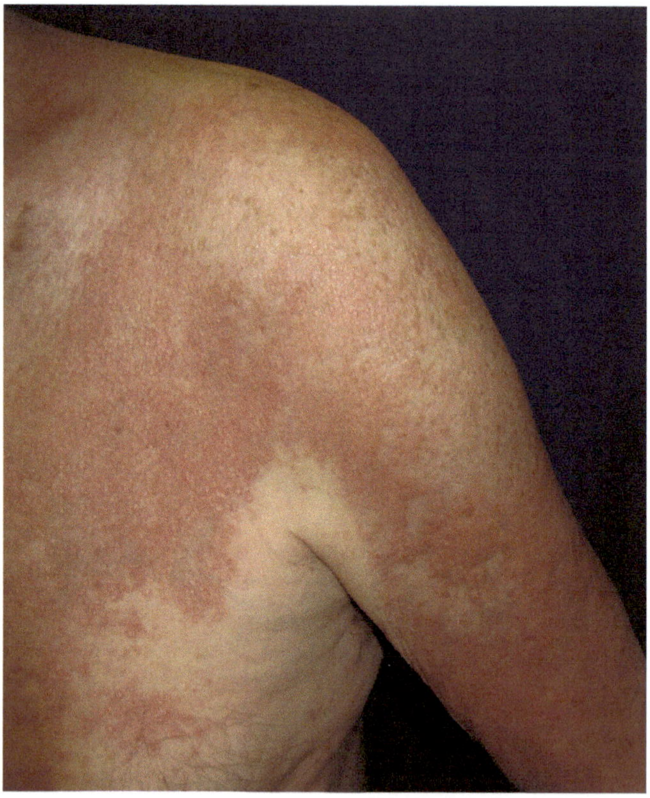

FIGURE 5.28 Reactive granulomatous dermatitis: Granuloma annulare-like.

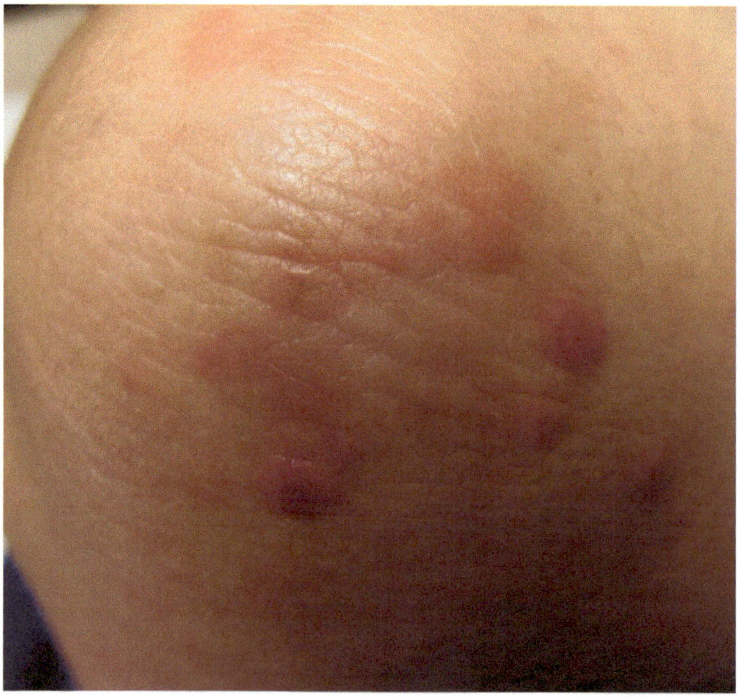

FIGURE 5.29 Reactive granulomatous dermatitis: Palisaded neutrophilic granulomatous dermatitis.

TABLE 5.4

Drugs that Cause RGD

• ACE inhibitors
• Anti-TNFα
• Calcium channel blockers
• Statins
• Hydrochlorothiazide
• Imipramine
• Topiramate
• Bosutinib

TABLE 5.5

Laboratory Evaluation of RGD

• Complete blood count with platelets and differential
• Renal function test
• Liver function test
• Urinalysis
• Complement 3/4
• Antinuclear antibody
• Antineutrophilic cytoplasmic antibodies
• Anti-Ro/SSA and anti-La/SSB antibodies
• Anti-topoisomerase (Scl 70) and anti-centromere antibodies
• Rheumatoid factor and anti-cyclic citrullinated antibody
• Cryoglobulin
• Thyroid function tests
• Anti-thyroglobulin antibody
• Anti-thyroid peroxidase antibody
• Anti-mitochondrial antibodies
• Serum protein electrophoresis/Serum immunofixation/Serum free light chains, and 24-hour Urine protein electrophoresis/Urine immunofixation (if >60 years)

BIBLIOGRAPHY

Kumar AB, Lehman JS, Johnson EF, et al. Reactive granulomatosis dermatitis as a clinically relevant and unifying term: A retrospective review of clinical features, associated diseases, histopathology and treatment for a series of 65 patients at Mayo Clinic. J Eur Acad Dermatol Venereol 2022;36(12):2443–2450.

Lagace M, Mainville L, Dionne MC. Reactive granulomatous dermatitis: A descriptive study of 10 patients. J Cutan Med Surg 2024;28(1):33–36.

Rosenbach M. Reactive granulomatous dermatitis: Lumping terms to split confusion. J Eur Acad Dermato Venereol 2022;36(12):2262–2263.

Rosenbach M, English JC 3rd. Reactive granulomatous dermatitis: A review of palisaded neutrophilic and granulomatous dermatitis. Interstitial granulomatous dermatitis, interstitial granulomatous drug reaction and a proposed reclassification. Dermatol Clin 2015;33(3):373–387.

Sarcoidosis

Etiopathogenesis

Sarcoidosis is a noncaseating granulomatous inflammatory condition that can affect any organ system. The exact etiology is unknown, but environmental factors (for firefighters, Navy personnel, and exposure to pesticides), genetic factors (HLA-DRB*1101, TNF gene), infections (mycobacterial,

Propionibacterium acne), and immune reactions to a still unknown antigen (Th1, Th2, Th17 helper, CD4+, CD8+ lymphocytes and TNF α, IL-2 IFN -γ, IL-17, IL-12, JAK-STAT cytokines), or combinations of the above-mentioned factors have been speculated as possible reasons for developing the disease.

Clinical Manifestations

Although black females are most commonly affected, all races and ethnic groups may develop the disease in a bimodal age distribution (20–39/65–69 years). Cutaneous manifestations are specific (due to granulomatous inflammation) or nonspecific (reactive) and are polymorphic. Nonspecific skin lesions include erythema nodosum, erythema multiforme, pruritus, and clubbing. Specific skin lesions (**Figures 5.30–5.42**) may be reddish-brown to apple-jelly-colored papules, plaques, nodules, subcutaneous nodules, infiltrative scars, and lupus pernio. Atypical sarcoidosis lesions reported include ulcerative and verrucous lesions, as well as acquired ichthyosis and scarring alopecia.

Systemic Manifestations

Sarcoidosis can infiltrate any organ system (**Figure 5.41**), with subsequent fibrosis and loss of function. Lung involvement presents with dyspnea and shortness of breath. Ocular involvement from uveitis may lead to blindness. Neurosarcoidosis may lead to facial nerve palsy, meningitis, encephalopathy, and mass effect. Infiltration of the heart may lead to arrhythmia, congestive heart failure, and sudden cardiac death. Endocrinopathies include hypothyroidism and hypercalcemia with subsequent nephrolithiasis. In addition, patients may experience anemia, fatigue, and depression. Sarcoidosis has also been associated with an increased risk of malignancy (testicular, lymphoma) and medication use (interferon-α).

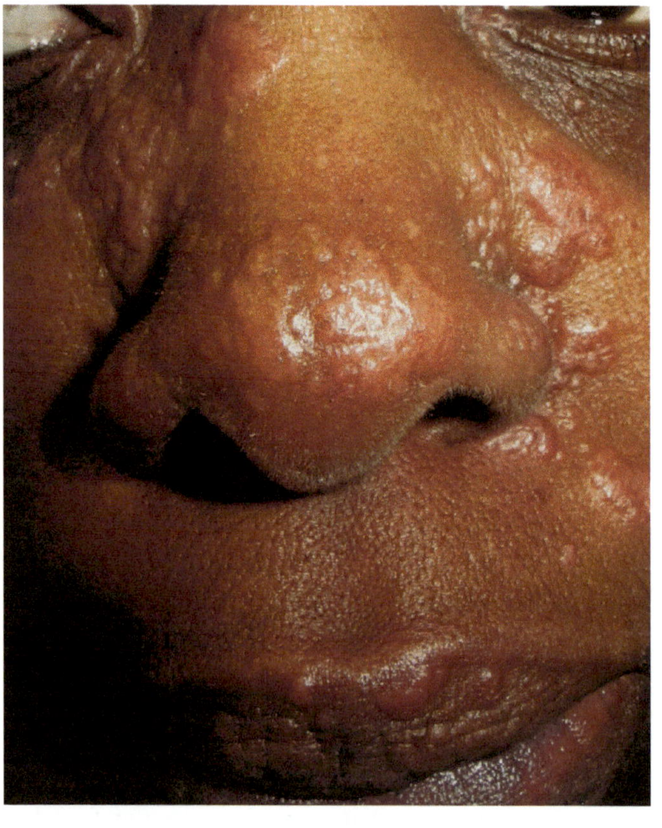

FIGURE 5.30 Sarcoidosis: Papulonodular.

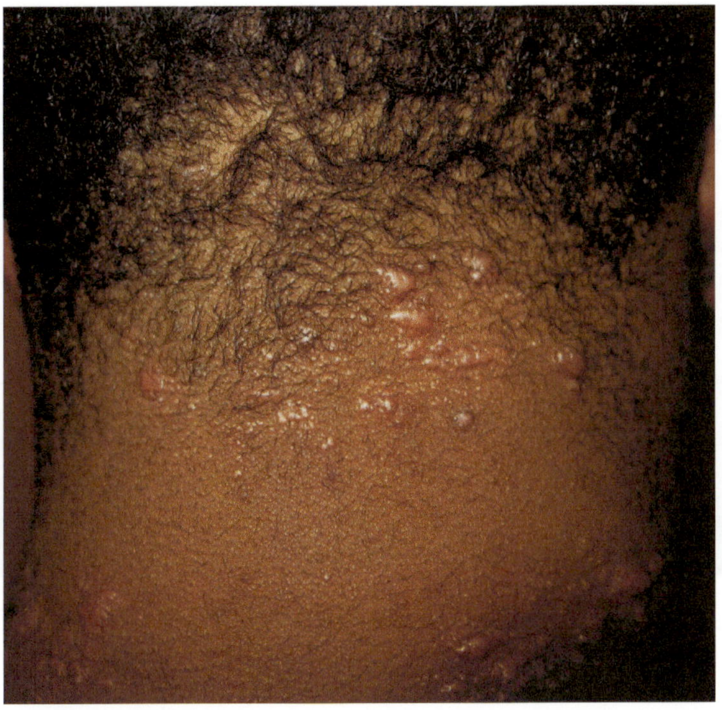

FIGURE 5.31 Sarcoidosis: Papulonodular.

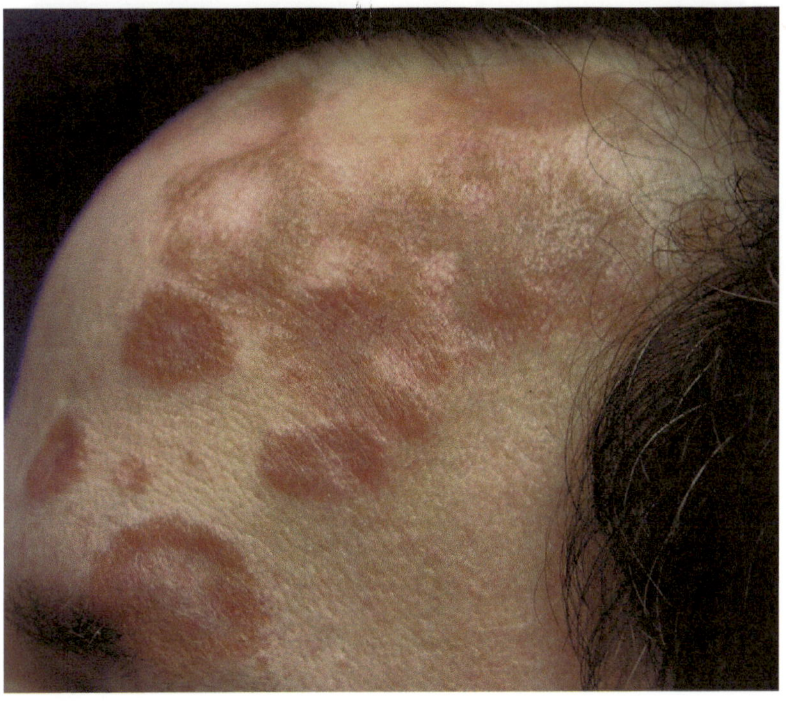

FIGURE 5.32 Sarcoidosis: Annular plaques.

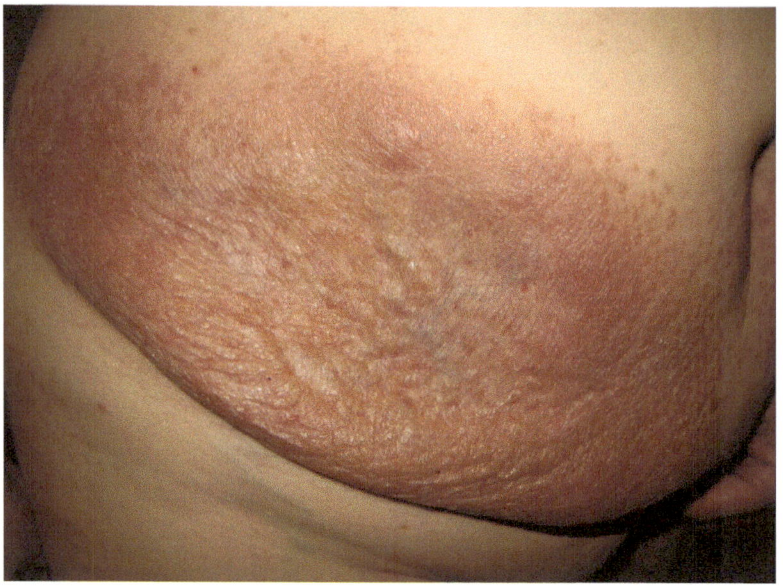

FIGURE 5.33 Sarcoidosis: Indurated plaque.

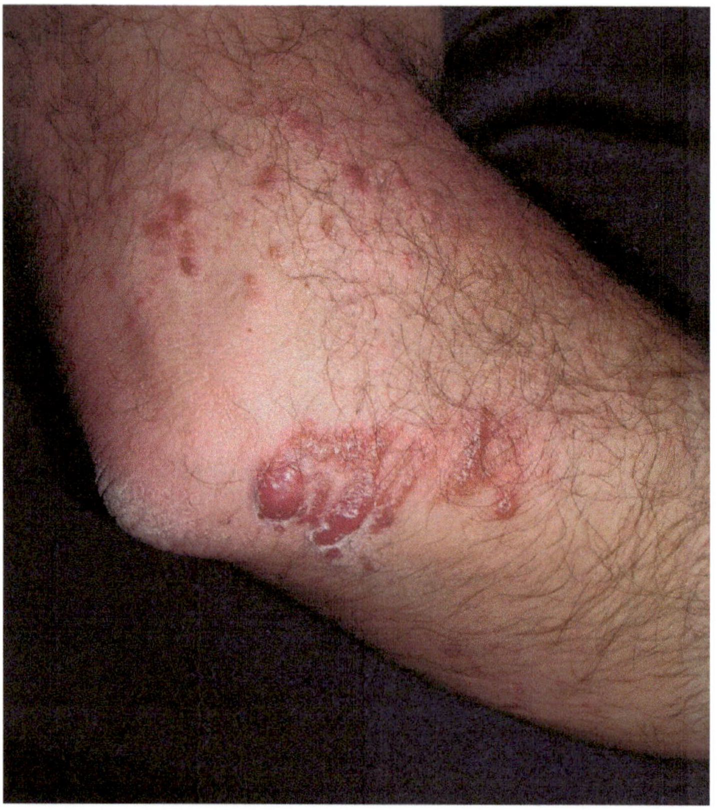

FIGURE 5.34 Sarcoidosis: Scar.

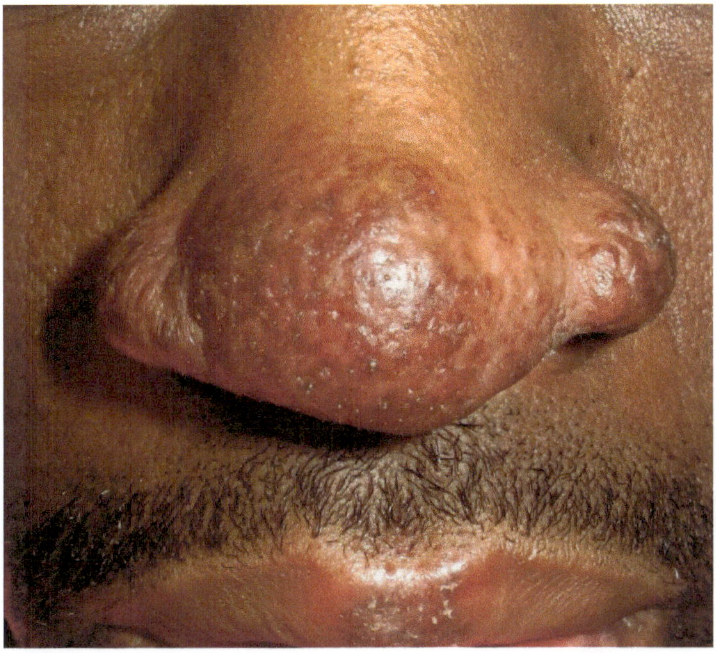

FIGURE 5.35 Sarcoidosis: Lupus pernio.

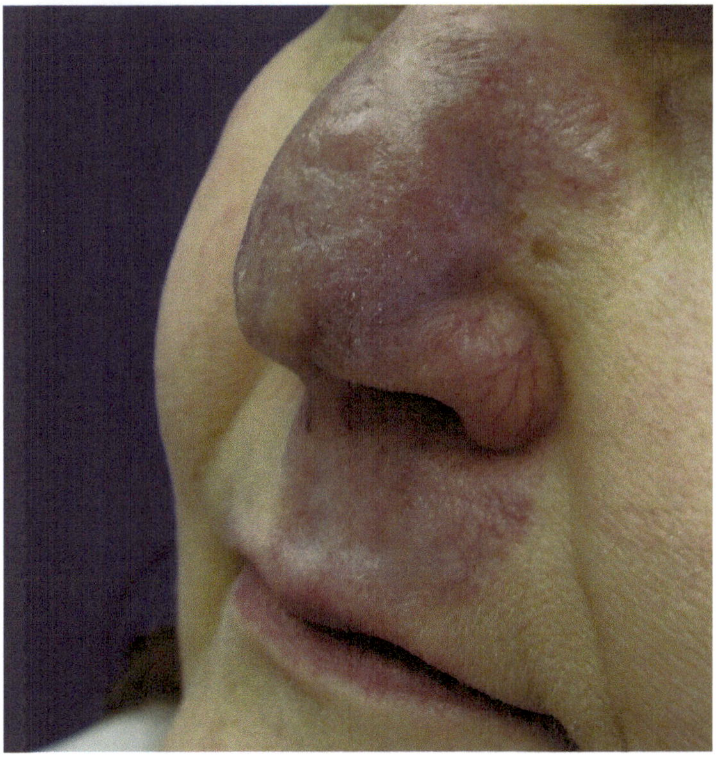

FIGURE 5.36 Sarcoidosis: Lupus pernio (angiolupoid variant).

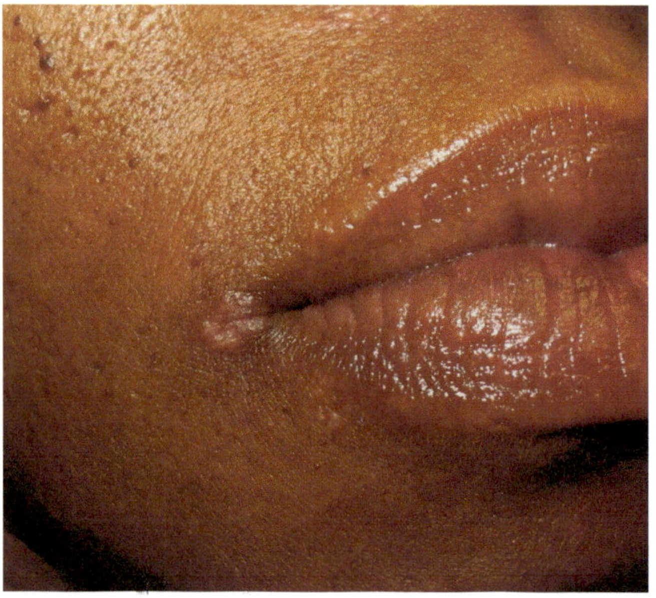

FIGURE 5.37 Sarcoidosis: Split papule.

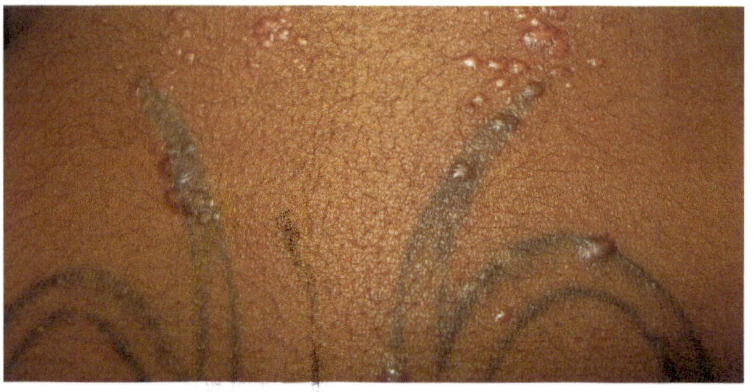

FIGURE 5.38 Sarcoidosis: Tattoo.

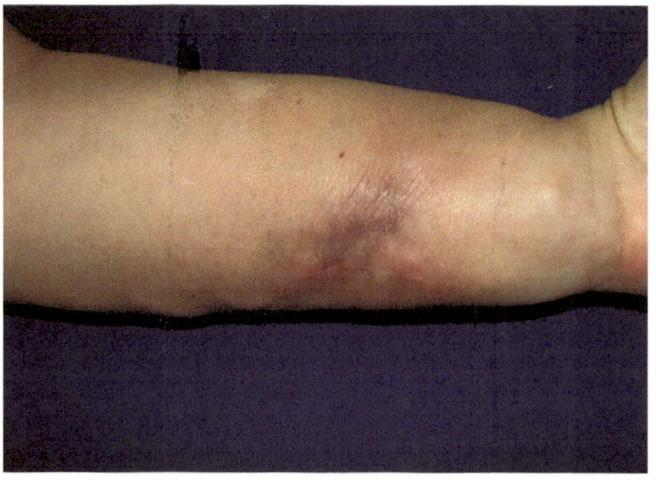

FIGURE 5.39 Sarcoidosis: Subcutaneous.

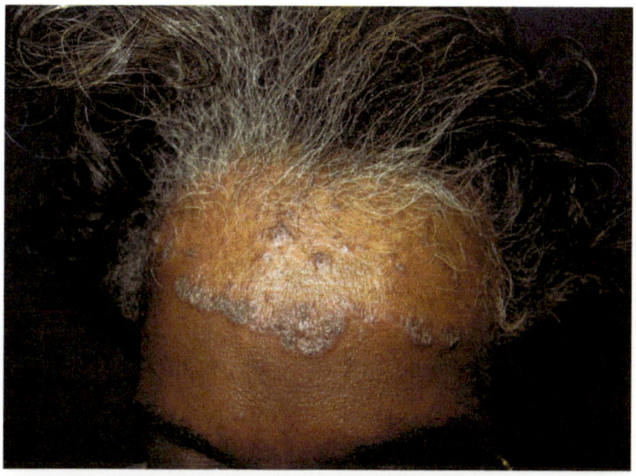

FIGURE 5.40 Sarcoidosis: Verrucous plaque causing alopecia.

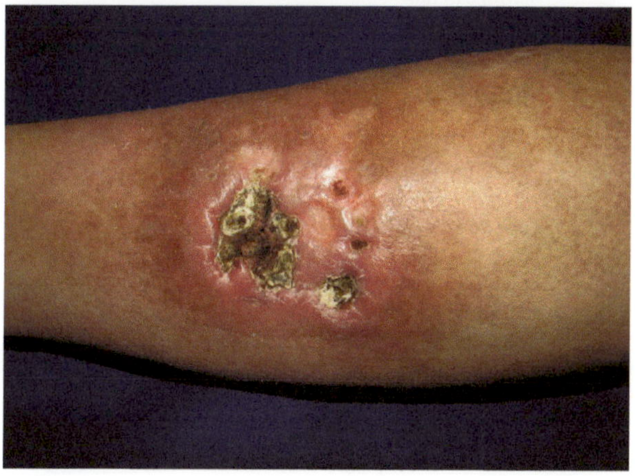

FIGURE 5.41 Sarcoidosis: Ulcerative.

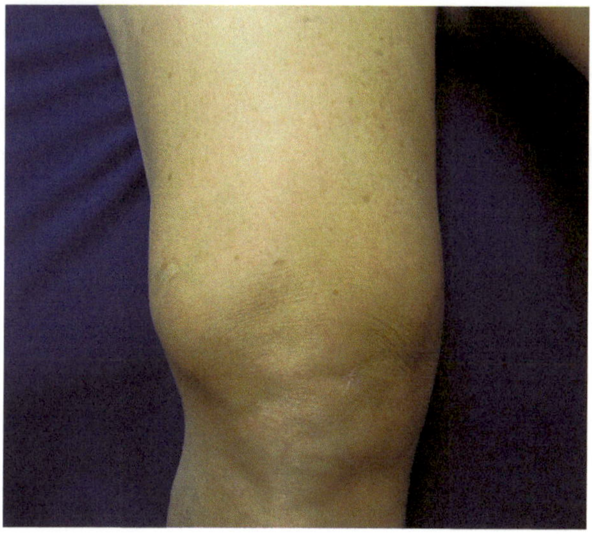

FIGURE 5.42 Sarcoidosis: Muscle.

Evaluation and Management

All patients diagnosed with biopsy-proven sarcoidosis need to be evaluated for systemic disease. A complete review of systems and physical exam are prudent, and a team approach with a dermatologist, internist, pulmonologist, cardiologist, and ophthalmologist is necessary. Initial evaluation is summarized in **Table 5.6**, which can be ordered prior to consultations. Each organ system responds to different therapies. Cutaneous sarcoidosis therapy consists of intralesional/oral steroids, minocycline, hydroxychloroquine, methotrexate, apremilast, anti-TNF and JAK inhibitors, or biologics.

TABLE 5.6

Evaluation of Patients with Cutaneous Sarcoidosis

Laboratory
• Complete blood count with platelets and differential
• Liver function tests
• Renal function tests
• Serum calcium
• Vitamin D
• Parathyroid hormone
• Thyroid function tests
• Urinalysis
Other diagnostic tests
• Chest X-ray
• High-resolution CT of lungs
• Positron emission tomography scan with computed tomography (PET-CT) scan
• Pulmonary function tests
• Electrocardiogram
• Echocardiogram
• Cardiac MRI
• Dilated eye exam

BIBLIOGRAPHY

Cooper D, Suau S. Sarcoidosis. Immunol Allergy Clin North Am 2023;43(3):583–591.

Drent M, Crouser ED, Grunewald J. Challenges of sarcoidosis and its management. N Eng J Med 2021;385(11):1018–1032.

Ezeh N, Caplan A, Rosenbach M, et al. Cutaneous sarcoidosis. Dermatol Clin 2023;41:455–470.

Williams JR, Frey C, Cohen GF. Cutaneous sarcoidosis in skin of color. J Drugs Dermatol 2023;22(7):695–697.

6

Immunobullous Disorders

Dermatitis Herpetiformis

Etiopathogenesis

Dermatitis herpetiformis (DH) is the cutaneous manifestation of gluten-sensitive enteropathy (GSE). Although it is generally accepted that all patients with DH have some degree of GSE, only 10%–15% of patients experience clinically significant symptoms. Patients with DH develop anti-tissue transglutaminase IgA (IgA TG 3) antibodies in the gut, which develop an affinity for epidermal transglutaminase and form complexes in the superficial dermis. There is a higher incidence of DH in male patients with certain human leukocyte antigen (HLA) haplotypes, including HLA DQ2 and HLA DQ8.

Clinical Manifestations

Patients with DH develop an intensely pruritic dermatitis, often out of proportion to their clinical findings, whose primary lesions consist of grouped, minute vesicles, although a widespread dermatitis can occasionally be present (**Figures 6.1–6.6**). On examination, it is common to see only excoriations. Anatomic areas favored by DH include the elbows, knees, scalp, and sacral area. DH patients are at risk of developing bullous pemphigoid and can present at that time with different bullae size and distribution.

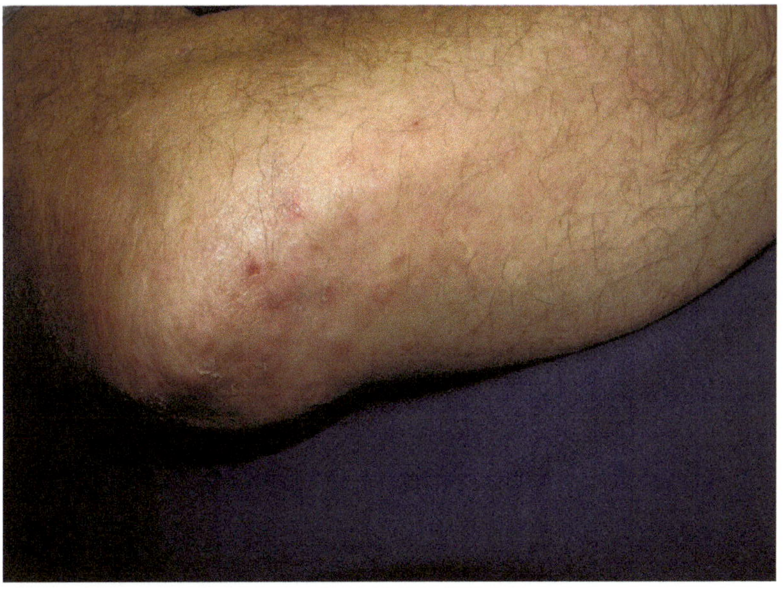

FIGURE 6.1 Dermatitis herpetiformis: Elbow.

DOI: 10.1201/9781003492665-6

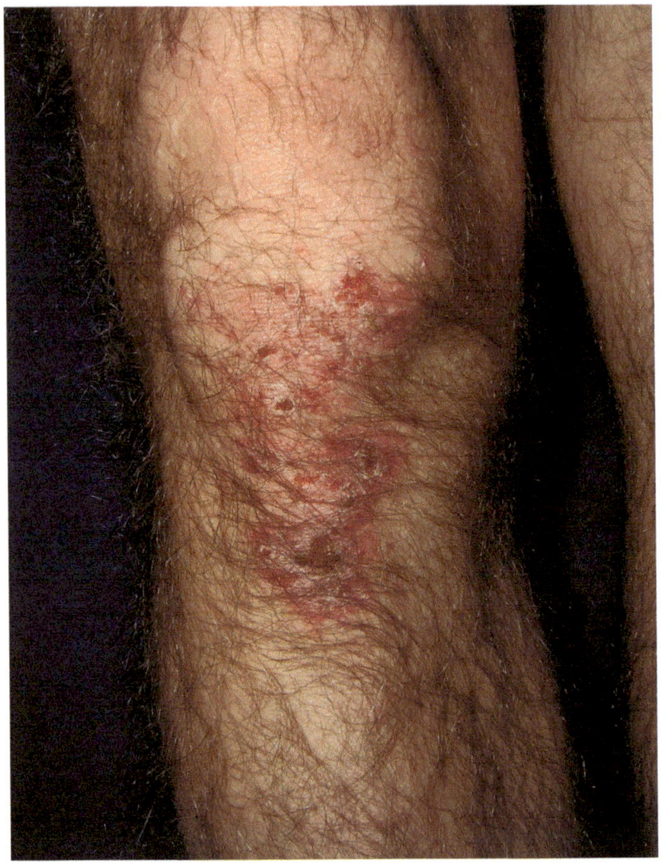

FIGURE 6.2 Dermatitis herpetiformis: Knee.

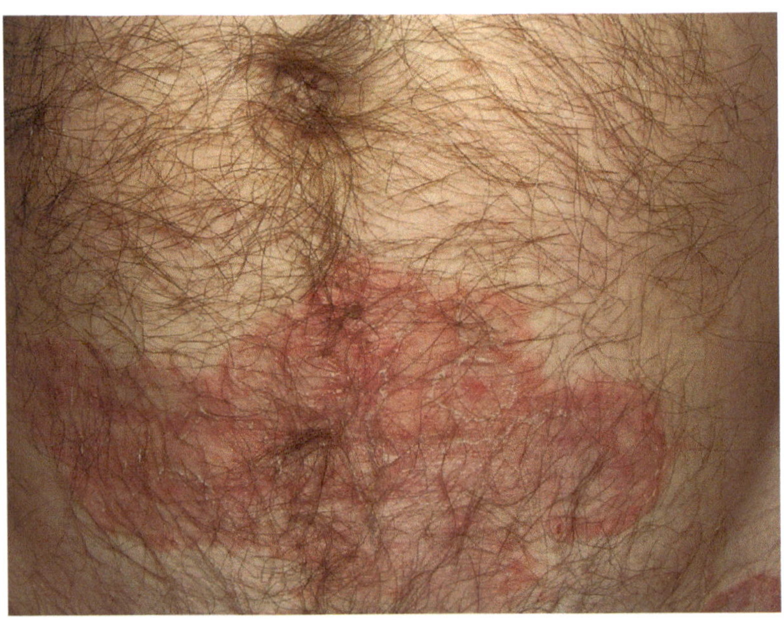

FIGURE 6.3 Dermatitis herpetiformis: Abdomen.

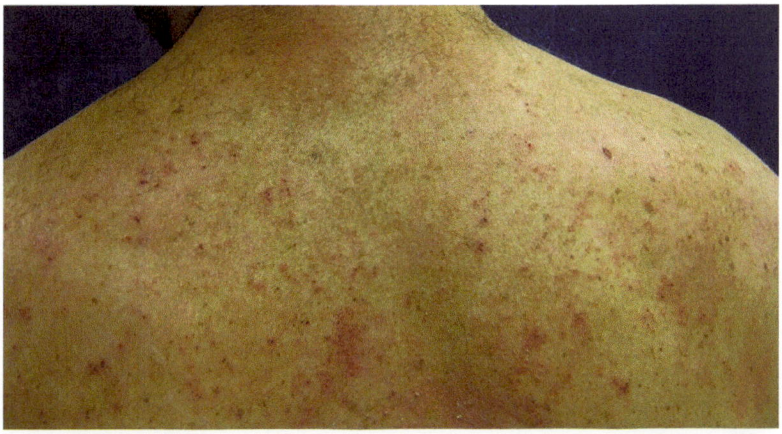

FIGURE 6.4 Dermatitis herpetiformis: Back.

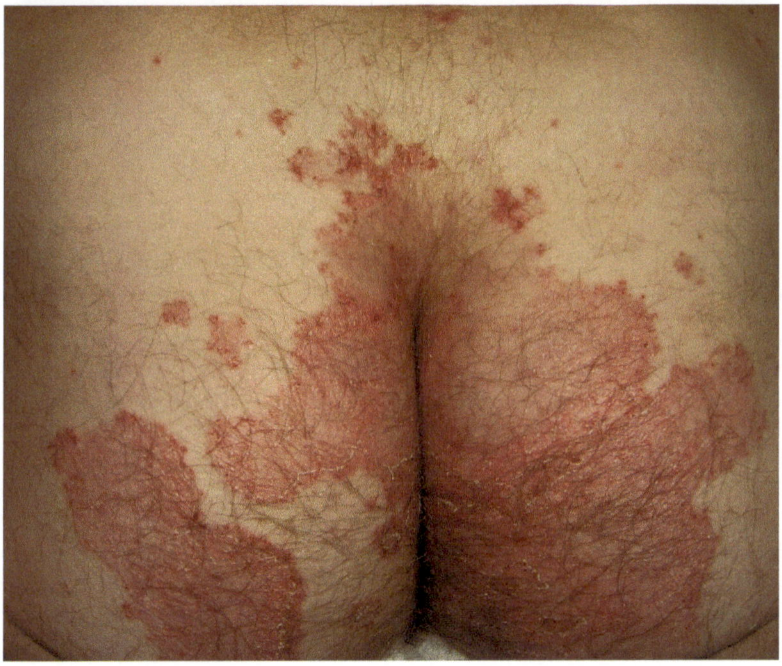

FIGURE 6.5 Dermatitis herpetiformis: Buttock.

Systemic Manifestations

Patients with DH have been reported to have a higher degree of other autoimmune diseases, most commonly involving the thyroid, but including diseases such as diabetes and Addison disease. Rarely, connective tissue diseases (scleroderma, Sjögren syndrome, lupus) have been reported concurrently with DH. Because of the presence of GSE, patients may also suffer from malabsorption, such as iron deficiency and pernicious anemia. Despite the increased lymphoma mortality in the first 5 years of follow-up, patients with DH overall have a lower mortality rate compared to that of the general population when on a gluten-free diet.

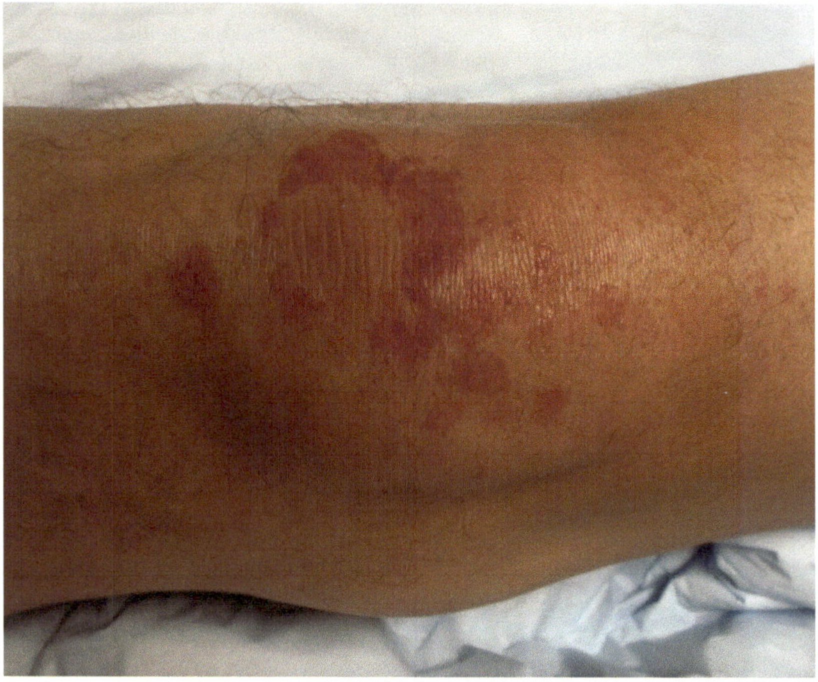

FIGURE 6.6 Dermatitis herpetiformis: Atypical petechial reaction (knee).

Evaluation and Management

The diagnosis of DH can be made by skin biopsy. Standard hematoxylin and eosin (H&E) biopsy should be taken from lesional skin and will classically demonstrate sterile neutrophilic microabscesses within the dermal papillae. Direct immunofluorescent testing, which is more sensitive, should be taken from skin approximately 1 cm from a vesicle and will demonstrate granular IgA present within the dermal papillae, with serum testing for transglutaminase antibodies [CELIAC]. A small-bowel biopsy can be performed to help confirm the diagnosis of GSE in selected patients but is not required to make the diagnosis. Workup for other autoimmune conditions can be performed in certain individuals based on history and clinical findings. This may include thyroid function tests (TFTs), anti-thyroglobulin antibodies (TG), anti-thyroid peroxidase antibodies (TPO), a.m. cortisol, anti-topoisomerase antibodies (anti-scl70), anticentromere antibodies (ACA), anti-Ro/SSA and anti-La/SSB antibodies (Ro/La), antinuclear antibodies (ANA), and anti-double stranded DNA (dsDNA) antibodies. The first-line therapy is to adhere to a life-long gluten-free diet. For severe cases, medical therapy for DH is dapsone and will provide immediate relief in a vast majority of patients. Alternative therapies reported include mycophenolate mofetil and rituximab.

BIBLIOGRAPHY

Antiga E, Maglie R, Quintarelli L, et al. Dermatitis herpetiformis: Novel perspectives. Front Immunol 2019;10:1290.

Nguyen CN, Kim SJ. Dermatitis herpetiformis: An update on diagnosis, disease monitoring and management. Medicina (Kaunas) 2021;57(8):843.

Reunala T, Hervonen K, Salmi T. Dermatitis herpetiformis: An update on diagnosis and management. Am J Clin Dermatol 2021;22(3):329–338.

Salmi TT. Dermatitis herpetiformis. Clin Exp Dermatol 2019;44(7):728–731.

Paraneoplastic Pemphigus

Etiopathogenesis

Pemphigus is an autoimmune disease in which patients develop antibodies to desmogleins, proteins present on the surface of keratinocytes. Binding of antibodies to these proteins leads to keratinocyte disassociation that manifests clinically as erosions, vesicles, and blisters, which can form on the skin or mucous membranes. In paraneoplastic pemphigus (PNP), which develops as a result of an underlying malignancy, antibodies are directed against other epithelial proteins in the plakin family in addition to the desmogleins. These proteins can be present on epithelial cells or can be components of the basement membrane zone. As a consequence of additional proteins being targeted, clinical manifestations can be more severe, and epithelial surfaces of other organs, especially the lungs, can be affected (paraneoplastic autoimmune multiorgan syndrome).

Clinical Manifestations

The vast majority of patients with PNP will have severe mucositis (**Figure 6.7**). The mucositis will typically be more severe than what is seen in pemphigus vulgaris, with more widespread involvement and larger areas of sloughing. The cutaneous lesions of PNP can be flaccid bullae or erosions (pemphigus vulgaris-like) as well as lesions resembling more inflammatory conditions, such as acute toxic epidermal necrolysis or chronic lichen planus or erythema multiforme (**Figures 6.8–6.11**).

Systemic Manifestations

PNP is associated with an underlying malignancy in almost all cases. The most common malignancies in adults are non-Hodgkin lymphomas (NHLs) or chronic lymphocytic leukemia (CLL), with occasional reports of thymomas, sarcomas, or other tumors. In children, Castleman disease is the most commonly reported malignancy, although adult cases of Castleman have been reported as well. Patients with lung involvement may develop progressive dyspnea leading to respiratory failure (bronchiolitis obliterans). Patients are also at risk for myasthenia gravis, and this diagnosis should be considered if patients develop dyspnea without evidence of bronchiolitis obliterans.

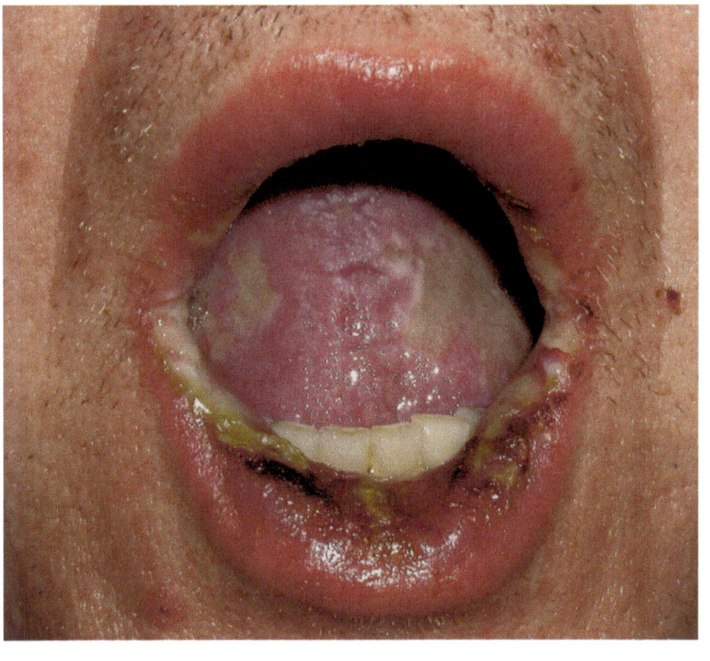

FIGURE 6.7 Paraneoplastic pemphigus: Stomatitis.

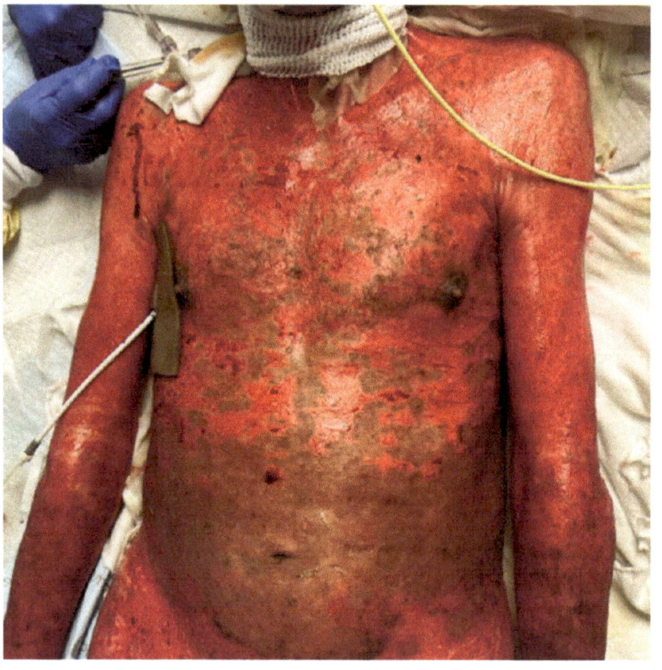

FIGURE 6.8 Paraneoplastic pemphigus: Acute toxic epidermal necrolysis-like.

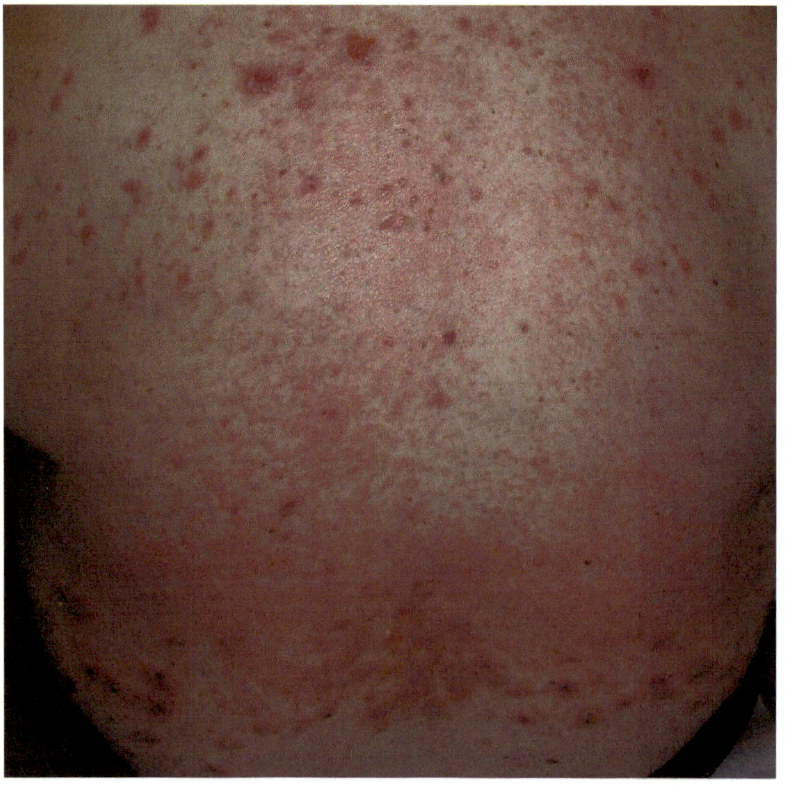

FIGURE 6.9 Paraneoplastic pemphigus.

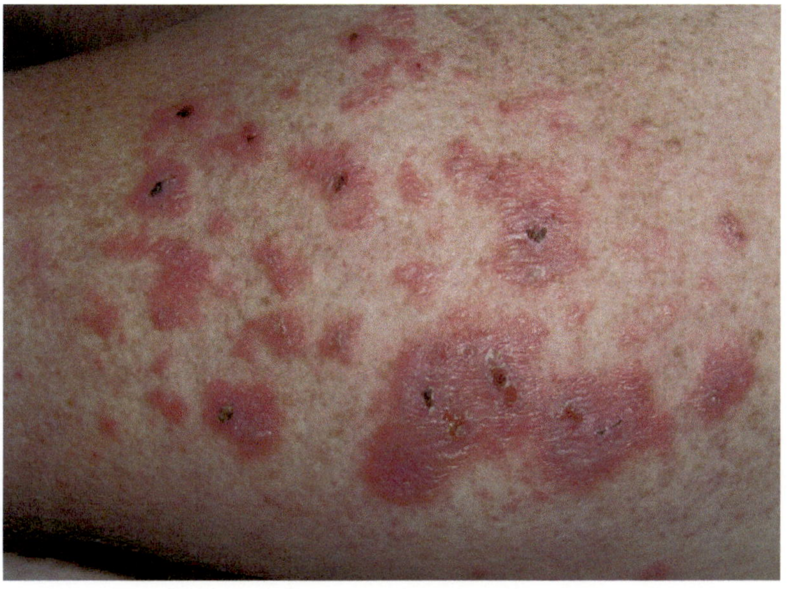

FIGURE 6.10 Paraneoplastic pemphigus: Erythema multiforme–like.

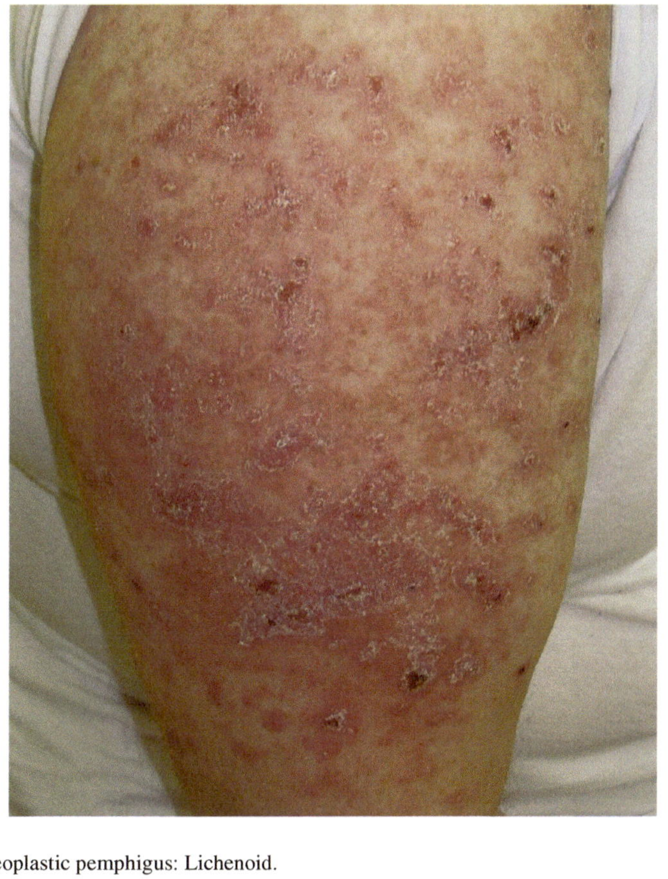

FIGURE 6.11 Paraneoplastic pemphigus: Lichenoid.

Evaluation and Management

The diagnosis of PNP requires a high level of suspicion, as the most specific tests are not widely available. Histologically, patients with PNP may have more interface changes in addition to the acantholysis that is seen with pemphigus vulgaris. Immunofluorescent findings may demonstrate reactants at the basement membrane zone (BMZ) in addition to the intercellular immunoreactants seen in pemphigus. Serum from PNP patients will react against substrates such as rodent bladder, and if immunoblotting or immunoprecipitation can be performed, antibodies against specific epithelial proteins can be demonstrated. If these more specific tests are not available and PNP is suspected, computed tomography (CT) of the chest, abdomen, and pelvis and a complete blood count (CBC) would be a reasonable workup. Pulmonary function testing should be prompt if there are respiratory complaints; in addition to treatment of the underlying malignancy, treatment of PNP includes systemic corticosteroids and other immunosuppressive agents, including rituximab. See **Table 6.1** for immunobullous disease with systemic associations.

TABLE 6.1

Immunobullous Disease with Systemic Associations

Disease	Clinical Findings	Histologic Findings	Immunofluorescent Findings	Associated Conditions
Dermatitis herpetiformis	Extremely pruritic vesicles, papules, erosions on elbows, knees, sacrum, scalp	Dermal papillary microabscesses	Granular IgA in the tips of the dermal papilla. Linear IgA is sometimes present as well	Gluten-sensitive enteropathy
Paraneoplastic pemphigus	Lichenoid or erythema multiforme (EM)-like plaques associated with flaccid bullae and erosions. Severe mucositis is often present	Acantholysis, intraepidermal, and/or subepithelial vesicles with associated interface or lichenoid inflammatory infiltrate	Intraepidermal and subepidermal deposition of IgG and/or C3	NHL, CLL, Castleman's disease

BIBLIOGRAPHY

Anderson HJ, Huang S, Lee JB. Paraneoplastic pemphigus/paraneoplastic autoimmune multiorgan syndrome: Part I. Clinical overview and pathophysiology. J Am Acad Dermatol 2024;91(1):1–10.

Huang S, Anderson HJ, Lee JB. Paraneoplastic pemphigus/paraneoplastic autoimmune multiorgan syndrome: Part II. Diagnosis and management. J Am Acad Dermatol 2024;91(1):13–22.

Paolino G, Didona D, Magliulo G, et al. Paraneoplastic pemphigus: Insight into the autoimmune pathogenesis, clinical features and therapy. Int J Mol Sci 2017;18(12):2532.

Svoboda SA, Huang S, Liu X, et al. Paraneoplastic pemphigus: Revised diagnostic criteria based on literature analysis. J Cutan Pathol 2021;48(9):1133–1138.

7

Lymphoproliferative Disorders

Cutaneous Lymphomas

Etiopathogenesis

Primary cutaneous lymphomas encompass a broad category of hematologic malignancies, with cutaneous T-cell lymphoma (CTCL) and cutaneous B-cell lymphoma (CBCL) accounting for more than 80% of all cases. Mycosis fungoides (MF) is the most common type of CTCL and represents nearly 50% of all primary cutaneous lymphomas. MF is a malignancy of CD 3+ CD4+, CD8- memory T cells. The most common age of presentation is ≥55 years, but MF has been reported in younger age groups. MF is usually an indolent malignancy with a prolonged course. Less than one-third of patients develop advanced disease. CBCLs account for 25%–29% of all primary lymphomas in the United States. It is very important to distinguish between primary CBCL and systemic B-cell lymphoma with cutaneous involvement because the prognosis and management differ greatly. The most common type of CBCL is primary cutaneous follicle center B-cell lymphoma (PCFCL). The median age at diagnosis is 60 years. Like CTCL, the majority of CBCL is indolent and may recur after treatment. Recurrence, however, does not portend a worse prognosis.

Clinical Manifestations

MF classically presents with erythematous, *cigarette paper* texture (**Figure 7.1**) to scaling, pruritic patches in the photoprotected, or *bathing trunk* distribution. These patches can evolve over time into plaques and tumors (**Figures 7.2–7.8**). It is common to see all three types of lesions on a patient at one time. MF can also be hypopigmented, and this variant is seen more commonly in children and in patients with darker skin types. Approximately 30% of patients present with skin tumors or erythroderma at disease onset. MF variants include folliculotropic, granulomatous, and pagetoid reticulosis. Sezary syndrome (SS), or leukemic CTCL, is characterized by large numbers of atypical circulating Sezary cells. Patients are often erythrodermic and have severe pruritus. Unlike classic MF, SS is not indolent. Less commonly, CTCL can present as subcutaneous panniculitis-like T-cell lymphoma, primary cutaneous gamma/delta T-cell lymphoma, adult T-cell leukemia/lymphoma, extranodal natural killer (NK)/T-cell lymphoma (nasal type), and others. CBCLs often present as nonspecific papules, plaques, or violaceous nodules on the skin. PCFCL has a predilection for the scalp, forehead (**Figure 7.9**), neck, and trunk), whereas primary cutaneous diffuse large B-cell lymphoma, leg type, is limited to the leg (**Figure 7.10**). The subtypes of CBCLs are listed in **Table 7.1**. Systemic B-cell lymphomas can present similarly (**Figures 7.11** and **7.12**) The differential diagnosis can be broad, and biopsy is usually required for diagnosis.

Systemic Manifestations

Given the chronicity of these conditions, systemic manifestations may negatively affect long-term quality of life. For patients with CTCL, pruritus is often the most prevalent and most studied symptom. Pain, insomnia, anxiety, and depression can also be significant. Systemic B-cell lymphoma may be asymptomatic or have fatigue, weight loss, and malaise.

DOI: 10.1201/9781003492665-7

Evaluation and Management

Patients with cutaneous lymphomas should be evaluated by a dermatologist with expertise in cutaneous lymphomas. The workup and management often include a multidisciplinary team approach with dermatologists, oncologists, dermatopathologists, and radiation oncology, as well as testing for T-cell gene rearrangements, flow cytometry for CTCL, and B-cell markers, and monoclonal expression of immunoglobulins (kappa or lambda) of CBCL.

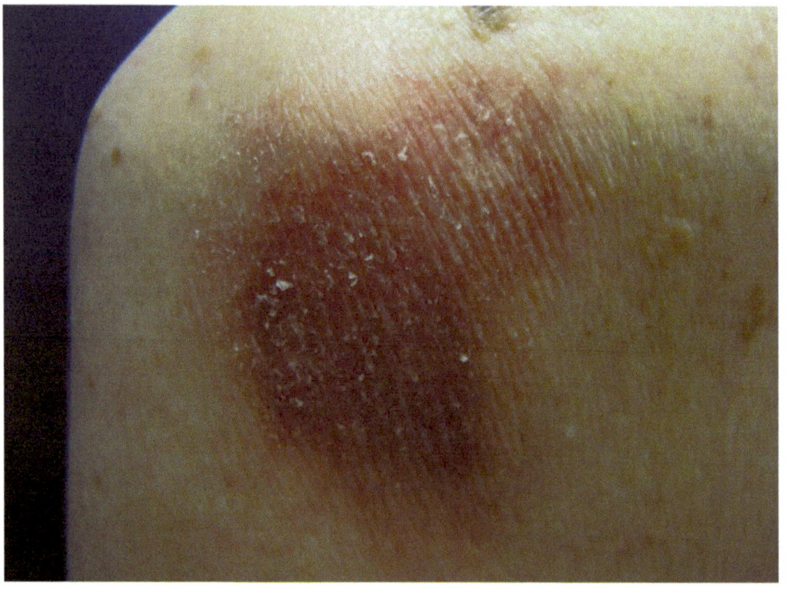

FIGURE 7.1 Cutaneous T-cell lymphoma: Cigarette paper texture.

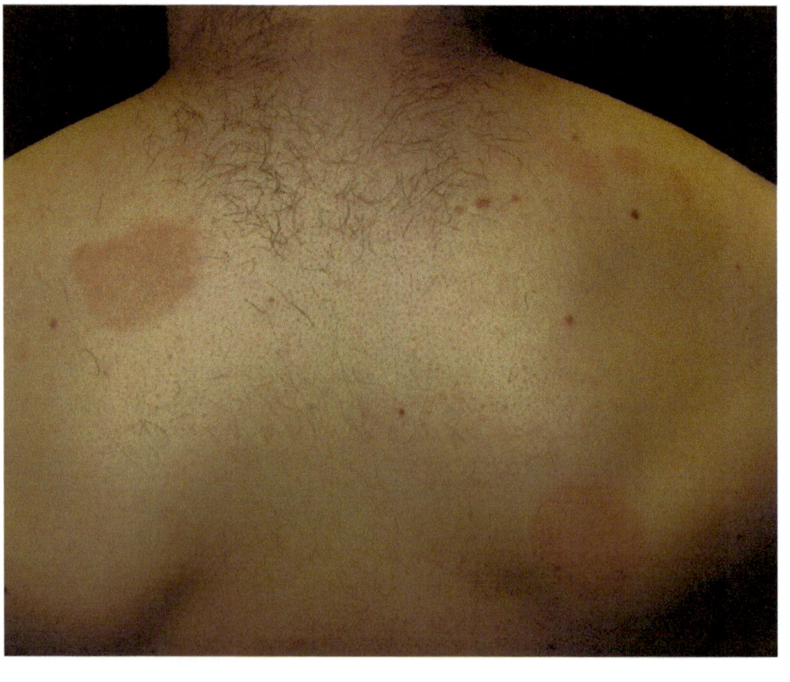

FIGURE 7.2 Cutaneous T-cell lymphoma: Patch stage.

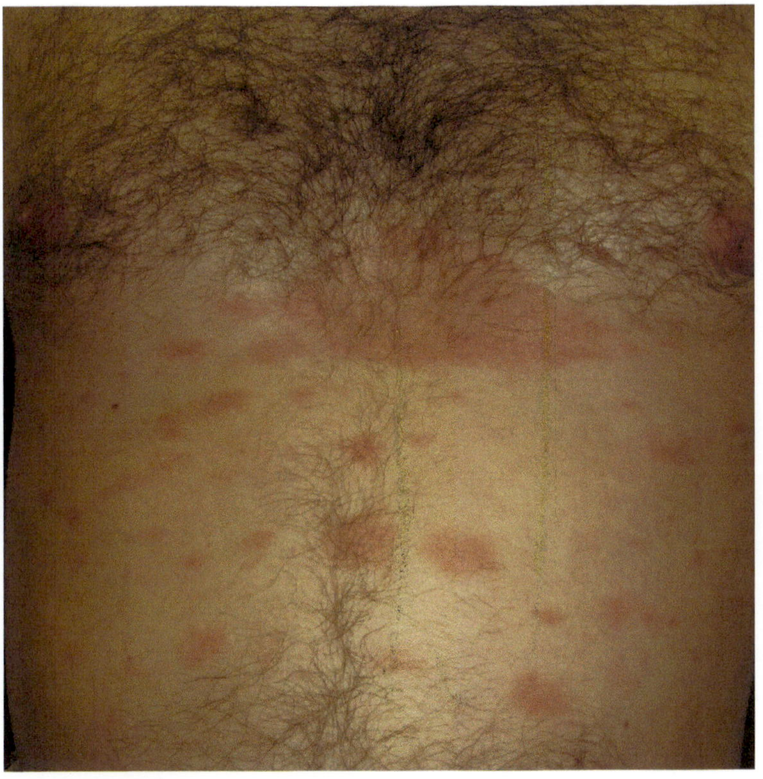

FIGURE 7.3 Cutaneous T-cell lymphoma: Patch stage.

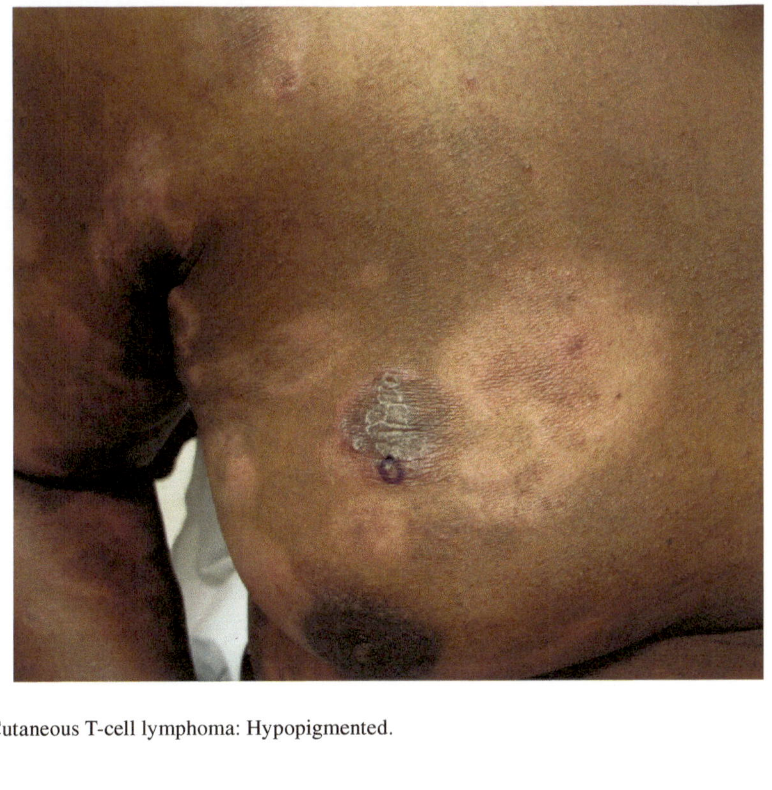

FIGURE 7.4 Cutaneous T-cell lymphoma: Hypopigmented.

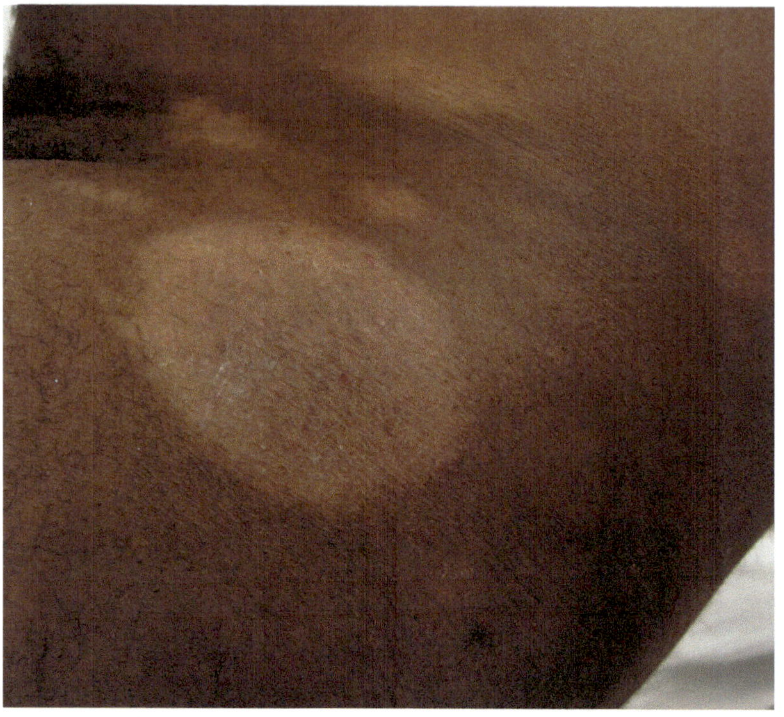

FIGURE 7.5 Cutaneous T-cell lymphoma: Hypopigmented.

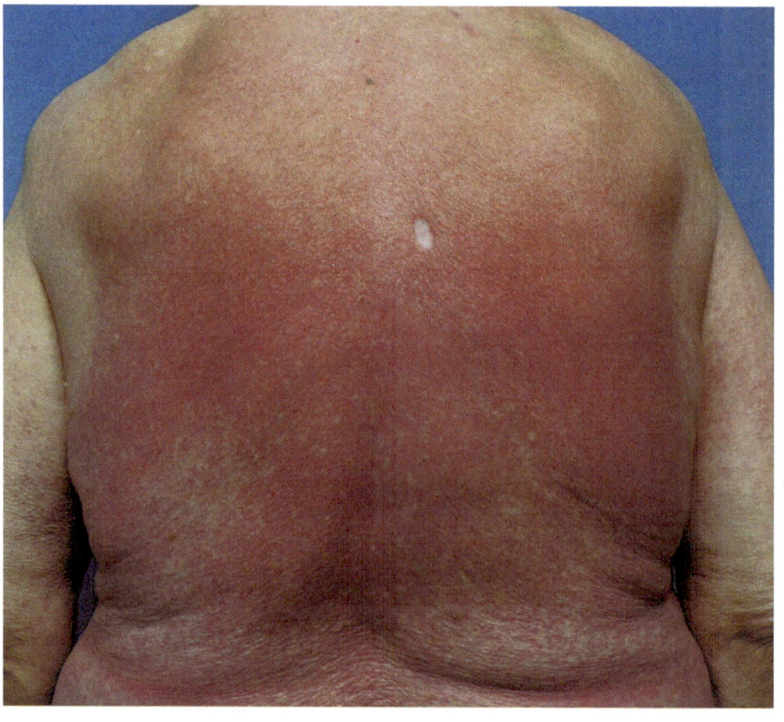

FIGURE 7.6 Cutaneous T-cell lymphoma: Poikilodermatous.

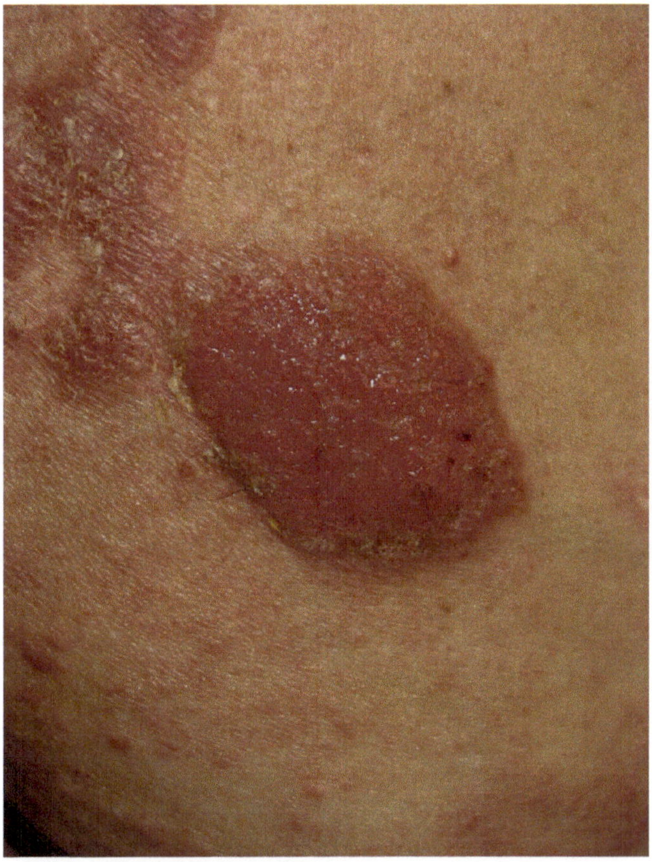

FIGURE 7.7 Cutaneous T-cell lymphoma: Early tumor stage.

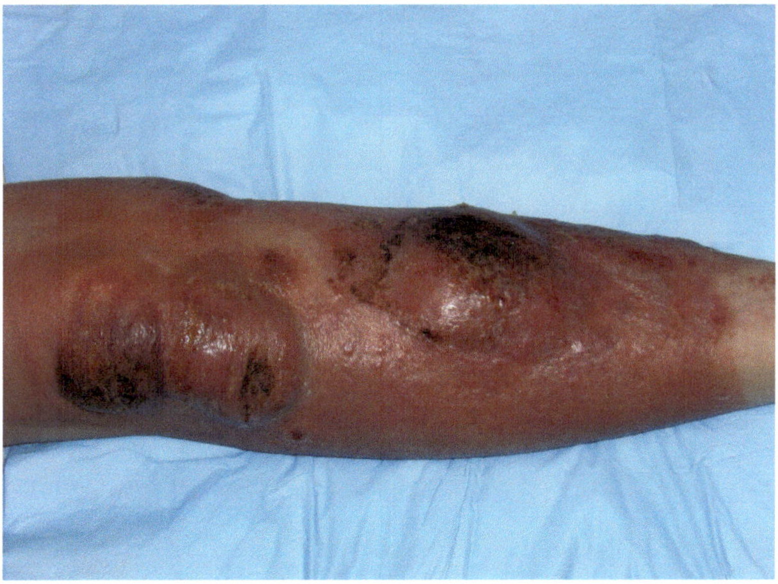

FIGURE 7.8 Cutaneous T-cell lymphoma: Advanced tumor stage.

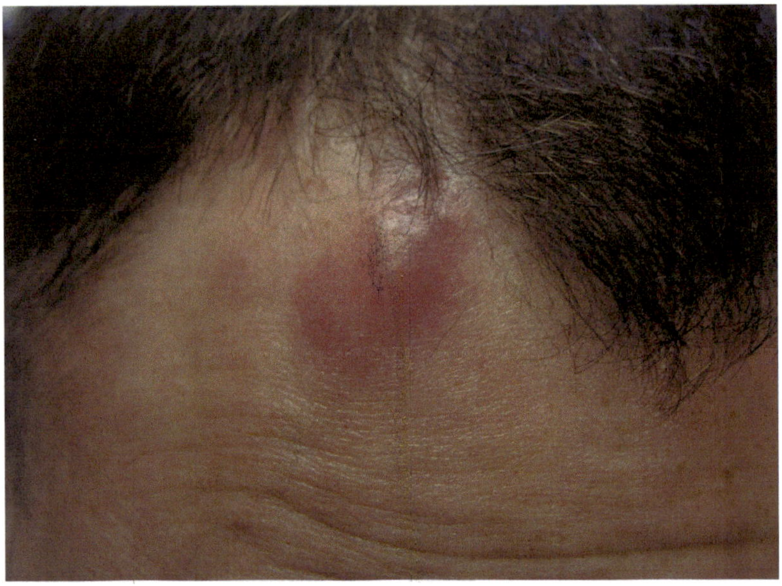

FIGURE 7.9 Primary cutaneous follicle center lymphoma.

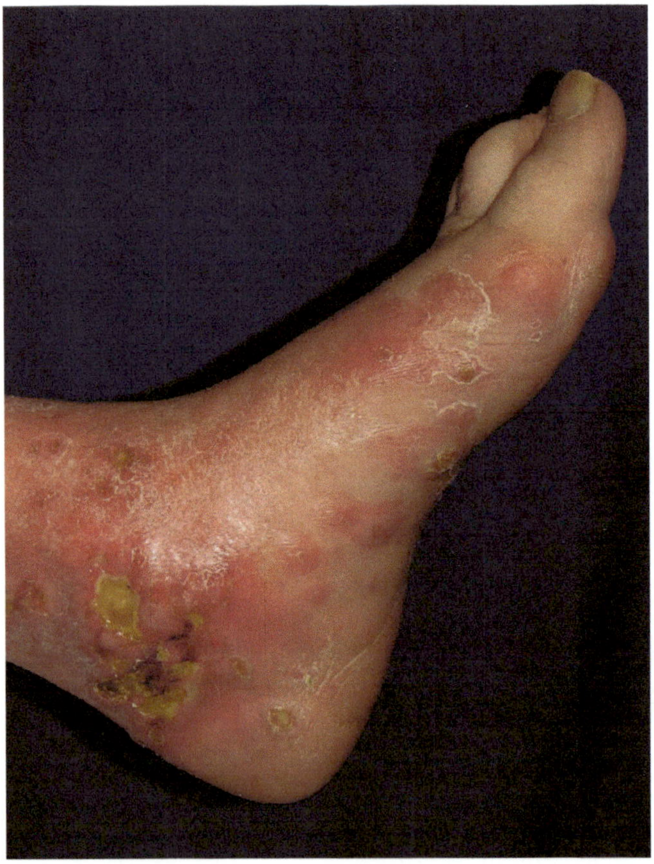

FIGURE 7.10 Primary cutaneous diffuse large B-cell lymphoma, leg type.

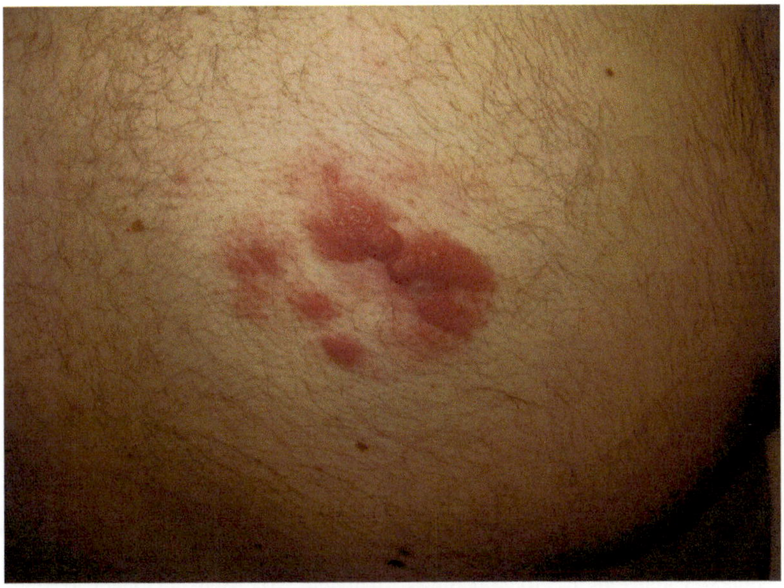

FIGURE 7.11 Systemic B-cell lymphoma with cutaneous involvement.

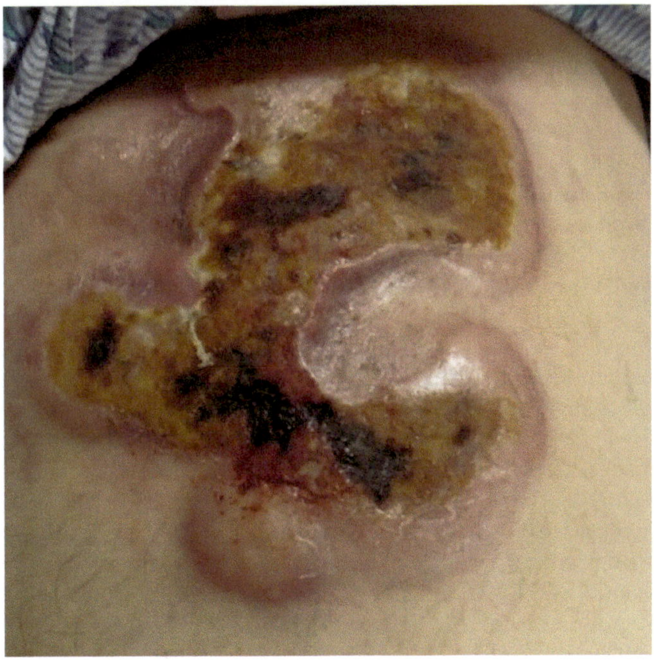

FIGURE 7.12 Systemic B-cell lymphoma with cutaneous involvement.

In general, for CTCL, patients with limited skin involvement and no evidence of internal disease can be treated with topical corticosteroids or other skin-directed therapies, including ultraviolet light and oral retinoids. More aggressive presentations may require biologic-response modifiers, histone deacetylase inhibitors, antibody-based strategies, or allogenic stem-cell transplantation. For patients with CBCL, excision of the lesion, local radiation treatment, and intralesional corticosteroids can be considered in the initial treatment plan. Reduction of immunosuppression is treatment for Epstein–Barr virus-positive mucocutaneous ulcer. Referral to a dermatology expert in cutaneous lymphoma or hematology/oncology for more advanced disease or more aggressive subtype cases is highly recommended to consider rituximab and anthracycline-based chemotherapy.

TABLE 7.1

Types of Primary Cutaneous B-Cell Lymphoma

Type	Clinical Course
Primary cutaneous marginal cell lymphoma (30%)	Indolent
Primary cutaneous follicle center lymphoma (50%)	Indolent
Primary cutaneous diffuse large B-cell lymphoma, leg type (20%)	Aggressive
Intravascular large B-cell lymphoma, skin-only variant	Less aggressive
Epstein–Barr virus-positive mucocutaneous ulcer	Indolent

BIBLIOGRAPHY

Hristov AC, Tejasvi T, Wilcox RA. Cutaneous T-cell lymphomas: 2023 update on diagnosis, risk stratification and management. Am J Hematol 2023;98(1):193–209.

Kempf W, Mittledorf C. Cutaneous T-cell lymphoma - An update 2021. Hematol Oncol 2021;39(Suppl 1):46–51.

Villasenor-Park J, Chung J, Kim EJ. Cutaneous B-cell lymphomas. Hematol Oncol Clin North Am 2024;38(5):111–1131.

Monoclonal Gammopathy

Etiopathogenesis

An abnormal clonal B-cell proliferation (plasma cells) with concomitant aberrant clonal immunoglobulin production is referred to as plasma cell dyscrasia, dysparaproteinemia, or monoclonal gammopathy (MG). Proliferation produces MG of undetermined significance (MGUS) to multiple myeloma, which has been postulated to be related to oncogene activation/dysregulation (neuroblastoma RAS viral [v-ras] oncogene homolog [NRAS] and V-Ki-ras2 Kirsten rat sarcoma viral oncogene homolog [KRAS] mutations, v-myc avian myelocytomatosis viral oncogene homolog [MYC] upregulation), tumor suppression gene mutations (p53), and cytokine dysregulation (IL-6). Distinction is based on bone marrow plasma cell percentage, amount of immunoglobulin (g/dl), and systemic manifestations. Skin diseases can be a direct result of MG, as in Group I: amyloidosis; monoclonal cryoglobulinemia; Waldenstrom macroglobulinemia; plasmacytomas; polyneuropathy, organomegaly, endocrinopathy, monoclonal gammopathy, and skin changes (POEMS), telangiectasia with elevated erythropoietin, MG, perirenal fluid collections, and intrapulmonary shunt (TEMPI). They can also be associated with MG, as in Group II: scleromyxedema (**Figures 1.105** and **1.135**), erythema elevatum diutinum (**Figure 7.13**), subcorneal pustular dermatosis (**Figure 7.14**), scleredema, necrobiotic xanthogranuloma (NXG), plane xanthoma, Schnitzler syndrome; anecdotal to MG, as in Group III: epidermolysis bullosa acquisita (**Figure 7.15**), neutrophilic dermatoses, and leukocytoclastic vasculitis); or a nonspecific finding, as in Group IV: pruritus, purpura of MG.

Clinical Manifestations

Amyloidosis classically presents with pinch purpura, macroglossia, and carpal tunnel syndrome. Type I monoclonal cryoglobulinemia presents with noninflammatory purpura on the ears, face, chest, and extremities. Waldenstrom macroglobulinemia may present with flesh-colored discrete papules called IgM storage papules. Plasmacytomas are nodular proliferations from underlying multiple myeloma. POEMS syndrome may present with glomeruloid hemangiomas and diffuse pigmentation. Associated skin diseases (**Table 7.2**) of note are scleromyxedema, erythema elevatum diutinum (EED), and subcorneal pustular dermatosis (scleredema, planar xanthoma, NXG, pyoderma gangrenosum, cutis laxa, and Schnitzler's Sweet syndromes are discussed in other chapters). Scleromyxedema presents with flesh-colored papules, sclerodermoid changes, and leonine facies from mucin deposition due to fibroblastic proliferation. EED, a form of chronic leukocytoclastic vasculitis, produces red to purple papules to plaques classically overlying joints. Subcorneal pustular dermatosis is a chronic/recurrent pustular eruption with serpiginous shapes and pus accumulation in the lower half of the bullae.

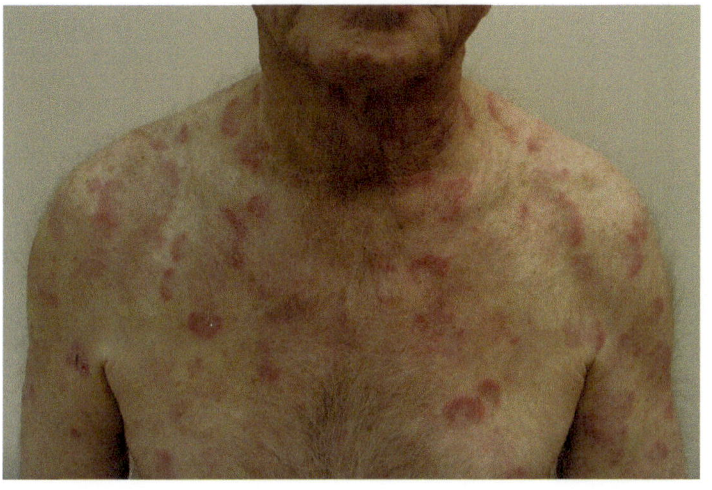

FIGURE 7.13 Erythema elevatum diutinum.

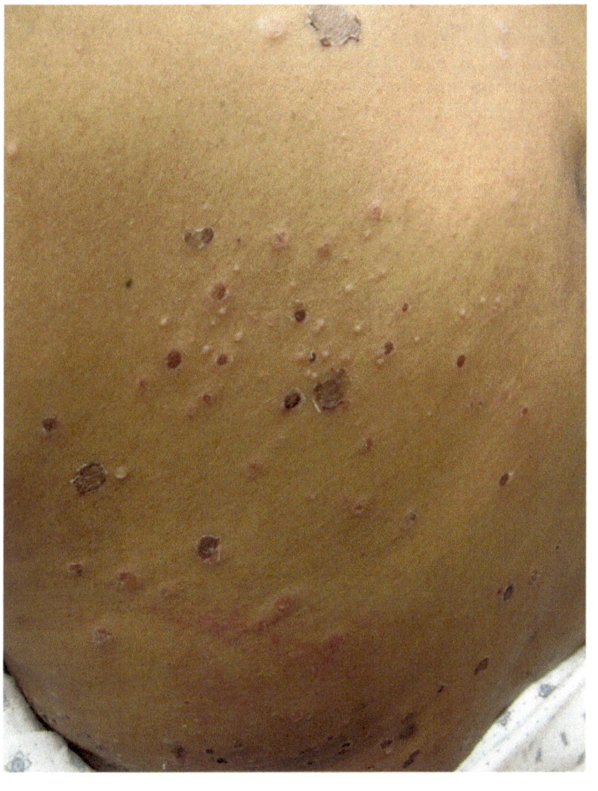

FIGURE 7.14 Subcorneal pustular dermatosis.

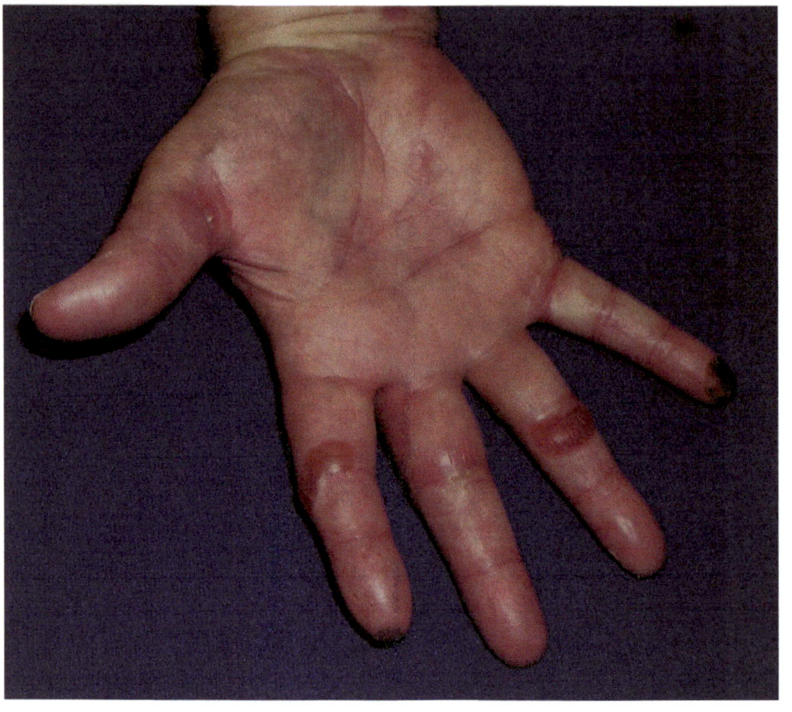

FIGURE 7.15 Epidermolysis bullosa acquisita.

TABLE 7.2

Monoclonal Gammopathy and Skin Disease

Monoclonal Gammopathy (Predominate)	Skin Disease
1. IgG	a. Diffuse normolipemic planar xanthoma
	b. Acquired C1-INH deficiency angioedema
	c. Sweet syndrome
	d. Acquired cutis laxa
2. IgG κ	a. NXG
	b. Xanthoma disseminate
	c. POEMS; TEMPI
3. IgG λ	a. Scleromyxedema
	b. Scleredema
4. IgM κ	a. Schnitzler syndrome
	b. Waldenstrom macroglobulinemia
	c. Cryoglobulinemia
5. IgA	a. EED
	b. Pyoderma gangrenosum
	c. Subcorneal pustular dermatosis
	d. Henoch–Schönlein purpura
6. Variable	a. Primary and myeloma-associated systemic amyloidosis
	b. Angioimmunoblastic lymphadenopathy with dysparaproteinemia
	c. Classic Kaposi sarcoma
	d. CTCL

Systemic Manifestations

Dysparaproteinemias may range from being asymptomatic to producing significant morbidity. A secondary hyperviscosity syndrome (fatigue, epistaxis, loss of visual acuity, headache, and stroke) may occur. In addition, bone pain, anemia, renal failure, elevated serum calcium, and recurrent bacterial infections are suggestive of multiple myeloma. Primary amyloidosis may develop peripheral neuropathies, congestive heart failure, and a nephritic syndrome. Waldenstrom macroglobulinemia, primary amyloidosis, and POEMS may have significant hepatosplenomegaly. Scleromyxedema may develop seizure, coma, cardiac arrhythmia, and dyspnea. EED patients develop significant arthritis.

Evaluation and Management

A history of generalized malaise with a wide range of skin findings should prompt concern for a possible underlying MG. Biopsy of skin findings may be specific, such as amyloid deposition around cutaneous vessels, mucin deposition with a fibroblastic proliferation of scleromyxedema, *onion skinning* around leukocytoclasia of EED, or nonspecific extravasated red blood cells. Once a skin disease associated with an MG is suspected, further investigation should include a complete blood count (CBC), renal function test (RFT), serum Ca2+, cryoglobulin (CRYO), serum protein electrophoresis/serum immunofixation electrophoresis (SPEP/SIFE), serum free light chains, 24-hour urine protein electrophoresis/urine immunofixation electrophoresis (UPEP/UIFE), bone marrow biopsy, and skeletal survey. MG that does not meet the full criteria for multiple myeloma requires routine monitoring, as MGUS has been shown to be a precursor to myeloma. Referral to hematology/oncology for the treatment of malignant states is suggested.

BIBLIOGRAPHY

Claveau JS, Wetter DA, Kumar S. Cutaneous manifestations of monoclonal gammopathy. Blood Cancer J 2022;12(4):58.

Cowan J, Green DJ, Kwok M, et al. Diagnosis and management of multiple myeloma: A review. JAMA 2022;327(5):464–477.

Lipsker D. Monoclonal gammopathy of cutaneous significance: Review of a relevant concept. J Eur Acad Dermatol Venereol 2017;31(1):45–52.

8

Metabolic and Nutritional Disorders

Adrenal Disease

Etiopathogenesis

Primary adrenal insufficiency (PAI), or Addison disease, is due to lack of production of cortisol and mineralocorticoids. PAI can be caused by infections (tuberculosis) or autoimmunity. Secondary adrenal insufficiency is due to hypothalamic/pituitary failure. Hyperpigmentation of the skin in PAI is due to subsequent increased pituitary secretion of proopiomelanocortin (POMC). Melanocyte-stimulating hormone is a cleaved peptide of POMC that stimulates production of melanin by melanocytes. Cushing syndrome is due to excess cortisol from a cortisol-producing adrenal tumor, excess adrenocorticotropic-hormone (ACTH)-producing pituitary tumor, ectopic ACTH-producing tumor, or due to iatrogenic glucocorticoids.

Clinical Manifestations

The hyperpigmentation of PAI can be diffuse and appreciable when the patient's skin tone is compared to other family members. Hyperpigmentation (**Figures 8.1–8.4**) may occur in the palmar creases, orogenital mucosa, areas of friction (flexural skin) or pressure (elbows and knees), and nails (longitudinal melanonychia or Bissell's lines). See **Table 8.1** for differential diagnosis. Cushing syndrome produces central obesity with fat pads, facial fullness/flushing, ecchymoses, hyperpigmentation, striae, thin skin, and hirsutism (**Figures 8.5** and **8.6**).

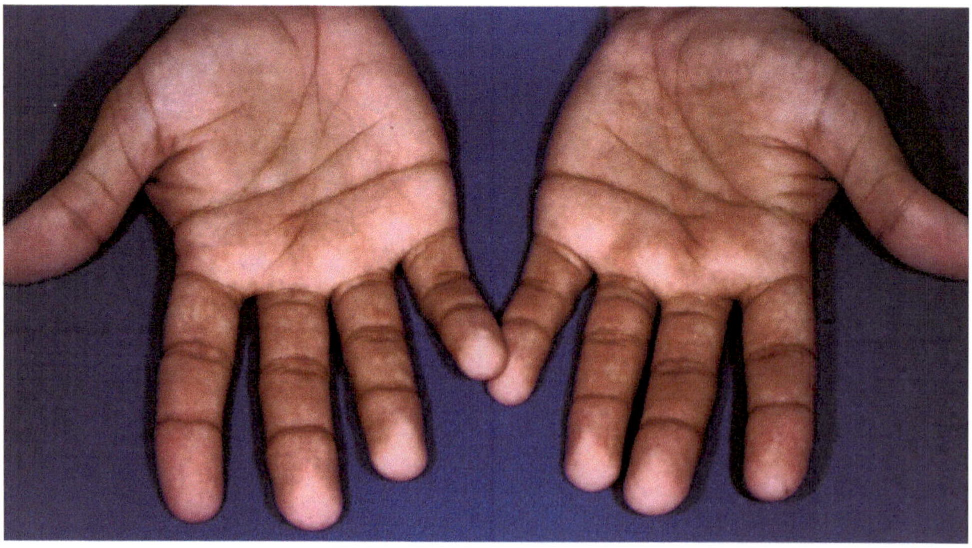

FIGURE 8.1 Primary adrenal insufficiency: Palmar skin line hyperpigmentation.

DOI: 10.1201/9781003492665-8

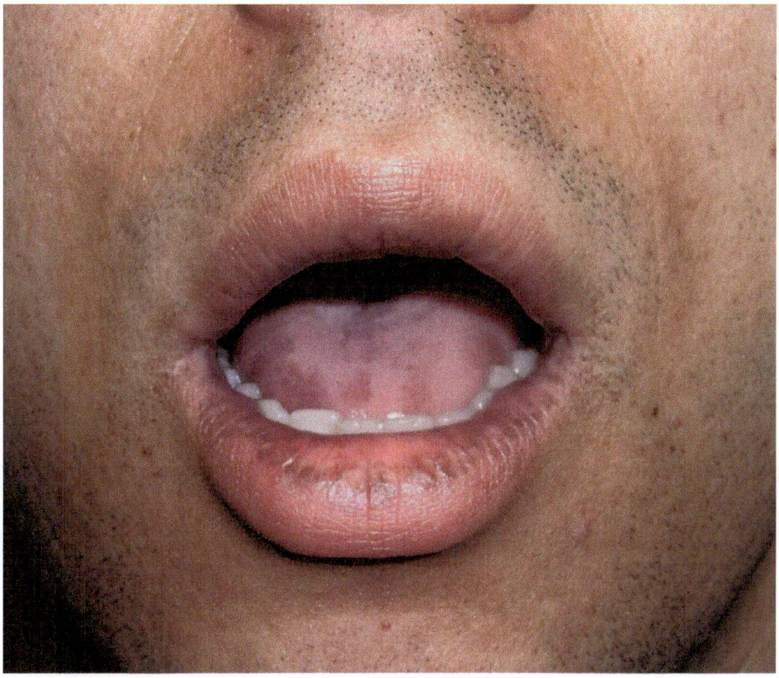

FIGURE 8.2 Primary adrenal insufficiency: Lip pigmentation.

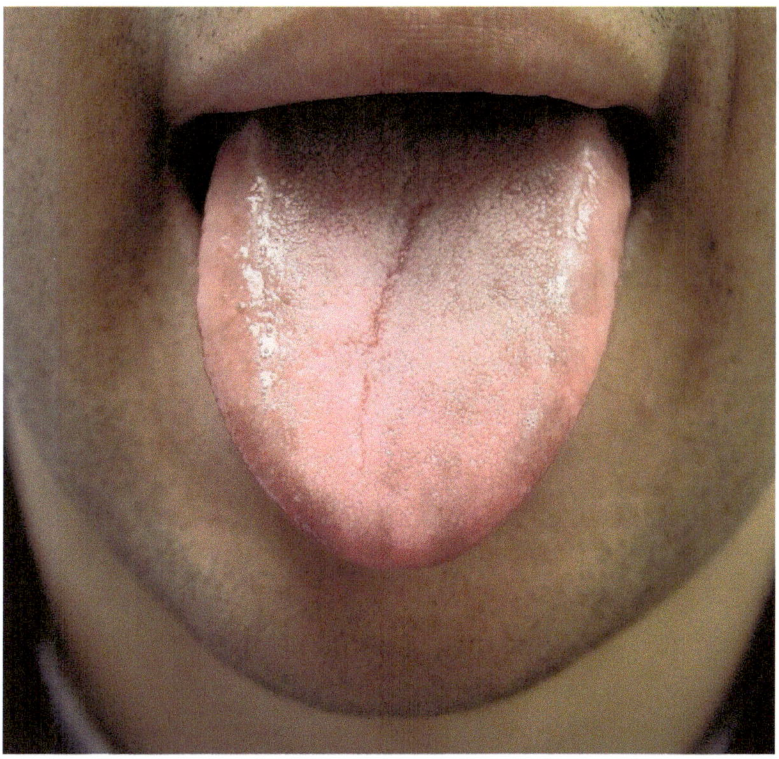

FIGURE 8.3 Primary adrenal insufficiency: Tongue hyperpigmentation.

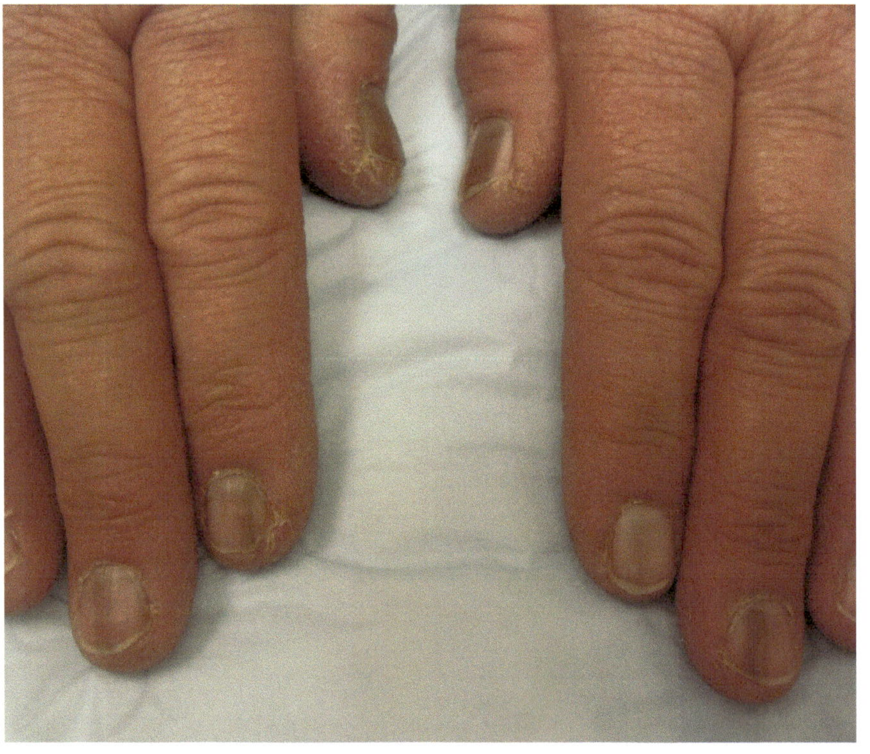

FIGURE 8.4 Primary adrenal insufficiency: Bissell's lines.

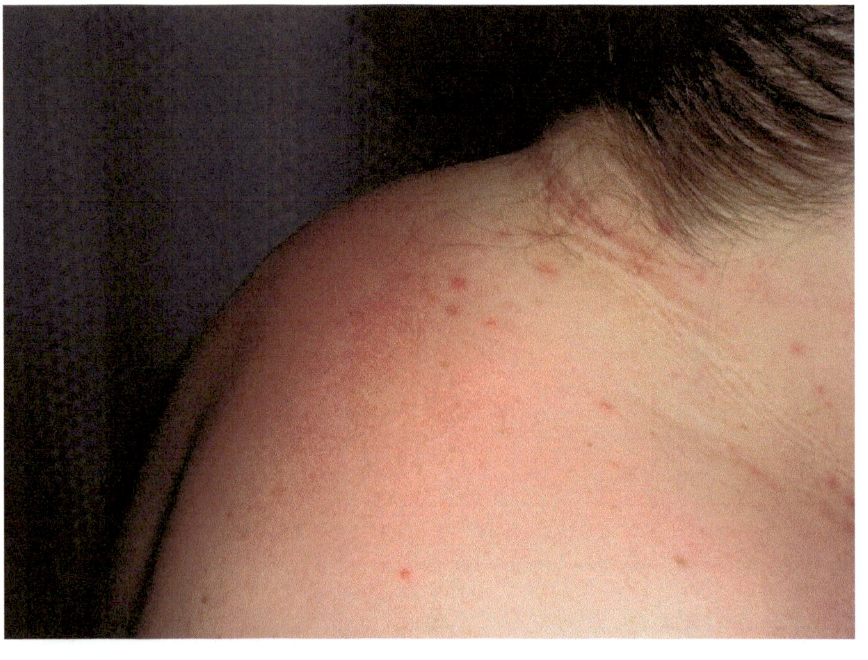

FIGURE 8.5 Cushing syndrome: Dorsal fat pad.

Systemic Manifestations

Patients with PAI can present with hypotension, hypoglycemia, hyponatremia, hyperkalemia, which manifest as fatigue, nausea, vomiting, weight loss, salt cravings, and fever. Autoimmune destruction of the adrenals can occur alone or as a spectrum of autoimmune diseases (polyglandular autoimmune syndromes I and II) that can include alopecia areata, vitiligo, diabetes mellitus, parathyroid/thyroid dysfunction, and mucocutaneous candidiasis. In Cushing syndrome, patients may experience fatigue, depression, menstrual irregularities, myopathy, early osteoporosis, diabetes, hypertension, and recurrent atypical infections (tuberculosis).

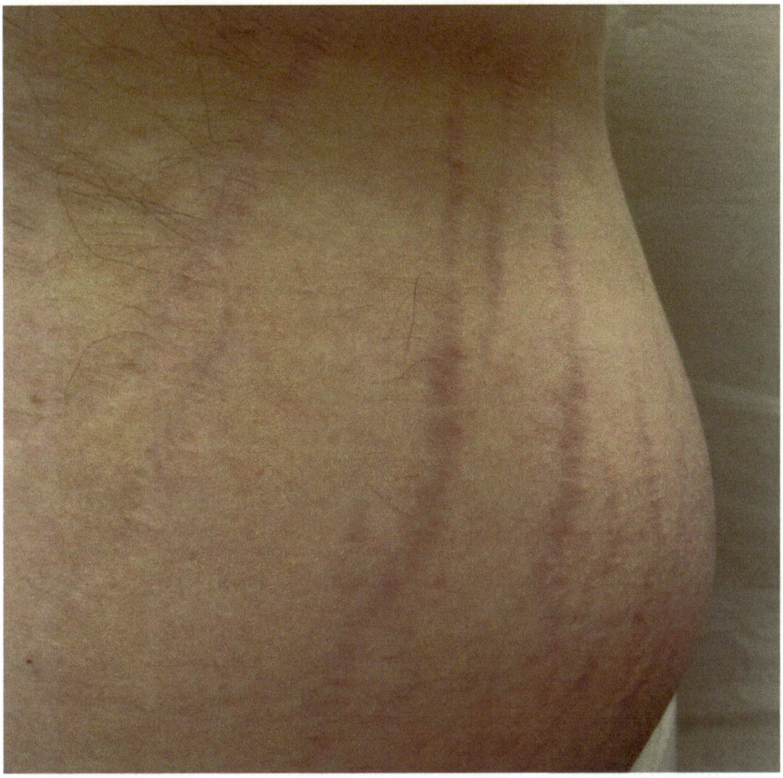

FIGURE 8.6 Cushing syndrome: Striae.

Evaluation and Management

History and physical examination with an inquisitive nature to the salient features of these diseases are essential. Consultation with endocrinology is recommended. PAI can be diagnosed by measuring morning cortisol, serum ACTH, aldosterone, renin, and performing a cosyntropin stimulation test with follow-up imaging of the adrenal glands. Treatment consists of glucocorticoid and mineralocorticoid replacement. Cushing syndrome screening may include a 24-hour urine-free cortisol, late-night salivary cortisol, and a dexamethasone suppression test. If screening tests are positive, plasma ACTH levels are needed. If suppressed, magnetic resonance imaging (MRI) imaging of the adrenals is required. If elevated, focused imaging of the pituitary and torso is recommended. Therapy may include surgery, medications to modulate pituitary ACTH secretion (pasireotide, cabergoline), or inhibit adrenal steroidogenesis (osilodrostat, metyrapone, etomidate, mitotane), or block peripheral glucocorticoid receptors (mifepristone), or combination therapy and discontinuation of exogenous steroids.

TABLE 8.1

Differential Diagnosis of Addisonian Pigmentation

Drugs
- Amiodarone
- Minocycline
- Hydroxychloroquine
- Clofazimine
- Cytotoxic and psychotropic agents

Autoimmunity
- Systemic Lupus erythematosus
- Dermatomyositis
- Systemic sclerosis

Nutritional deficiency
- Vitamin B12
- Folic acid
- Niacin
- Vitamin A

Endocrine disorders
- Thyrotoxicosis
- Cushing syndrome

Other
- Argyria
- Arsenic
- POEMS (polyneuropathy, organomegaly, endocrinopathy, monoclonal gammopathy, and skin changes)
- Cronkite Canada syndrome
- Neoplastic/Paraneoplastic
- Hemochromatosis
- Renal failure

BIBLIOGRAPHY

Charoensri S, Auchus RJ. A contemporary approach to the diagnosis and management of adrenal insufficiency. Endocrinol Meta (Seoul) 2024;39(1):73–82.

Fleseriu M, Varlamov EV, Hinojosa-Amaya JM, et al. An individualized approach to the management of Cushing disease. Nat Rev Endocrinol 2023;19(10):581–599.

Verma D, Sarkar R, Mendiratta V, et al. Addisonian pigmentation – The great mimicker - A review. Indian J Dermatol 2024;69(5):422.

Diabetic Dermopathy

Etiopathogenesis

There are several skin conditions that can be seen in association with diabetes mellitus. Some of these conditions, such as acanthosis nigricans, scleredema, and necrobiosis lipoidica, are addressed in Chapters 1 and 5. Dermatologic entities that are reviewed in this section include neuropathic ulcers, bullous diabeticorum, diabetic dermopathy, and Huntley's papules. A combined sensory and motor neuropathy, common in diabetes mellitus (DM), predisposes patients to the development of neuropathic ulcers. The pathophysiology of bullous diabeticorum, Huntley's papules, and diabetic dermopathy are not well understood.

Clinical Manifestations

Neuropathic ulcers (**Figures 8.7** and **8.8**) occur on weight-bearing areas of the skin and are usually well circumscribed, painless, with surrounding callus formation. Severe diabetic neuropathy accompanies the development of these ulcers. Diabetic dermopathy (**Figure 8.9**) appears as multiple, small, brownish atrophic plaques on the anterior lower legs. Huntley's papules occur on the dorsal aspect of the fingers as hyperkeratotic, cobblestone-like papules (**Figure 8.10**). Diabetic bullae appear as rapidly developing noninflammatory blisters that occur most frequently on the feet or lower extremities (**Figures 8.11** and **8.12**). Lipohypertrophy and lipoatrophy occur because of insulin injection site reactions.

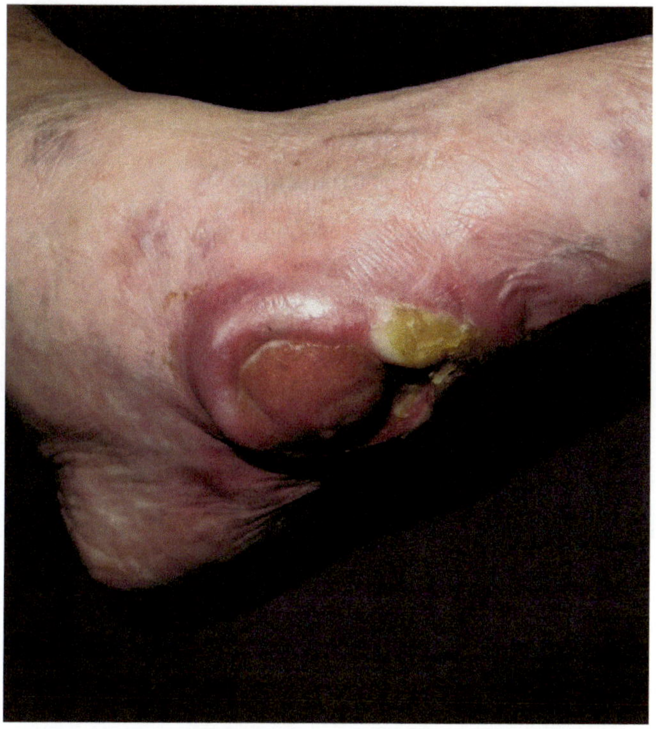

FIGURE 8.7 Diabetes: Neurotrophic ulcer of foot.

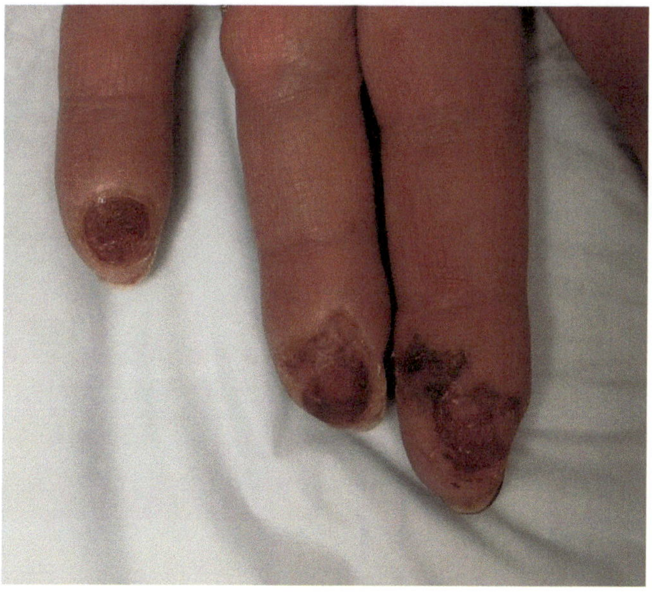

FIGURE 8.8 Diabetes: Neurotrophic ulcers of finger tips.

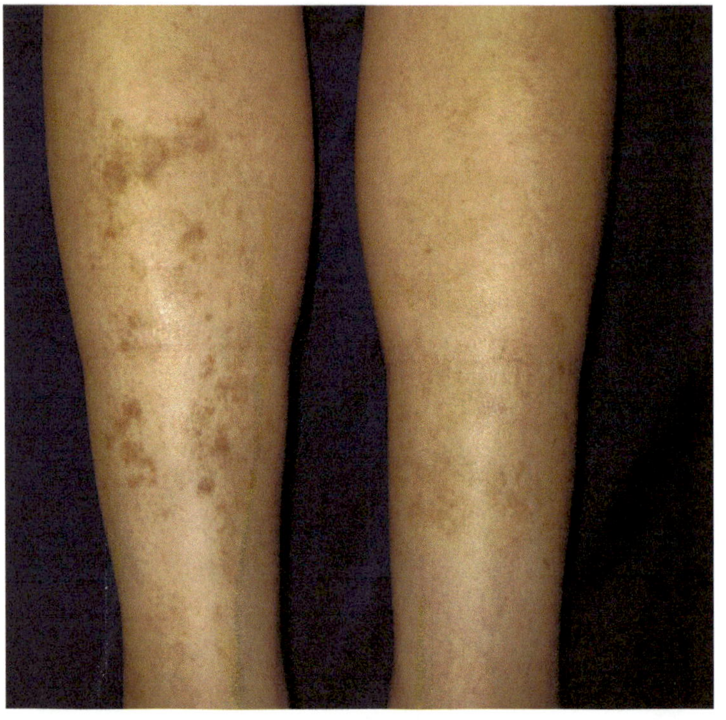

FIGURE 8.9 Diabetes: Diabetic dermopathy.

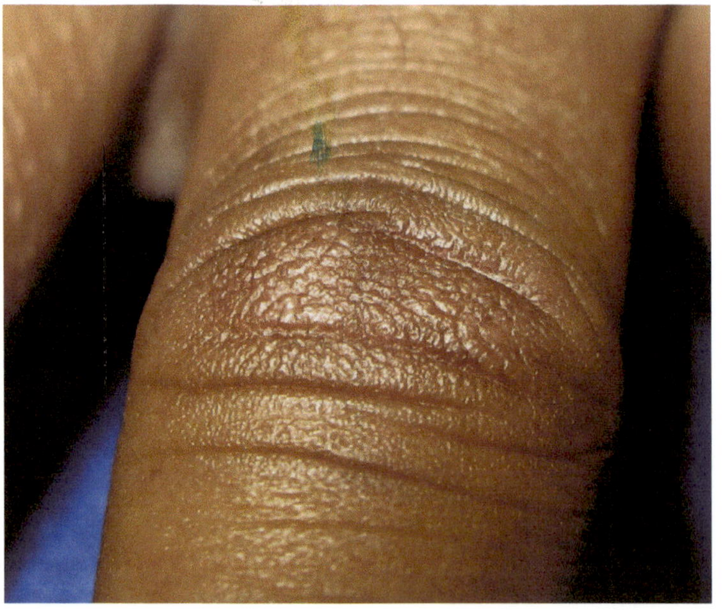

FIGURE 8.10 Diabetes: Huntley's papules.

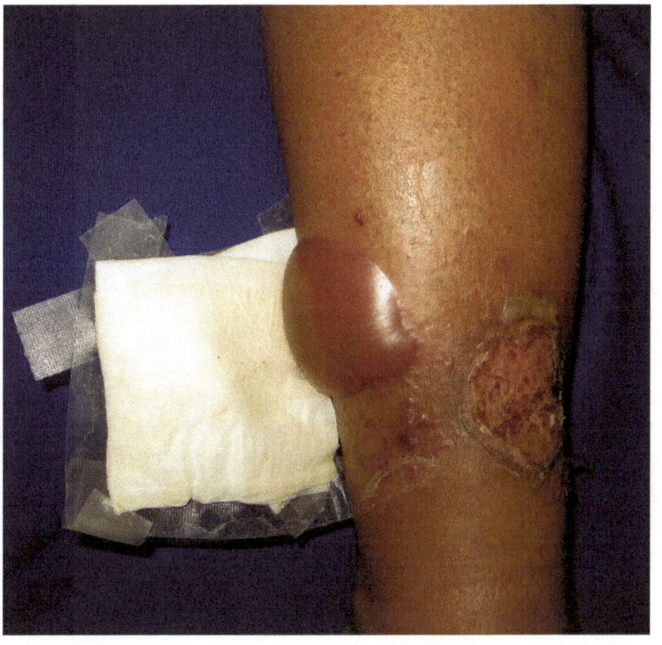

FIGURE 8.11 Diabetes: Diabetic bullae.

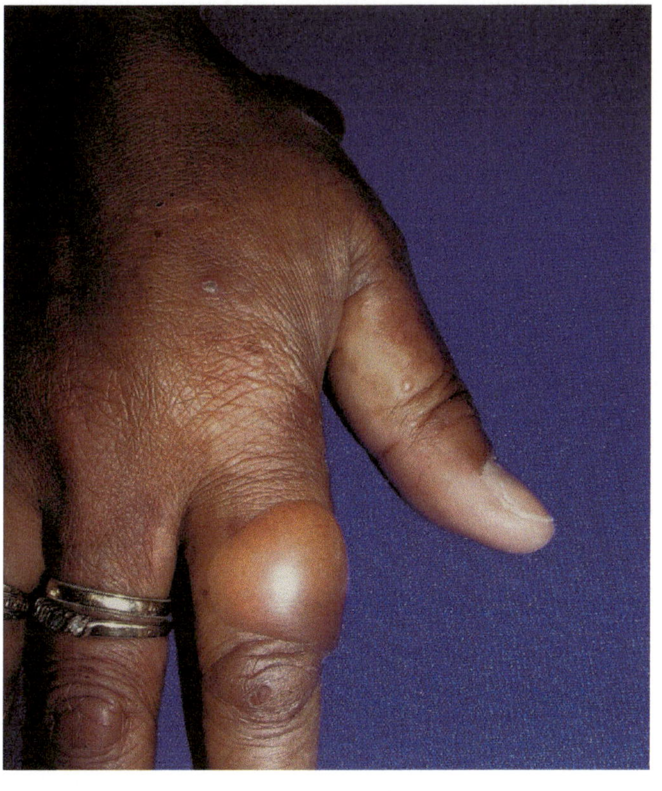

FIGURE 8.12 Diabetes: Diabetic bullae.

Systemic Manifestations

Diabetes, especially if it is poorly controlled, can adversely affect multiple organ systems, including the kidneys, liver, and nervous and circulatory systems. In a patient without a known history of diabetes, symptoms such as polyuria, polydipsia, and polyphagia may be elicited. Cutaneous findings may be the initial finding of diabetes, and can lead to early diagnosis and institution of therapy. Diabetic dermopathy is a sign of associated neuropathy, retinopathy, nephropathy, and cardiovascular disease.

Evaluation and Management

In a patient suspected of having diabetes, diagnosis can be made by having an elevated hemoglobin A1c (HA1c) (>6.5%), an elevated fasting blood glucose (FBG) (>126 mg/dL), or an elevated glucose following an oral glucose tolerance test. Management of diabetes includes both lifestyle changes and medical therapy. In some patients, tight glycemic control can improve the appearance of the skin lesions, whereas in other instances, skin lesions may persist despite effective DM management. For diabetic dermopathy and Huntley's papules, there are no well-established effective therapies. Neuropathic ulcers are managed with surgical debridement, paring of hyperkeratotic tissue, aggressive wound care, application of orthotics that alleviate pressure on focal areas of the sole and educational interventions. Diabetic bullae can be managed conservatively, with aspiration of the blister fluid and topical wound care.

BIBLIOGRAPHY

Alshammari L, O'Halloran P, McSorley O, et al. The effectiveness of foot care educational interventions for people living with diabetes mellitus: An umbrella review. J Tissue Viability 2023;32(3):406–416.

Hines A, Alavi A, Davis MPD. Cutaneous manifestations of diabetes. Med Clin North Am 2021;105(4):681–697.

Petersmann A, Muller-Wieland D, Muller UA, et al. Definition, classification and diagnosis of diabetes mellitus. Exp Clin Endocrinol Diabetes 2019;127(S 01):S1–S7.

Gout

Etiopathogenesis

All patients with gout have elevated levels of serum uric acid at some point in their disease. This can be due to an increased production or decreased excretion of uric acid, or both. Disease manifestations of gout are due to the deposition of monosodium urate crystals in various tissues. Activation of NOD-like receptor protein 3 (NLRP3) inflammasomes by these crystals leads to interleukin (IL)1-β induced inflammation. Gout can manifest as flares of acute gouty arthritis, separated by intercritical periods and tophaceous gout. Tophaceous gout usually occurs in patients who have had gout for several years and whose disease is poorly controlled, although there are reports of tophaceous gout as the initial clinical manifestation of disease.

Clinical Manifestations

Cutaneous tophaceous gout (**Figures 8.13–8.18**) manifests as hard, flesh-colored or yellow-white papulonodules in the skin. Areas that are more commonly affected include the skin overlying joints, such as the elbow and interphalangeal joints. Tophi can also develop on the pinna. Lesions of tophaceous gout are typically asymptomatic, but occasionally skin breakdown can occur in the area of the tophi, leading to perforation, ulceration, inflammation, and possible infection. Deposition of the tophi may rarely appear miliarial (disseminated papules) or as an indurated, painful erythema due to gouty panniculitis in the subcutaneous tissue.

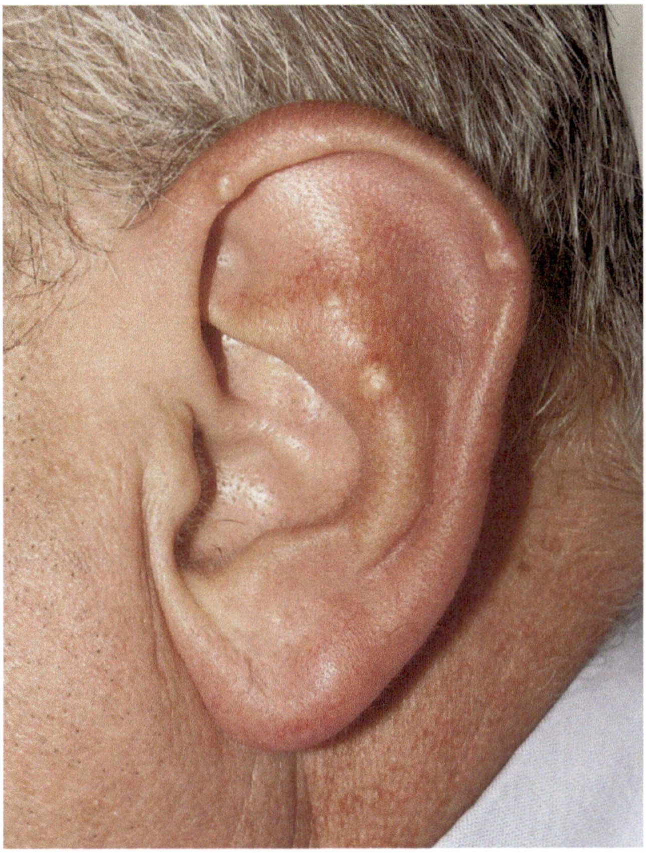

FIGURE 8.13 Tophaceous gout: Helix.

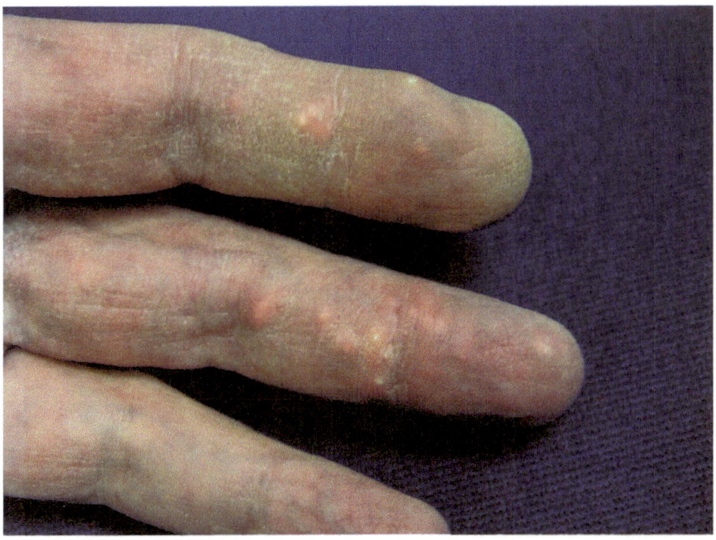

FIGURE 8.14 Tophaceous gout: Miliarial.

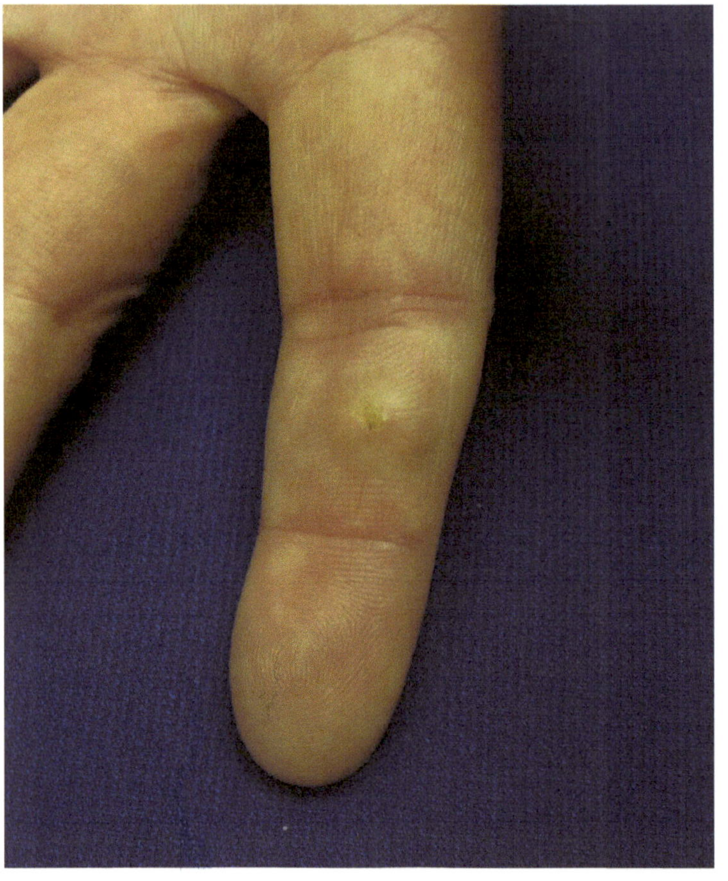

FIGURE 8.15 Tophaceous gout: Perforating.

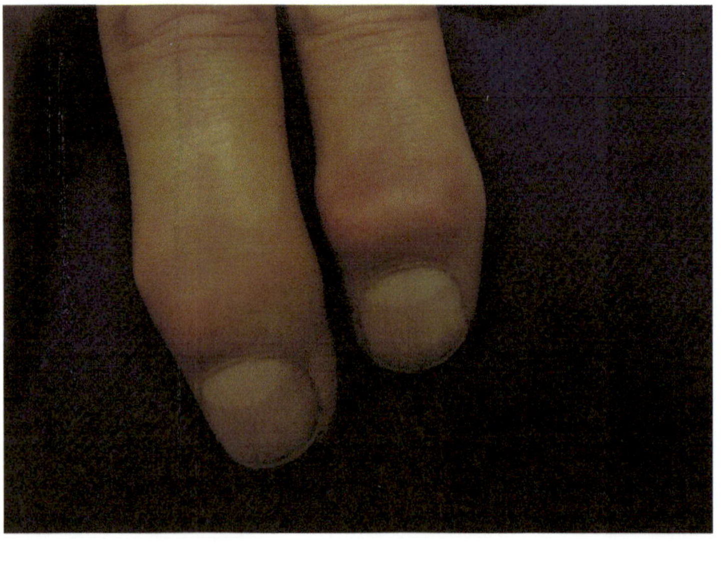

FIGURE 8.16 Tophaceous gout: Mimicking Heberden's nodes of osteoarthritis.

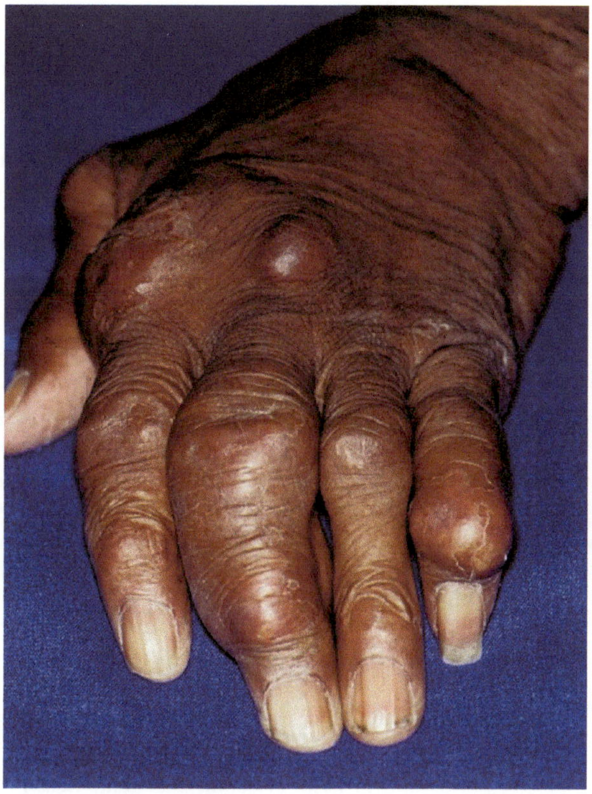

FIGURE 8.17 Tophaceous gout: Disfiguring.

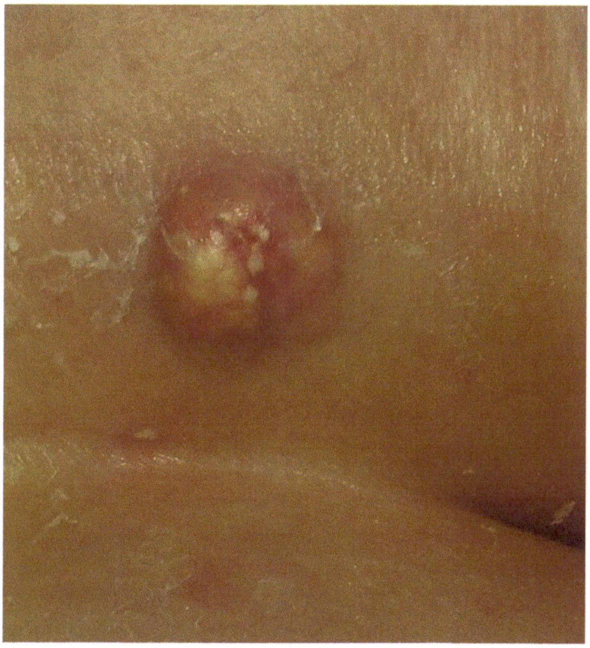

FIGURE 8.18 Tophaceous gout: Nodular.

Systemic Manifestations

Prior to the development of tophaceous gout, most patients will experience one or more episodes of acute gouty arthritis, which occurs as an acutely painful, inflamed joint. Symptoms arise quickly and will resolve over a few days in most cases. Patients with gout have higher rates of ischemic heart disease, diabetes, and hypertension. Increased uric acid in the urine can lead to uric acid nephrolithiasis and chronic kidney disease. In addition to the skin, tophaceous gout can deposit in the tendons, in bursa, and within the synovial tissue.

Evaluation and Management

Tophaceous gout is diagnosed by the demonstration of uric acid crystals in the skin. Histology may demonstrate crystal-like spaces with varying levels of surrounding histiocytic inflammation. Use of a nonaqueous media, such as 100% ethanol, can increase the likelihood that the crystals will survive processing and are strongly birefringent under polarized microscopy. Evaluating serum and urine uric acid levels is also recommended. Management of gout can be achieved by lifestyle modification (weight loss) combined with pharmacotherapy (allopurinol, febuxostat, pegloticase, rasburicase, colchicine, glucocorticoids, nonsteroidal anti-inflammatories (NSAIDs), probenecid, IL-1 inhibitors). If tophaceous gout significantly impairs function, surgical excision can be performed.

BIBLIOGRAPHY

Dalbeth N, Gosling AL, Gaffo A, et al. Gout. Lancet 2021;397(10287):1843–1855.

Danve A, Sehra ST, Neogi T. Role of diet in hyperuricemia and gout. Best Pract Res Clin Rheumatol 2021;35(4):101723.

Punzi L, Galozzi P, Luisetto R, et al. Gout: One year in review 2023. Clin Exp Rheumatol 2024; 42(1):1–9.

Pellagra

Etiopathogenesis

Pellagra is the term given to the clinical manifestations of niacin (vitamin B3) +/- tryptophan deficiency, known by the classic "three *D*s" mnemonic: dermatitis, diarrhea, and dementia. Although epidemics of niacin deficiency have been reported in the past, isolated niacin deficiency is not common and is usually part of a spectrum of overall nutritional deficiencies (see **Table 8.2**) or associated with human immunodeficiency virus (HIV) infection, Sjögren's syndrome, alcoholism, carcinoid syndrome, and malabsorption due to gastrointestinal disease such as Crohn's disease. Medications can also interfere with niacin processing (**Table 8.3**).

Clinical Manifestations

The dermatitis that is seen in pellagra is considered a photodermatosis (photodistributed and symmetric). Patients initially present with edema and erythema of affected areas, with progression to skin thickening, hyperkeratosis (*flaky paint*–like) (**Figure 8.19**), and hyperpigmentation. Affected areas frequently include the dorsum of the hands and feet, face, and anterior upper chest and neck (Casal necklace [**Figure 8.20**]). Genital lesions can also occur as part of the oculo-oro-genital syndrome that can be seen in other vitamin B complex deficiencies. Niacin deficiency can also cause glossitis (**Figure 8.21**).

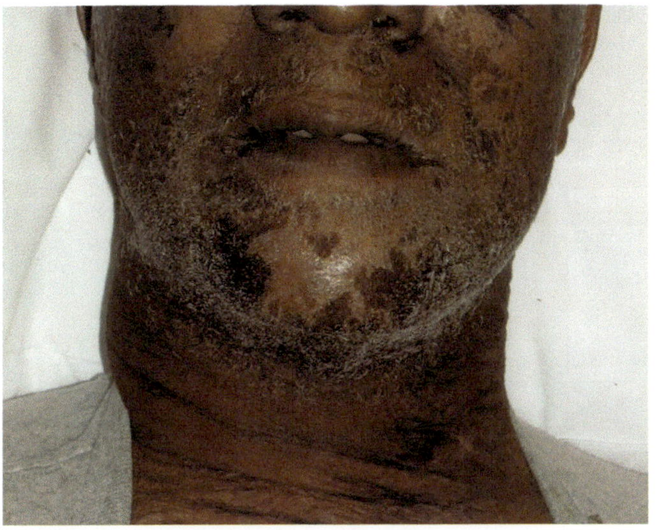

FIGURE 8.19 Pellagra: Flaky paint.

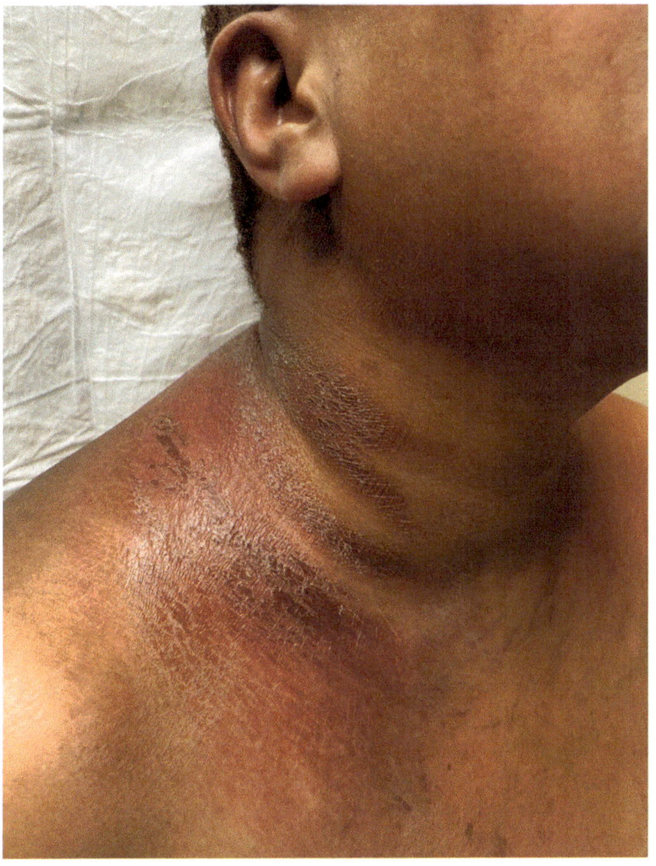

FIGURE 8.20 Pellagra: Casal's collar.

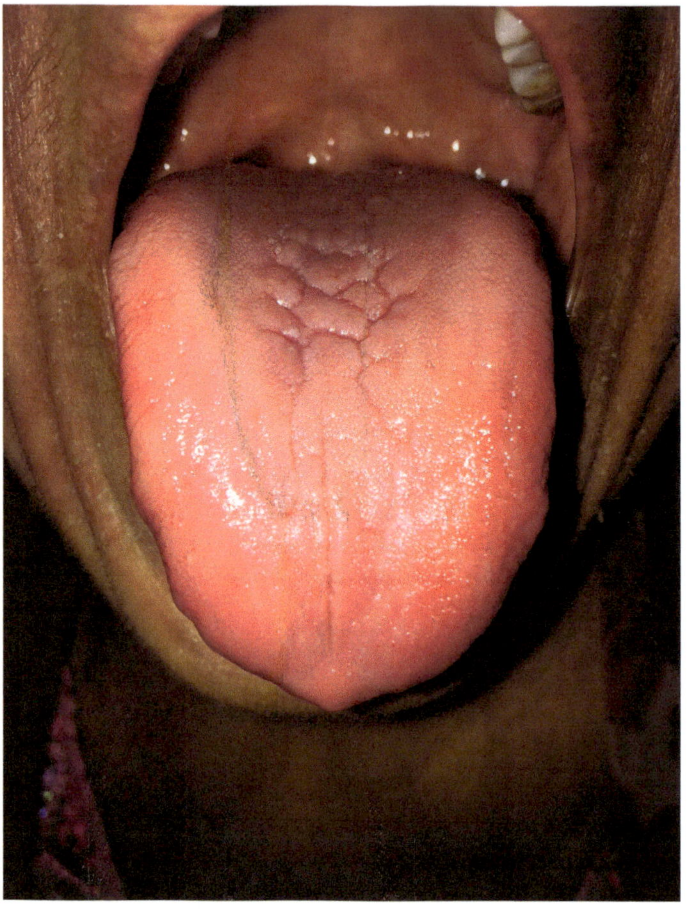

FIGURE 8.21 Pellagra: Glossitis.

Systemic Manifestations

Gastrointestinal manifestations include abdominal pain, nausea, vomiting, and diarrhea. The neurological findings of pellagra include irritability, mental dullness, and disorientation. A sensorimotor neuropathy can be detected in some patients.

Evaluation and Management

Given that isolated niacin deficiency is rare, a full nutritional evaluation should be undertaken in patients with signs and symptoms of pellagra. The diagnosis of pellagra is often made by history and physical examination. Histologic findings of the rash are nonspecific. Hyperkeratosis can be seen in the stratum, with the epidermis displaying necrosis, pallor, and ballooning. Lesions can be inflammatory in the early stages, but no specific pattern of inflammation is diagnostic. Measurement of urinary metabolites may assist in the diagnosis. Treatment is directed at the underlying disorder, if present, as well as supplementation with nicotinamide or increase in consumption of meat, milk, eggs, and plant products such as soybeans, sunflower seeds, sesame seed, or oats. Interestingly, diets that are predominantly corn may lead to pellagra.

TABLE 8.2

List of B Vitamins

Vitamin	Name
B1	Thiamine
B2	Riboflavin
B3	Niacin
B5	Pantothenic acid
B6	Pyridoxine
B7	Biotin
B9	Folate
B12	Cyanocobalamin

TABLE 8.3

Drugs That Cause Niacin Deficiency

Immunosuppressants
- Azathioprine
- 6-mercaptopurine
- 5-flourouracil

Anti-tuberculosis drugs
- Isoniazid
- Pyrazinamide
- Ethionamide

Other
- Anti-convulsants
- Phenobarbital
- Estrogens
- Chloramphenicol

BIBLIOGRAPHY

Holubiec P, Leonczyk M, Staszewski F, et al. Pathophysiology and clinical management of pellagra – A review. Folia Med Cracov 2021;61(3):125–137.

Prabhu D, Dawe RS, Mponda K. Pellagra a review exploring causes and mechanisms, including isoniazid-induced pellagra. Photodermatol Photoimmunol Phoyomed 2021;37(2):99–104.

Yano H, Kingo M. Pruritic rash and diarrhea. JAMA 2021;325(11):1103–1104.

Porphyria Cutanea Tarda

Etiopathogenesis

The term *porphyria* refers to a group of diseases whose manifestations are the result of abnormalities in the enzymes responsible for the synthesis of the heme molecule. Defects in the enzymes, whether through an inherited or acquired defect, lead to increased levels of precursor molecules in the skin. After subsequent activation of these molecules by wavelengths of light in the visible spectrum, damage to the skin can occur. The most common type of porphyria is porphyria cutanea tarda (PCT), which is the only porphyria that can occur as an acquired condition and is due to the inhibition of liver uroporphyrinogen decarboxylase. Due to elevated liver iron content and oxidative stress, the production of iron-generated free oxygen radicals oxidize uroporphyrinogen leading to a uroporphomethene inhibitor of uroporphyringogen decarboxylase.

Clinical Manifestations

Patients with PCT can present with multiple skin findings. Most commonly, patients will present with bullae, erosions, and skin fragility in sun-exposed regions of the skin (**Figure 8.22**). This most commonly occurs on the dorsal hands. Milia, hypertrichosis, and sclerodermoid changes can also occur (**Figures 8.23** and **8.24**).

Systemic Manifestations

PCT occurs most often spontaneously (Type 1) in adulthood or as a familial autosomal dominant condition (Type 2) in childhood. Type 1 acquired disease is associated with liver dysfunction due to alcoholism, chronic hepatitis C and HIV infection, hemochromatosis, estrogen use, tobacco smoking, and exposure to other hepatotoxins. Hepatocellular carcinoma has also been reported in association with PCT. PCT patients have a poor survival rate compared to healthy controls and have an increased risk of premature death due to malignancies, liver disease, and drug and alcohol overdose.

Evaluation and Management

If porphyria is suspected, elevated levels of porphyrins can be detected in urine, serum, or stool. In PCT, total serum porphyrins can be detected while the skin manifestations are present. In patients who have been diagnosed with PCT, the workup should include testing for HIV and hepatitis C, genetic testing for hemochromatosis, and ultrasound (US) or computed tomography (CT) scan can be performed to rule out cirrhosis and hepatocellular carcinoma. Skin biopsy will reveal a cell-poor bullae, and direct immunofluorescence will be negative, distinguishing it from epidermolysis bullosa acquisita (which may present with acral bullae). If serum porphyrins are negative and skin biopsy is consistent with porphyria, a diagnosis of drug-induced pseudoporphyria (**Figure 8.25**, **Table 8.4**) should be considered. In PCT, phlebotomy remains a mainstay of therapy. Low dose antimalarials can be administered in patients who are not phlebotomy candidates. Avoidance of triggering factors is an important part of management in the acute porphyrias, as well as photoprotection.

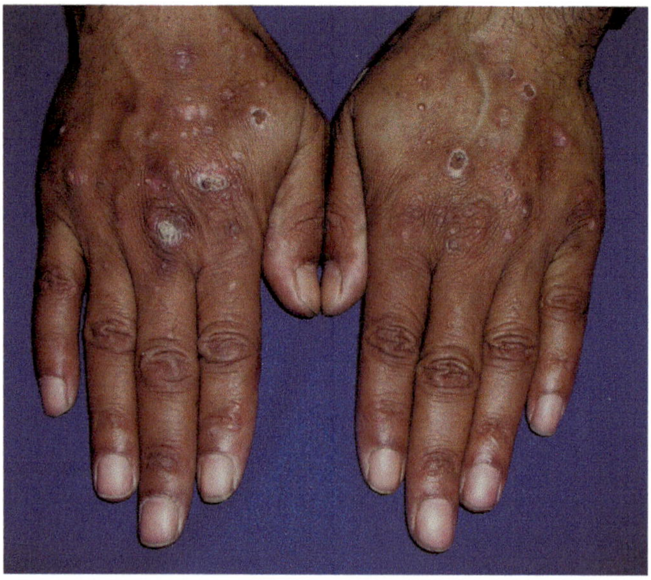

FIGURE 8.22 Porphyria cutanea tarda: Erosions.

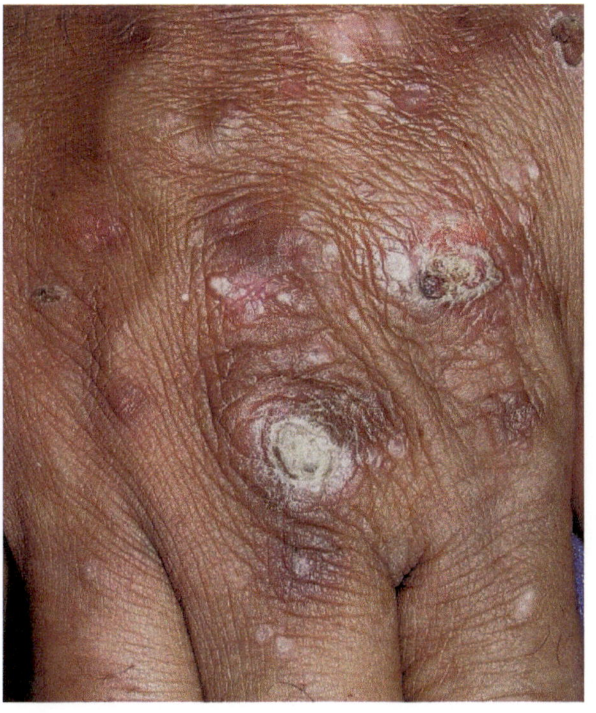

FIGURE 8.23 Porphyria cutanea tarda: Milia.

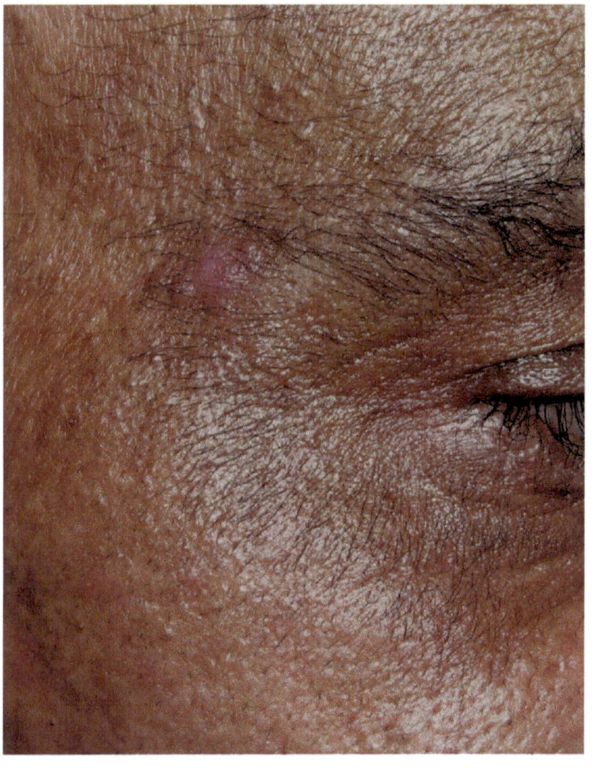

FIGURE 8.24 Porphyria cutanea tarda: Hypertrichosis.

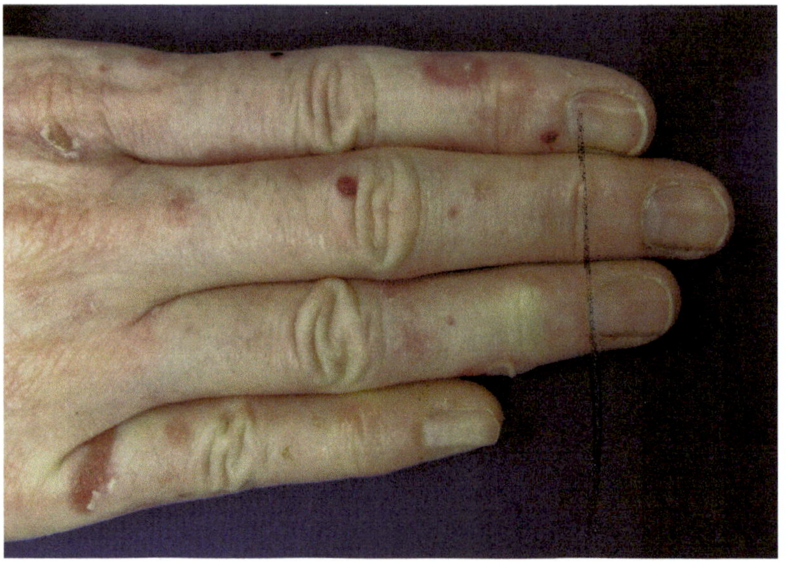

FIGURE 8.25 Pseudoporphyria: Medication-induced.

TABLE 8.4

Drug-Induced Pseudoporphyria

Agent
• Amiodarone
• Etretinate
• Furosemide
• Hydrochlorothiazide/Triamterene
• Isotretinoin
• Imatinib
• Naprosyn
• Nalidixic acid
• Olanzapine
• Tetracycline
• Voriconazole

BIBLIOGRAPHY

Aardsand AK, To-Figueras J, Whatley S, et al. Practical recommendations for biochemical and genetic diagnosis of the porphyrias. Live Int 2024;45(3):e16012.

Di Bartolomeo L, Irrera N, Maurizio Compo G, et al. Drug-induced photosensitivity: Clinical types of phototoxicity and photoallergy and pathogenetic mechanisms. Front Allergy 2022;3:876695.

Leaf RK, Dickey AK. Porphyria cutanea tarda: A unique iron-related disorder. Hematology Am Soc Hematol Educ Program 2024;2024(1):450–456.

Sarkany RPE, Phillips JD. The clinical management of porphyria cutanea tarda: An update. Liver Int 2024;44(9):2191–2196.

Thyroid Disease

Etiopathogenesis

Thyroid hormone has a direct effect on the epidermis, dermis, and adnexa. The hormone function is mediated by cutaneous thyroid hormone receptors with subsequent conversion of the prohormone T4 by cutaneous deiodinases to active T3 and the activation of keratin, hairless, and ZAKI-4 genes. The lack of T3 results in an enhanced cornified envelope, subsequent decreased keratinocyte shedding, abnormal sterol synthesis, increased dermal hyaluronic acid and carotene, as well as decreased hair/nail growth cycles, and eccrine gland secretions. In contrast, elevated T3 results in the opposite effects except in Graves' disease when autoimmune-induced glycosaminoglycans deposition occurs.

Clinical Manifestations

Hypothyroidism classically produces generalized myxedema (pale, cool, boggy skin), palmoplantar keratoderma, vilitigo, and xerotic (**Figure 8.26**) to acquired ichthyotic skin that may easily bruise. Dry, brittle, slow-growing hair producing scalp/eyebrow alopecia and dystrophic nails are a common complaint, while xanthoderma (**Figure 8.27**) and xanthomas are rare. Hyperthyroidism classically causes warm, moist, soft, hyperpigmented, flushed, thin skin with fine, soft hair/nails, alopecia, and eyelid edema. When due to Graves' disease (**Figures 8.28–8.32**), pretibial myxedema (thyroid dermopathy), acropachy (clubbing and periostosis), exophthalmos, onycholysis (Plummer's nails), and koilonychia may develop.

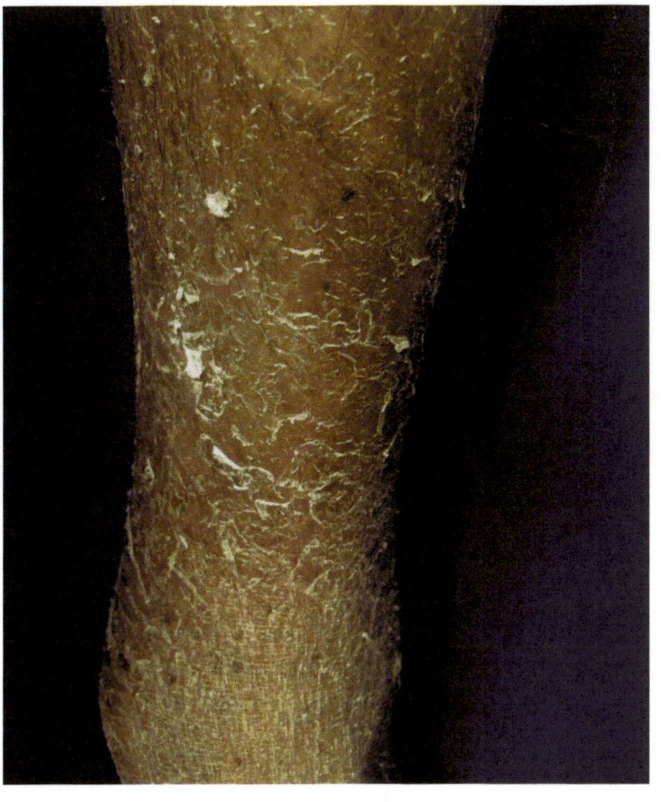

FIGURE 8.26 Hypothyroidism: Xerosis.

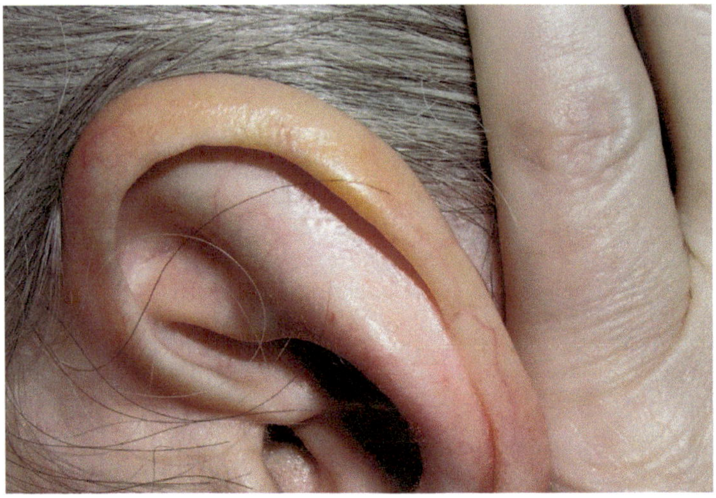

FIGURE 8.27 Hypothyroidism: Xanthoderma and myxedema (finger).

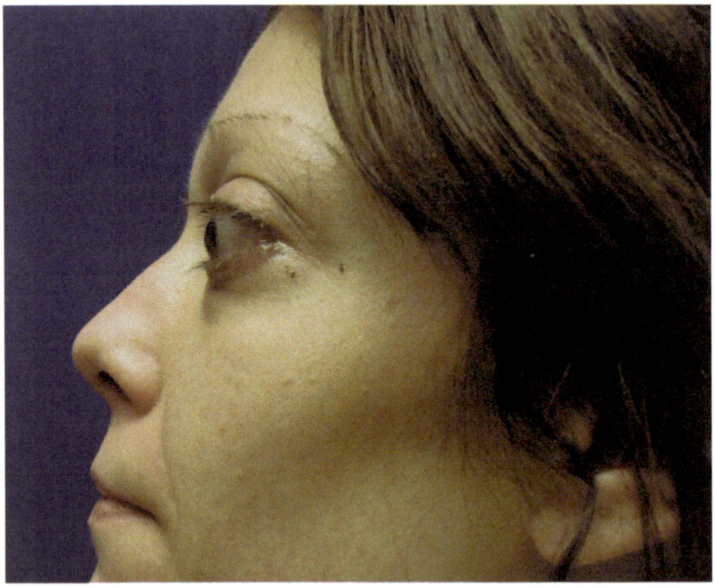

FIGURE 8.28 Hyperthyroidism: Exophthalmos.

Systemic Manifestations

Hypothyroidism patients may develop cold intolerance, fatigue, constipation, weight gain, polyarthritis, mental sluggishness, impotence, and amenorrhea. Profound disease may manifest with arrhythmias (bradycardia) and pleural and cardiac effusions. Hyperthyroidism patients develop heat intolerance, emotional instability, hyperhidrosis, hypertension, tremors, muscle weakness, and arrhythmias (tachycardia to atrial fibrillation). Both disease processes may cause thyromegaly.

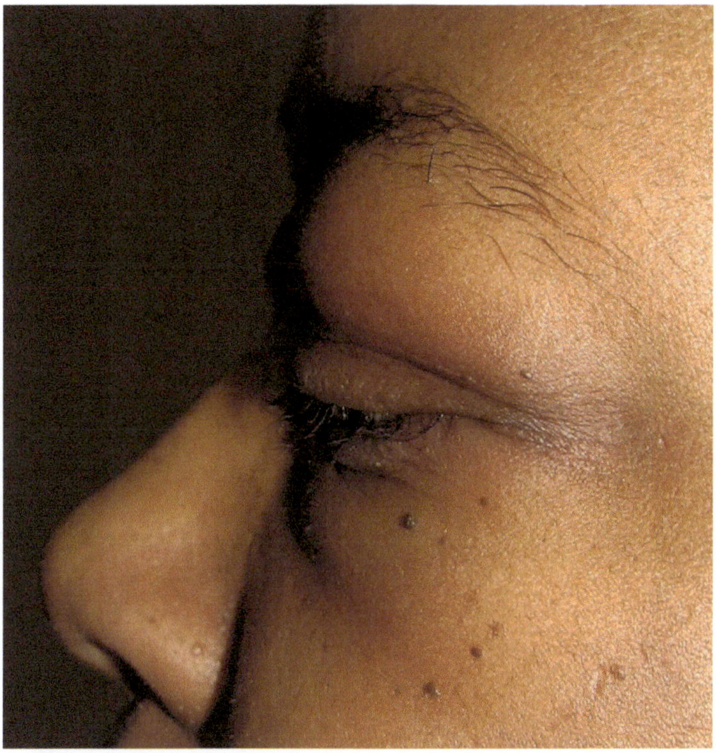

FIGURE 8.29 Hyperthyroidism: Eyelid edema.

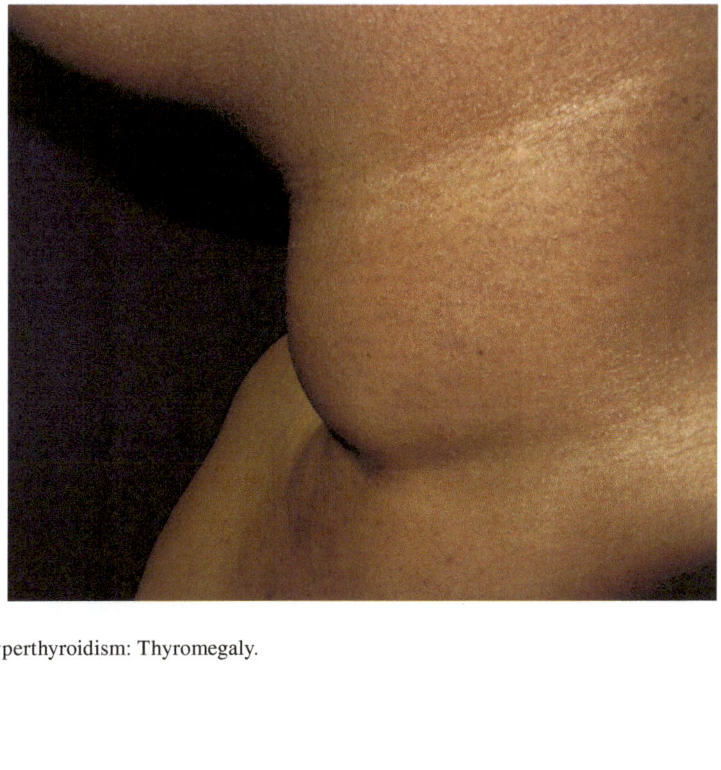

FIGURE 8.30 Hyperthyroidism: Thyromegaly.

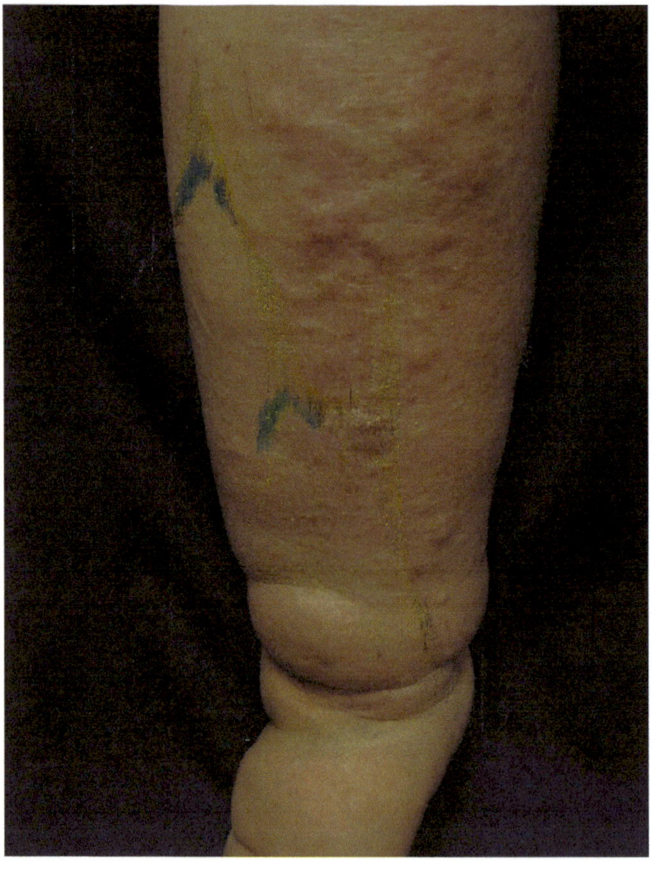

FIGURE 8.31 Hyperthyroidism: Pretibial myxedema.

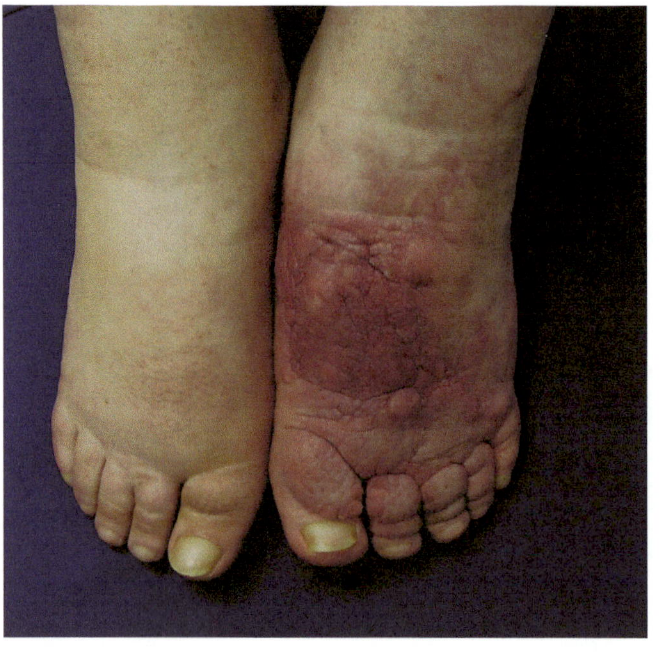

FIGURE 8.32 Hyperthyroidism: Acral myxedema.

Evaluation and Management

Physical examination should include assessment of skin color, texture, and turgor. Palpating the thyroid gland for thyromegaly is prudent. Clinical suspicion can be confirmed by evaluating the hypothalamus, pituitary, and thyroid gland axis. This can be accomplished by laboratory testing for thyroid stimulating hormone (TSH), free T4, anti-thyroglobulin antibodies (TG), anti-thyroid peroxidase antibodies (TPO) for autoimmune-induced hypothyroidism, and anti-thyroid stimulating hormone receptor antibodies for autoimmune-induced hyperthyroidism. Thyromegaly should be evaluated with US to look for changes of thyroiditis, goiter, and nodules by evaluating the gland size, echogenicity, echotexture, margins, and vascularity. Referral to endocrinology is appropriate for management. Treating with replacement thyroxine for hypothyroidism and ablation therapy for hyperthyroidism with subsequent replacement therapy should help resolve most skin manifestations. However, exophthalmos may require surgical decompression, and myxedema may need compression therapy to improve.

BIBLIOGRAPHY

Alexander LF, Patel NJ, Caserta MP, et al. Thyroid ultrasound: Diffuse and nodular disease. Radiol Clin Noth Am 2020;58(6):1041–1057.

Cohen B, Cadesky A, Jaggi S. Dermatologic manifestations of thyroid disease: A literature review. Front Endocrinol (Lausanne) 2023;14:1167890.

Rosenberg A, Lipner SR. Nail changes associated with thyroid disease. Cutis 2022;110(2):E8–E12.

Vargas-Uricoechea H. Molecular mechanisms in autoimmune thyroid disease. Cells 2023;12(6):918.

Zinc Deficiency

Etiopathogenesis

Zinc deficiency can be due to either an inherited or acquired condition. Inherited zinc deficiency occurs as a result of decreased absorption of zinc from the small intestine due to defects in a zinc transporter protein. Acquired zinc deficiency can occur as a result of decreased absorption, which can occur in patients with cystic fibrosis or Crohn's disease. It can also result from decreased dietary intake of zinc, which can occur in patients with anorexia nervosa, alcoholism, HIV, or inadequate parenteral nutrition or consumption of low-nutrient foods.

Clinical Manifestations

Zinc deficiency presents as a psoriasiform or eczematous dermatitis that occurs around the mouth, in the genital region (**Figures 8.33** and **8.34**), and on the hands and feet. This is referred to as an acrodermatitis enteropathica-like eruption. With continued disease, generalized skin involvement can occur with subsequent erosive to bullous lesions, hair changes (brittleness and alopecia), and nail dystrophy (Beau's lines and paronychia). Differentiating clinical features of this from necrolytic migratory erythema, a pancreatic α-cell glucagon-secreting tumor, is often difficult in generalized eruptions. Necrolytic acral erythema presents as a limited acral psoriasiform dermatitis in the setting of zinc deficiency, hepatitis C infection, or both simultaneously (**Figures 8.35–8.37**). Zinc deficiency can be seen coexisting with protein, niacin, thiamine, and biotin deficiencies.

Systemic Manifestations

Pulmonary symptoms of shortness of breath, cough, and recurrent pneumonia suggest cystic fibrosis. Prior history of gastrointestinal pain, bleeding, and diarrhea favors associated inflammatory bowel disease. Diarrhea is the most common extracutaneous finding associated with zinc deficiency. Patients may experience photophobia and anorexia. Weight loss and development of diabetes are more suggestive of necrolytic migratory erythema. In general, patients with multiple nutrient deficiencies are at a high risk for mortality.

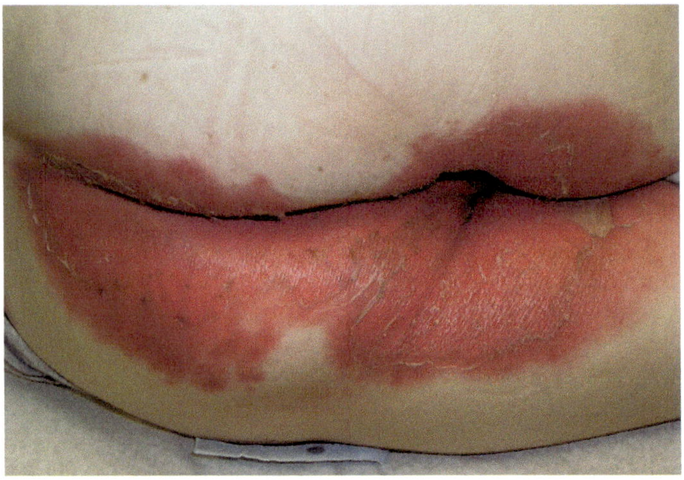

FIGURE 8.33 Zinc deficiency: Alcoholism.

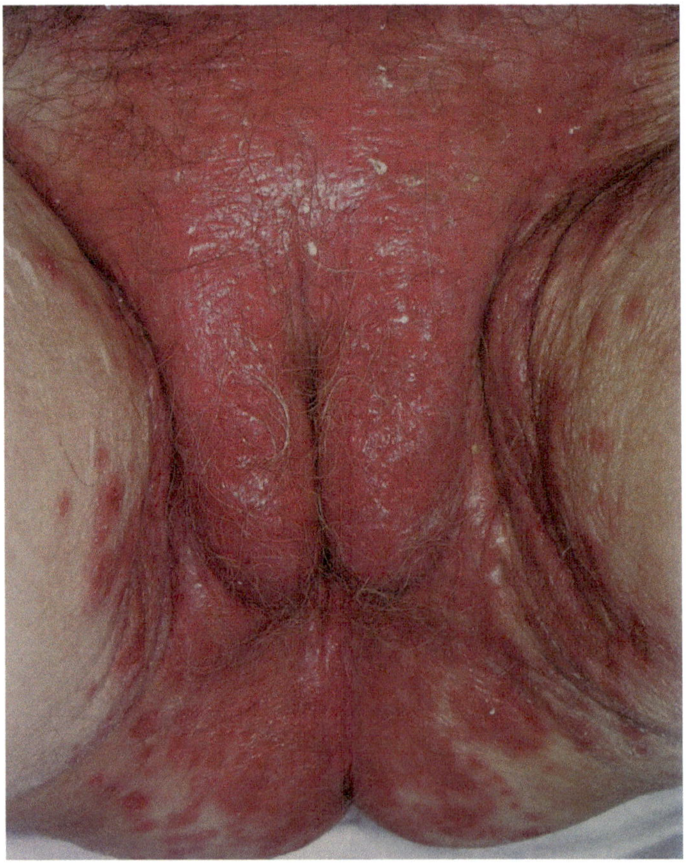

FIGURE 8.34 Zinc deficiency: Crohn's disease.

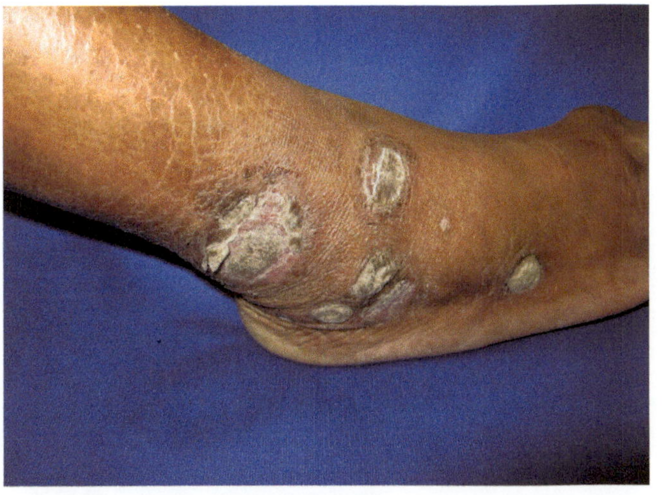

FIGURE 8.35 Necrolytic acral erythema: Zinc deficiency.

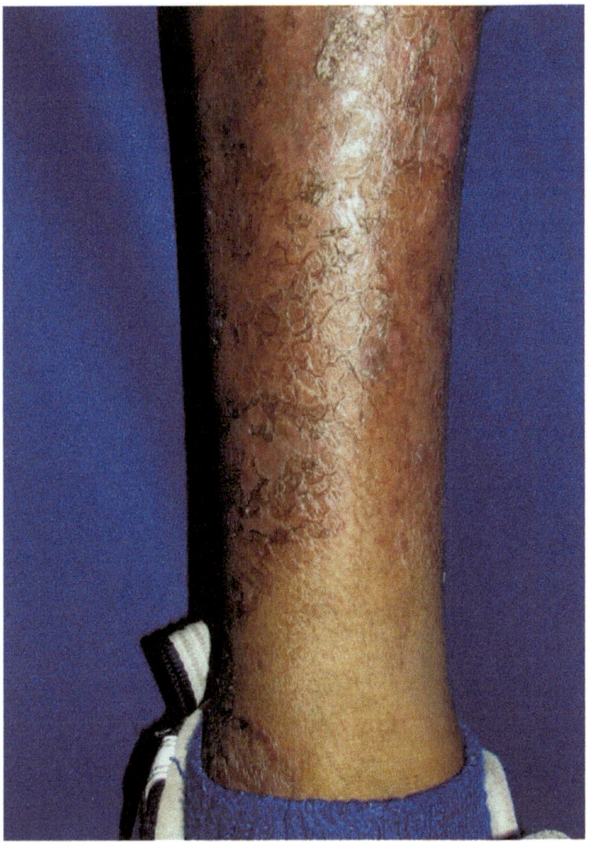

FIGURE 8.36 Necrolytic acral erythema: Hepatitis C and zinc deficiency.

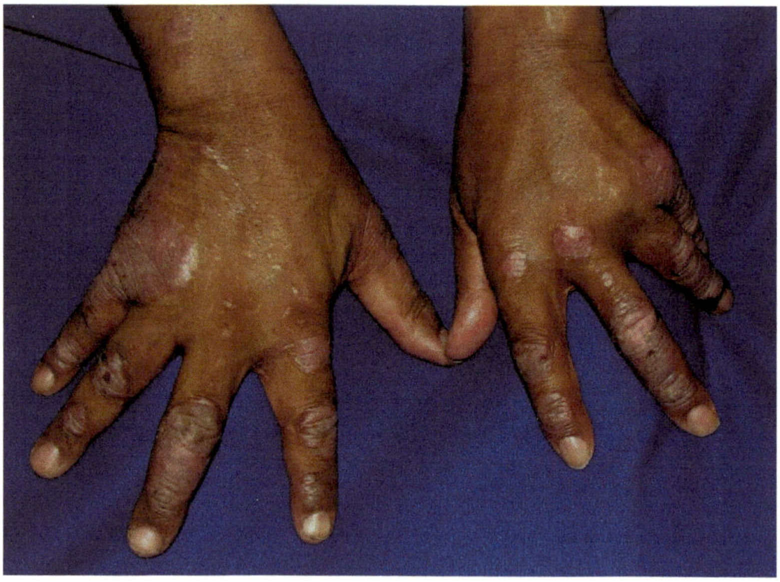

FIGURE 8.37 Necrolytic acral erythema: Hepatitis C and zinc deficiency.

Evaluation and Management

Plasma zinc values should be obtained in any patient suspected of having a zinc deficiency, with the understanding that in some cases, the plasma level may not reflect the true body stores of zinc. Plasma levels of alkaline phosphatase may be low because it is a zinc-dependent enzyme. Skin biopsy specimens demonstrate findings that can be present in any nutritional deficiency (keratinocyte pallor, ballooning degeneration of keratinocytes, and keratinocyte necrosis). Obtaining a glucagon level will differentiate necrolytic migratory erythema. If lesions are acral, evaluating Hep C is prudent. If positive, hepatitis C polymerase chain reaction (PCR) viral load is needed to determine if infection is active. Treatment involves zinc supplementation, which can vary from 1 to 3 mg/kg/day, depending on the nature and severity of the deficiency. Monitoring zinc levels every 3–6 months is recommended. Consider referral to gastroenterology as indicated.

BIBLIOGRAPHY

Al-Khafaji Z, Brito S, Bin B. Zinc and zinc transporters in dermatology. Int J Mol Sci 2022;23(24):16165.

Lee JJ, Mater S, Morilllo-Hernandez C, et al. Clinical outcomes of hospitalized adult patients with dermatologic manifestations of protein malnutrition and zinc deficiency. JAMA Dermatol 2019;155(8):975–977.

Ogawa Y, Kinoshita M, Shimada S, et al. Zinc and skin disorders. Nutrients 2018;10(2):199.

9

Neutrophilic and Eosinophilic Disorders

Bowel-Associated Dermatoses–Arthritis Syndrome

Etiopathogenesis

Bowel-associated dermatoses–arthritis syndrome (BADAS) is a disease affecting the skin and joints, which can occur in up to 20% of patients who have had a bowel bypass procedure performed. There have also been cases reported in patients with other gastrointestinal (GI) pathology, such as inflammatory bowel disease (ulcerative colitis, Crohn's disease) or diverticulitis. The skin and joint symptoms are believed to be the result of immune complexes that are formed in the gut as a consequence of a T-cell and B-cell immune complex response to gut bacterial pathogen-associated molecular patterns with interleukin-1 (IL-1) and IL-10.

Clinical Manifestations

A prodrome of flu-like symptoms (fever, chills, malaise) precedes the development of the skin lesions by 12–36 hours. The morphology of the skin lesions seems to progress with time from an erythematous macule to a pustule, pseudovesicle, or nodule over the course of 1–2 days (**Figures 9.1–9.4**). Lesions are typically less than a few centimeters in diameter, are located on the trunk and extremities, and can be asymptomatic, pruritic, or painful. The lesions are similar to those of Sweet syndrome and, in some cases, early pyoderma gangrenosum or neutrophilic dermatosis of the dorsal hands. The arthritis in BADAS typically affects the small peripheral joints of the extremities, occurs symmetrically, and is not associated with any significant radiologic abnormality.

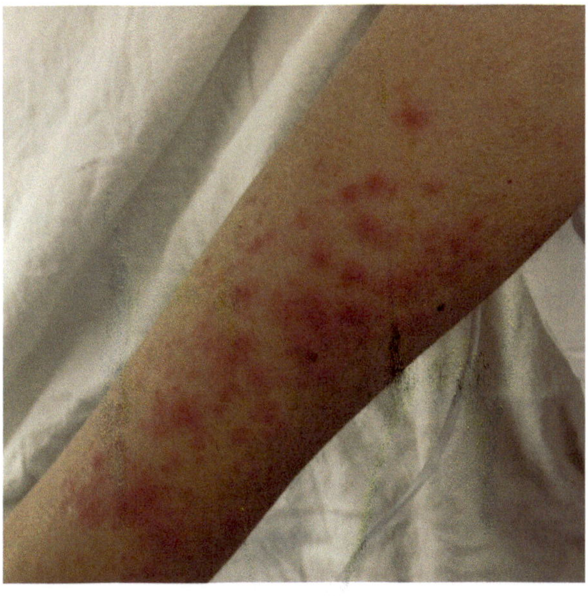

FIGURE 9.1 Bowel-associated dermatoses–arthritis syndrome: Crohn's disease.

DOI: 10.1201/9781003492665-9

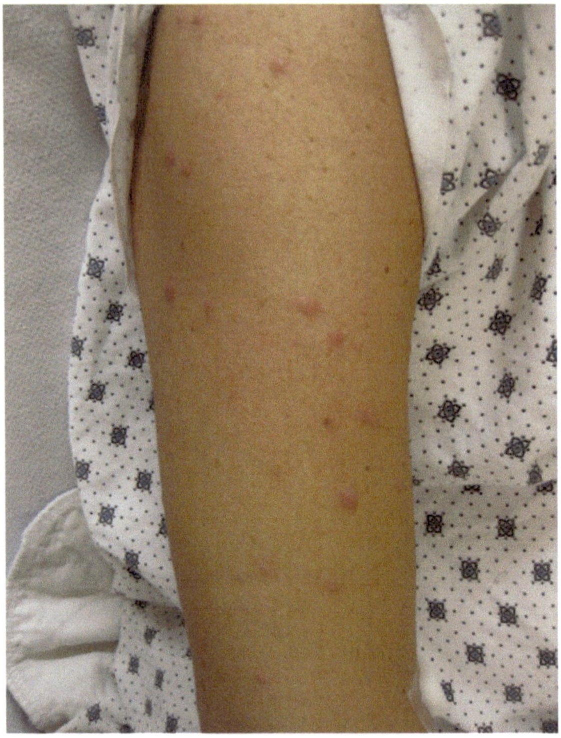

FIGURE 9.2 Bowel-associated dermatoses–arthritis syndrome: Crohn's disease.

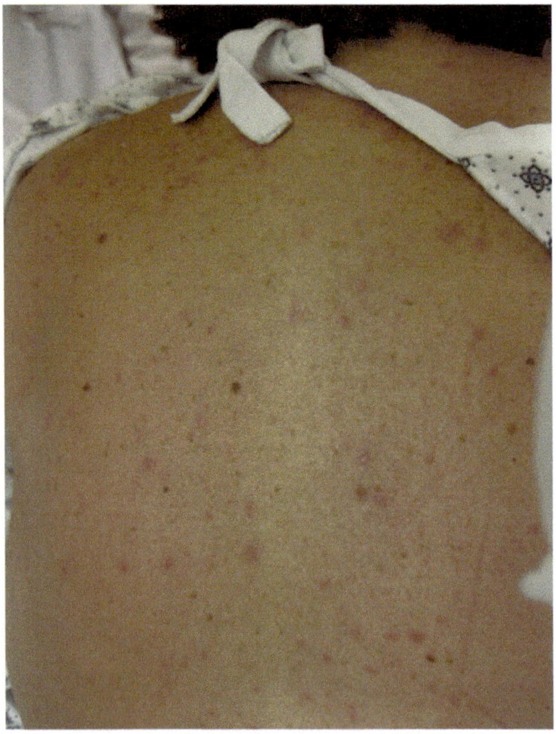

FIGURE 9.3 Bowel-associated dermatoses–arthritis syndrome: Crohn's disease.

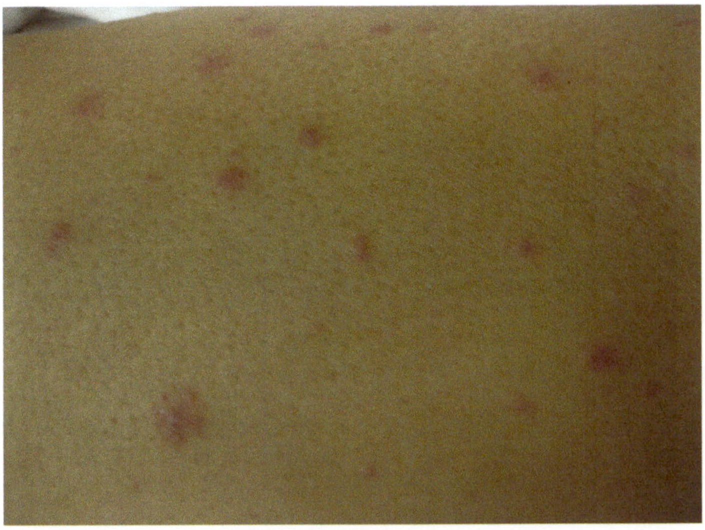

FIGURE 9.4 Bowel-associated dermatoses–arthritis syndrome: Crohn's disease.

Systemic Manifestations

BADAS falls under the spectrum of neutrophilic dermatoses, and the systemic diseases associated with BADAS in patients who have not had a bowel bypass procedure are similar to those reported with the other neutrophilic dermatoses, including inflammatory bowel disease or diverticulitis. The disease may have a relapsing-remitting course in 50% of cases.

Evaluation and Management

The diagnosis of BADAS is made clinically. The histopathology of the skin lesions is most commonly described as similar to Sweet syndrome—an abundant dermal infiltrate of neutrophils with dermal edema and no evidence of vasculitis, although reports of histology demonstrating vasculitis or subcorneal pustulosis exist. Reversal of the blind loop or treatment of the underlying GI disease is curative in many instances. In patients who cannot undergo surgical reversal, systemic corticosteroids are consistently effective. Systemic antibiotics (metronidazole and tetracyclines) and nonsteroidal immunosuppressive agents (mycophenolate mofetil, azathioprine, cyclosporine, infliximab, ustekinumab, and ruxolitinib) have been used.

BIBLIOGRAPHY

Armolo IF, Simeoli D, Maronese CA, et al. The bowel-associated arthritis-dermatosis syndrome (BADAS): A systematic review. Metabolites 2023;13(7):790.

Czjjkowski R, Lipska P, Watola W, et al. Bowel-associated dermatosis-arthritis: A narrative review. Postepy Dermatol Alergol 2023;40(3):355–361.

Flor D, Goncalves A, Morgado F, et al. Bowel-associated dermatosis-arthritis syndrome: A report of a rare case. Cureus 2024;16(10):e71217.

Hypereosinophilic Syndrome

Etiopathogenesis

Hypereosinophilic syndrome (HES) is defined by the presence of an absolute eosinophil count greater than 1500/mm^3 in two examinations at least a month apart, and evidence of end-organ dysfunction attributed to eosinophilia. A Fip1-like 1/platelet-derived growth factor receptor-α (FIP1L1-PDGFRA) mutant fusion gene was detected in a subset of patients with hypereosinophilia, and patients with this and other mutant genes are diagnosed with myeloid HES. Lymphocytic HES refers to patients in which a clonal T-cell population is present, which produces eosinophilia through the release of cytokines such as IL-5. Other subtypes include associated HES, overlap HES, familial HES, and idiopathic HES.

Clinical Manifestations

More than half of patients with HES present with skin findings. Unfortunately, cutaneous lesions of HES are nonspecific (pruritic urticarial papules, plaques, or nodules [**Figures 9.5–9.7**]). Widespread induration of the skin with erythroderma can occur rarely. Erosive and ulcerative mucosal lesions can occur in severe cases and portend a poorer prognosis.

Systemic Manifestations

Multiple organ systems can be targeted by eosinophilia. Patients with cardiac involvement can present with the signs and symptoms of restrictive cardiomyopathy. Other organ systems that can be affected include the lung, GI, central nervous system (CNS), and kidney. In patients with the myeloproliferative subtype of HES, fever, weight loss, and night sweats can be present.

Evaluation and Management

The first step in determining if a patient has HES is to rule out secondary causes of eosinophilia (**Table 9.1**). Once secondary causes of hypereosinophilia have been excluded, consultation with hematology-oncology for bone marrow biopsy, gene studies (FIP1L1:PDGFRA, Breakpoint Cluster Region-Abelson [BCR:ABL1], and translocation/mutations involving platelet-derived growth factor receptor-β [PDGFRB], Janus kinase 2 (JAK2), fibroblast growth factor receptor 1 [FGFR1], KIT), flow cytometry, and T-cell receptor (TCR) studies to determine T-cell clonality should be performed to determine if the patient satisfies the criteria for either myeloproliferative HES or lymphoproliferative HES. Other tests may include CBC, comprehensive metabolic panel (CMP), serum immunoglobulin E (IgE) and IgM, tryptase, Vit B12, echocardiogram, pulmonary function tests, pan computed tomography (pan CT) scan, or positron emission tomography scan with computed tomography (PET-CT) scan. The therapeutic algorithm that should be used depends on the disease subtype, with imatinib mesylate used as a first-line therapy for patients with the FIP1L1-PDGFRA mutation. Systemic corticosteroids can be used in patients with lymphocytic HES. Other therapies reported as effective in either form of HES or in patients with idiopathic HES include hydroxyurea, interferon, dapsone, and immunosuppressive agents. Mepolizumab, an anti-IL5 antibody, is the only biologic approved for use at present. A bone marrow transplant can be performed in severe, refractory cases.

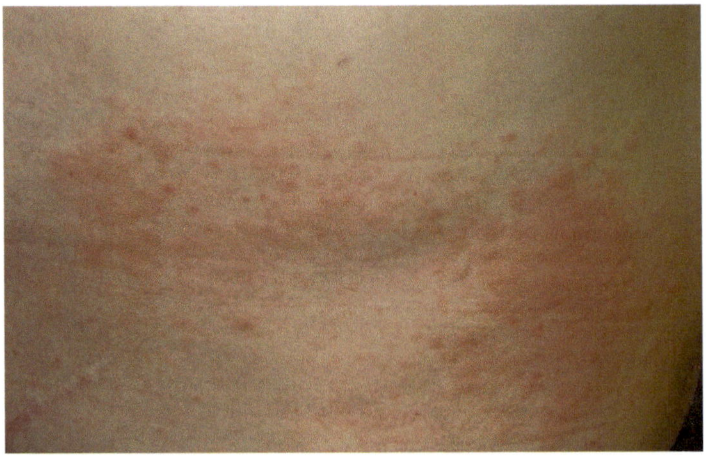

FIGURE 9.5 Hypereosinophilic syndrome: Nonspecific urticarial lesions.

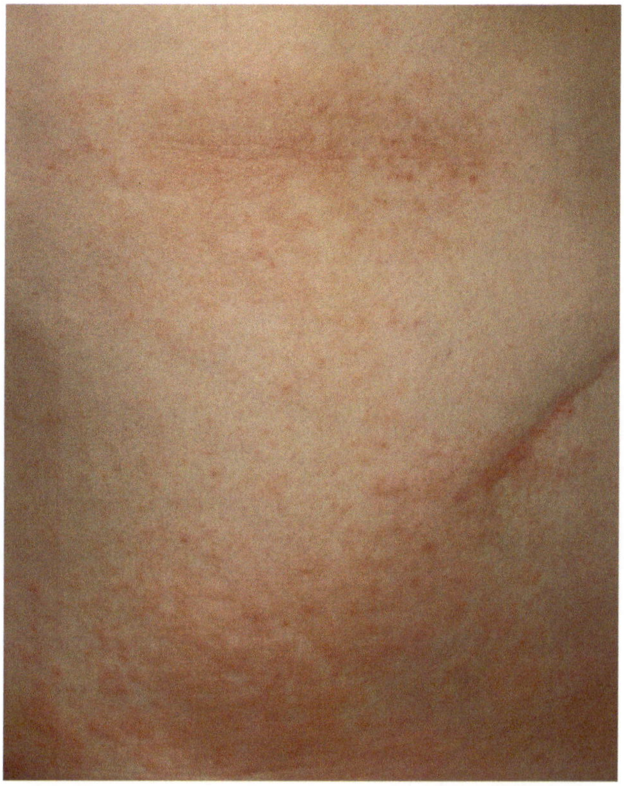

FIGURE 9.6 Hypereosinophilic syndrome.

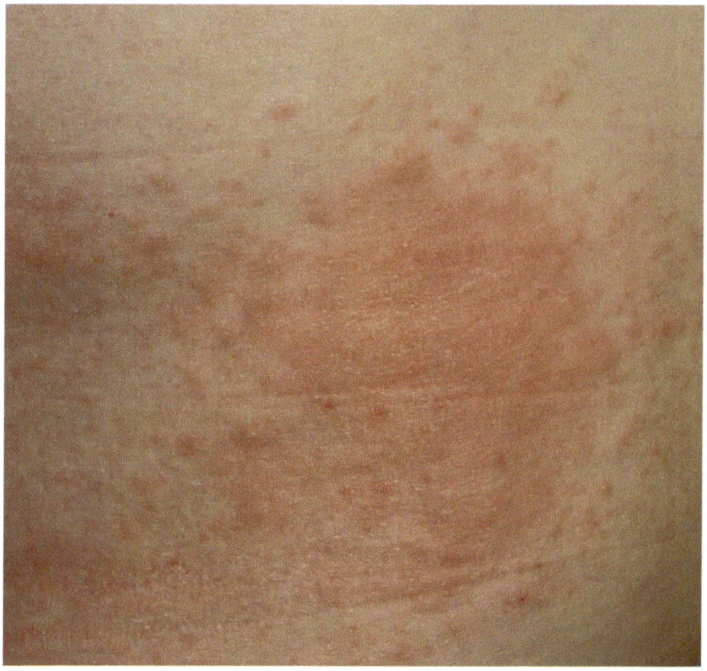

FIGURE 9.7 Hypereosinophilic syndrome.

TABLE 9.1

Causes of Hypereosinophilia

Atopy
• Atopic Dermatitis
• Asthma
• Chronic sinusitis
Drug hypersensitivity
• Drug reaction with eosinophilia and systemic symptoms
Infection/Infestation
• Fungal
• Viral
• Helminth
• Protozoal
• Ectoparasite
Autoimmune disease
• IgG4 disease
• Sarcoidosis
• Inflammatory bowel disease
• Eosinophilic fasciitis
• Eosinophilic granulomatous polyangiitis
Malignancy
• Leukemia/Lymphoma
• Solid Adenocarcinoma
Hypereosinophilic D/O
• Myeloid
• Lymphocytic
• Overlap
• Associated
• Familial
• Idiopathic

BIBLIOGRAPHY

Ezekwe E, Weskamp AL, Pittman LM, et al. Biologics in hypereosinophilic syndrome and eosinophilic granulomatous with angiitis. Immuno Allergy Clin North Am 2021;44(4):629–644.

Klion AD. Approach to the patient with suspected hypereosinophilic syndrome. Hematology Am Soc Hematol Educ Program 2022;2022(1):47–54.

Requena G, van den Bosch J, Akuthota P, et al. Clinical profile and treatment in hypereosinophilic syndrome variants: A pragmatic review. J Allergy Clin Immunol Pract 2022;10(8):2125–2134.

Pyoderma Gangrenosum

Etiopathogenesis

Pyoderma gangrenosum (PG) is a rare neutrophilic dermatosis that can be associated with a number of systemic diseases. The pathogenesis of the disease is unclear, but may involve an abnormal immune response from Th17 T cells and release of proneutrophilic cytokines (CXCL1, 2, 8, 16, and tumor necrosis factor alpha (TNF-α), IL-1, IL -12, IL- 15, IL-17 IL-23, IL-36) with subsequent disordered neutrophil chemotaxis. PG is commonly classified into five types): ulcerative (**Figures 9.8–9.10**), vegetative, pustular, bullous, and peristomal (**Figure 9.11**). Rarer types of PG include a superficial granulomatous form as well as post-surgical procedure PG (**Figure 9.12**) medication-induced PG (filgrastim) (**Figure 9.13**), and syndromic [genetic] PG.

Clinical Manifestations

The classic clinical presentation of PG is that of an initial pustule that rapidly grows into a painful ulceration with violaceous, undermined borders. Lesions occur on the lower extremities most commonly but any anatomic site can be affected. Crater-like openings and cribriform scarring are more specific findings in PG ulcers, but are often not present. Pathergy has been described in PG, with lesions occurring at sites of trauma, such as surgical scars or venipunctures, but this is unfortunately not a specific finding.

Systemic Manifestations

PG is associated with systemic diseases in about 50%–60% of cases. Inflammatory bowel disease is the most common disease reported in association with PG, but PG associated with inflammatory arthropathies, hematologic malignancies, and other autoimmunity disorders have also been described. In addition to skin lesions, patients with PG may rarely have neutrophilic infiltrates in other organs, such as the lungs, liver, bone, and muscle.

Evaluation and Management

Many conditions can present with cutaneous ulceration, and it is important to rule out these other entities when making a diagnosis of PG. Although pathergy can occur, a biopsy of a pustule or the edge of a lesion is important to rule out other causes of ulceration, including vasculitis, vascular occlusion, leukemia cutis, and infection. Tissue culture for bacteria, fungal, and mycobacterium should also be performed in all patients. Histology will demonstrate a dense neutrophilic infiltrate without evidence of vasculitis. Workup of the patient for inflammatory arthropathies, inflammatory bowel disease, hepatitis, and hematologic malignancies should be undertaken. This includes erythrocyte sedimentation rate (ESR), C-reactive protein (CRP), human leukocyte antigen (HLA-B27), joint radiographs, esophagogastroduodenoscopy (EGD)/colonoscopy (CS), liver function tests (LFT), hepatitis B (Hep B), anti-hepatitis C antibodies (Hep C) panel, complete blood count (CBC), serum protein electrophoresis/serum immunofixation electrophoresis (SPEP/SIFE), urine protein electrophoresis/urine immunofixation electrophoresis (UPEP/UIFE), rheumatoid factor, and anti-cyclic citrullinated peptide (anti-CCP). Therapies can include topical, intralesional, or systemic corticosteroids. For recalcitrant cases, other immunosuppressive therapies have been described, including cyclosporine, mycophenolate mofetil, azathioprine, tacrolimus, dapsone, intravenous immunoglobulin (IVIG), and biologic therapies (see **Table 9.2**).

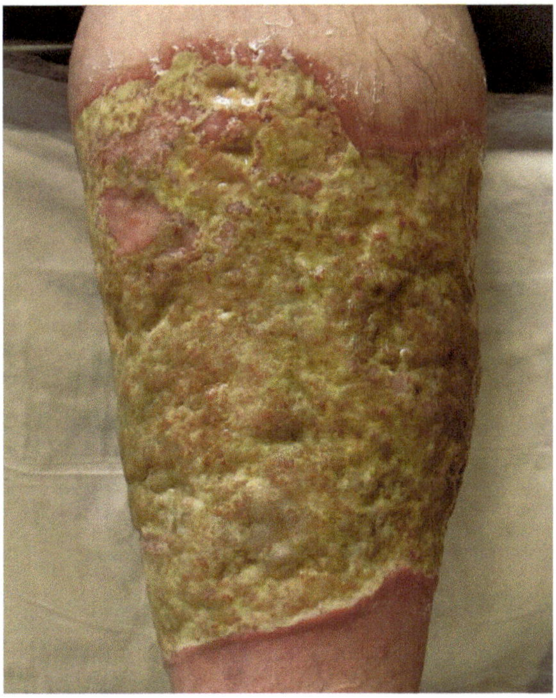

FIGURE 9.8 Pyoderma gangrenosum: Inflammatory arthropathy.

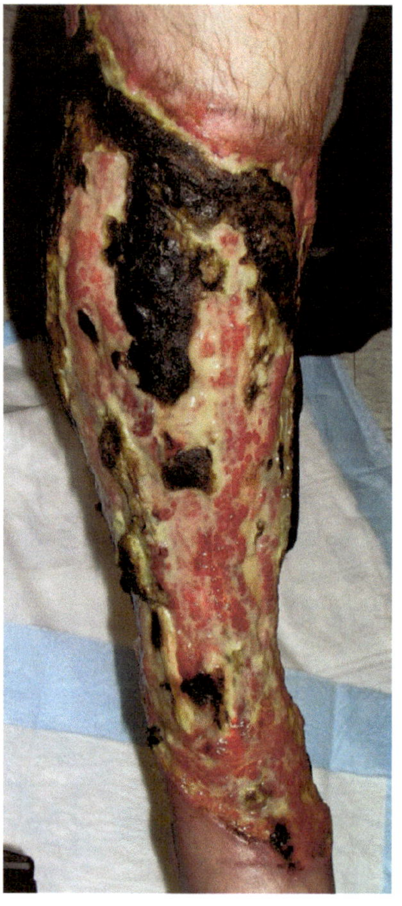

FIGURE 9.9 Pyoderma gangrenosum: Chronic pancreatitis.

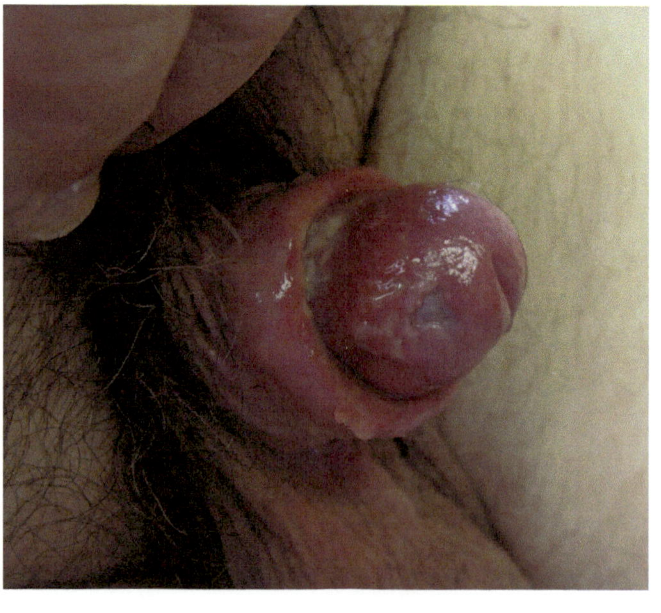

FIGURE 9.10 Pyoderma gangrenosum: Penis (inflammatory bowel disease).

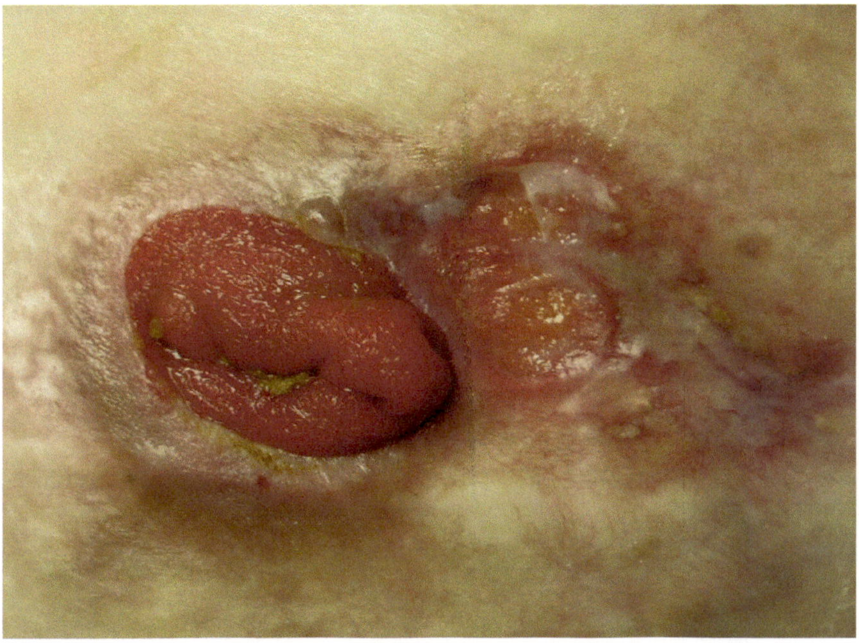

FIGURE 9.11 Pyoderma gangrenosum: Peristomal (ulcerative colitis).

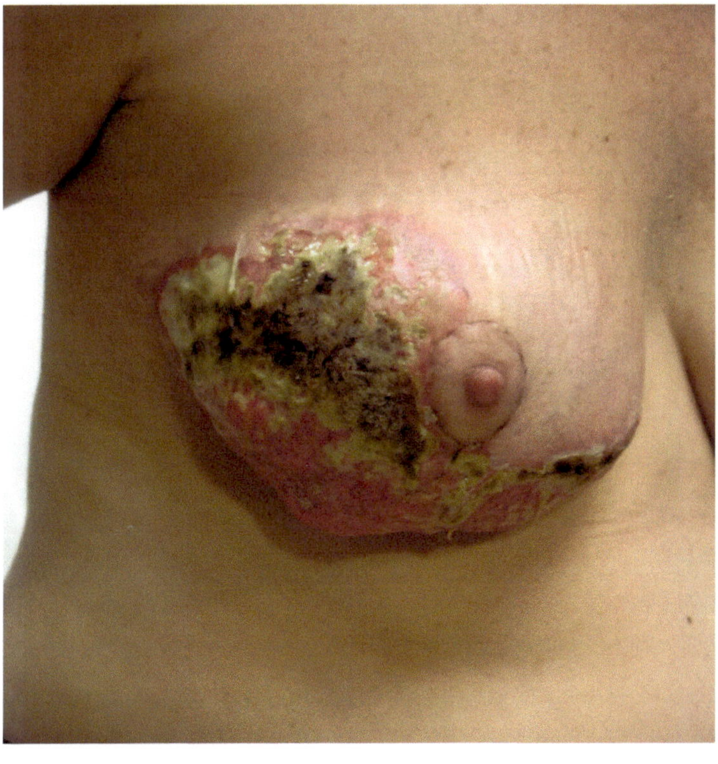

FIGURE 9.12 Pyoderma gangrenosum: Post-reconstruction for breast cancer.

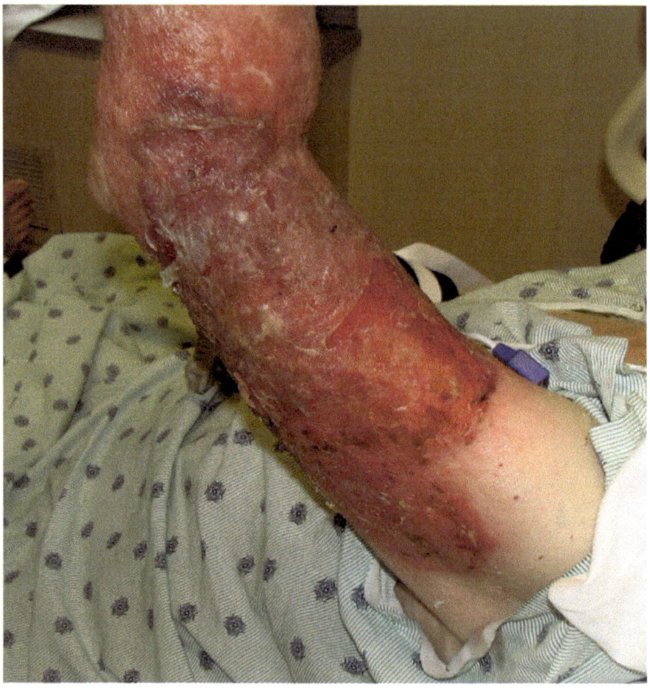

FIGURE 9.13 Pyoderma gangrenosum: Superficial type from filgrastim (G-CSF) injection.

TABLE 9.2

Biologic and Small Molecule Therapies for Pyoderma Gangrenosum

Drug	MOA
Infliximab	Anti-TNFα
Adalimumab	Anti-TNFα
Secukinumab	Anti-IL-17A
Risankizumab	Anti-IL-23
Anakinra	Anti- IL-lβ
Canakinumab	Anti- IL-lβ
Apremilast	Anti-PDE4
Tofacitinib	Anti-JAK 1/3
Ruxolitinib	Anti-JAK1/2
Baricitinib	Anti-JAK1/2
IVIG	Antibodies

BIBLIOGRAPHY

Flora A, Kozera E, Frew JW. Pyoderma gangrenosum: A systemic review of the molecular characteristic of disease. Exp Dermatol 2022;31(4):498–515.

Maronese CA, Pimentel MA, Li MM, et al. Pyoderma gangrenosum: An updated literature review on established and emerging pharmacological treatments. Am J Clin Dermatol 2023;23:615–634.

Zaino ML, Schadt CR, Callen JP, et al. Pyoderma gangrenosum: Diagnostic criteria, subtypes, systemic associations and work-up. Dermatol Clin 2024;42(2):157–170.

Sweet Syndrome

Etiopathogenesis

Acute febrile neutrophilic dermatosis, also known as Sweet syndrome, is a neutrophilic dermatosis. Classic or idiopathic Sweet syndrome occurs most commonly following an infection (hepatitis C, human immunodeficiency virus (HIV), COVID-19), although cases associated with internal diseases such as inflammatory bowel disease (Crohn's disease, ulcerative colitis) or other autoimmune conditions (lupus, Behcet's) have been reported. Malignancy-associated Sweet syndrome can occur with hematologic (acute myelogenous leukemia) and solid tumor malignancies (cervical, colorectal, gastric, lung). Drug-induced Sweet syndrome can be caused by medications such as granulocyte-macrophage colony-stimulating factor (GM-CSF), filgrastim, azathioprine, minocycline, trimethoprim-sulfamethoxazole, or chemotherapeutic agents.

Clinical Manifestations

Cutaneous lesions of Sweet syndrome occur abruptly as tender, erythematous papules, plaques, nodules, or bullae that can occur anywhere on the skin (**Figures 9.14–9.16**) and pyrexia. A pseudo-vesicular-like appearance is common. Lesions in locations such as the mucosa, eye, and internal organs are rare. A distinctive presentation known as neutrophilic dermatosis of the dorsal hands (**Figure 9.17**) is considered to be a localized form of Sweet syndrome. Finally, a subcutaneous variant of Sweet syndrome can occur, with lesions appearing as tender, indurated, erythematous plaques with a less fluctuant appearance. Hemorrhagic Sweet has a purpuric or necrotic appearance and is associated with hematologic malignancies. Histological variants include histiocytoid, cryptococcoid, eosinophilic, lymphocytic, and subcutaneous.

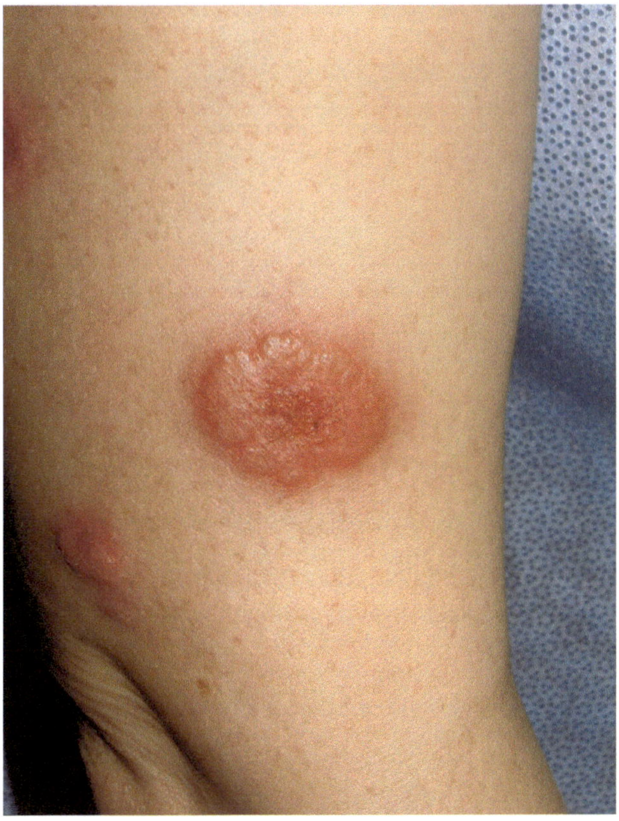

FIGURE 9.14 Sweet syndrome.

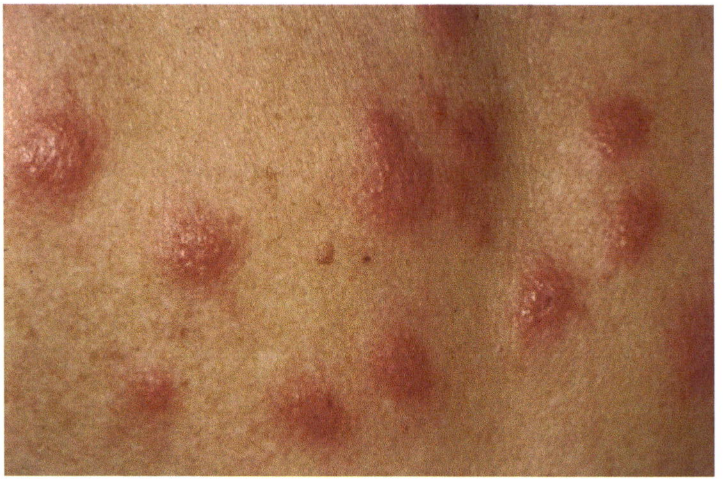

FIGURE 9.15 Sweet syndrome.

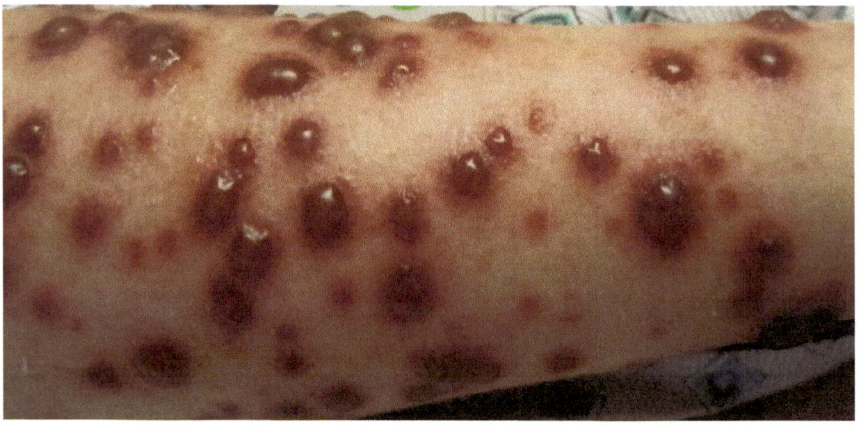

FIGURE 9.16 Sweet syndrome.

Systemic Manifestations

Patients with Sweet syndrome often have associated symptoms including fever, arthritis, conjunctivitis, and myalgias, which can occur as a prodrome or at the same time as the development of the skin lesions. Patients will often have an elevated ESR and leukocytosis. In addition to infections and inflammatory bowel disease, patients may have other autoimmune disorders such as rheumatoid arthritis (RA), systemic lupus erythematosus (SLE), or Sjögren syndrome. In malignancy-associated Sweet syndrome, leukemias (acute myeloid leukemia [AML], chronic myeloid leukemia [CML]) and solid tumor malignancies, especially genitourinary malignancies, may be present. As with pyoderma gangrenosum, extracutaneous involvement is seen with Sweet syndrome (eye, lung).

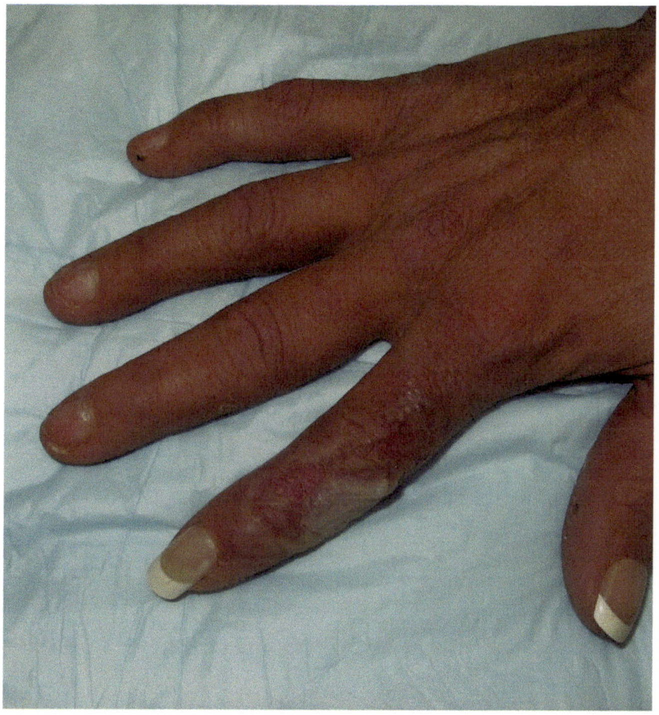

FIGURE 9.17 Neutrophilic dermatoses of the dorsal hand.

Evaluation and Management

The diagnosis of Sweet syndrome is made based on an appropriate history and the demonstration of certain histologic findings within the skin lesions. Histology demonstrates an abundant neutrophilic infiltrate in the dermis and dermal edema without evidence of vasculitis. Workup may include a CBC, bone marrow biopsy, SPEP/SIFE, and UPEP/UIFE with additional testing based on history and physical examination (CS for a patient with abdominal pain and bloody diarrhea). Age-appropriate malignancy screening should be performed, with additional workup based on risk factors, physical examination, and patient history. Sweet syndrome responds consistently to systemic corticosteroids. If disease persists despite steroid therapy or if the steroid dose is unable to be decreased, other therapies include dapsone, colchicine, or other steroid-sparing immunosuppressants and biologics.

BIBLIOGRAPHY

Delaleu J, Lepelletier C, Calugareanu A, et al. Neutrophilic dermatoses. Rev Med Interne 2022;43(12):727–738.

Edlyne Orfaly V, Shakshouk H, Heath M, et al. Sweet syndrome: A review of published cases. Dermatology 2023;239(4):664–669.

Joshi TP, Friske S, Hsiou DA. New practical aspects of sweet syndrome. Am J Clin Dermatol 2022;23(3):301–318.

Index

I

J

K

L

M

N